Pharmacy Law and Practice

SCHOOL OF MEDICINE & DENTISTRY
ST. BARTHOLOMEW'S
WEST SMITHFIELD
24HR RENEW

Pharmacy Law and Practice

Fourth Edition

Jonathan Merrills
BPharm, BA, BA (Law), FRPharmS
Barrister (Middle Temple)

and

Jonathan Fisher, QC
BA, LLB (Cantab)
Barrister (Grays Inn)
One of Her Majesty's Counsel

ELSEVIER

AMSTERDAM • BOSTON • HEIDELBERG • LONDON • NEW YORK • OXFORD
PARIS • SAN DIEGO • SAN FRANCISCO • SINGAPORE • SYDNEY • TOKYO

Elsevier
Radarweg 29, PO Box 211, 1000 AE Amsterdam, The Netherlands
The Boulevard, Langford Lane, Kidlington, Oxford OX5 1GB, UK

First edition 2006

First edition 1995 (Blackwell Science)   Reprinted 1998, 1999 (Blackwell Science)
Reprinted 1996 (Blackwell Science)   Third edition 2001 (Blackwell Science)
Second edition 1997 (Blackwell Science)   Fourth edition 2006 (Elsevier B.V.)

Library of Congress Cataloging in Publication Data
A catalog record for this book is available from the Library of Congress

British Library Cataloguing in Publication Data
A catalogue record for this book is available from the British Library

ISBN-13: 978-0-444-52201-6
ISSN-10: 0-444-52201-8

Printed and bound in the Netherlands

06 07 08 09 10   10 9 8 7 6 5 4 3 2 1

Contents

Preface

When we wrote the first edition, our objective was to describe the law rather than just list the Acts, regulations and cases that make up the law applying to community pharmacy.

That is still our objective. There has been an avalanche of new laws affecting pharmacy practice, all of which has had to be considered. The result is that the fourth edition is once again a complete rewrite. As always there has had to be a compromise between including everything we would have liked, and producing a readable text.

Once again we have concentrated on the laws which apply to community pharmacy and we have extended into other areas only where we consider it relevant to the community pharmacist. Although community pharmacists sometimes deal with agricultural products and veterinary medicines, we have generally left out the detailed laws in these areas. Instead we have included from those laws, sections which affect day-to-day practice as a pharmacist.

We have sought to produce an accessible text for both the community pharmacist and the pharmacy student. Any errors are ours – we hope there are none.

New challenges continue to confront the community pharmacist and we hope that this book will be a useful companion in meeting those challenges.

The law is stated as at 1 December 2005. We have tried to indicate where changes are likely in the new future.

Jon Merrills
Jonathan Fisher, QC

Chapter 1

The National Health Service

The National Health Service (NHS) has been described as the most magnificent feature of the United Kingdom's post–Second World War landscape. The National Health Service Act 1946, which created the NHS as we know it, was extensive in scope. It covered the funding of the service, and created a national network of hospitals operating in a tiered management structure. Benefits were extended to the whole of the population, which was provided free of charge with medicines and the services of hospitals, doctors, dentists and opticians.

The National Insurance Act 1911

Before 1911 the provision of medical care was haphazard. There were some voluntary health insurance schemes, often based on a particular industry. By 1900 about 7 million people in the country were covered. In return for flat rate payments they had the services of a doctor and were provided with free medicines.

In 1911 the then Prime Minister, Lloyd George, introduced a compulsory health insurance scheme. It was based on a German scheme which had been introduced in 1883 by Bismarck.

The National Health Insurance Act 1911 covered all employees below a certain income level. The employee paid into a scheme run by a trade union, a friendly society or a commercial insurance company. In return, when the employee was ill he or she received cash, the free services of a doctor and the necessary medicines.

Dispensing by pharmacists

The 1911 Act gave statutory recognition to the principle, long advocated by pharmacists, that the dispensing of prescriptions should be carried out under normal conditions only by, or under the supervision of, pharmacists. It applied this principle to the large class of the community which received their medicines under the provisions of the Act.

The National Health Service Act 1946

There remained a number of problems with the provision of health services. The hospitals varied in quality of buildings and quality of care. Many were run by charities. Only those persons who actually paid the insurance were covered for treatment. There was no provision for dependants. The problems, especially those of the hospitals, were highlighted during the Second World War. The new Socialist government of 1946 immediately implemented the National Health Service Act 1946, which brought the NHS into being on 5 July 1948.

Section 1 of the Act, which has now been superseded, states the following:

(1) It shall be the duty of the Minister of Health to promote the establishment in England and Wales of a comprehensive health service designed to secure improvement in the physical and mental health of the people of England and Wales and the prevention, diagnosis and treatment of illness, and for that purpose to provide or secure the effective provision of services in accordance with the following provisions of this Act

(2) The services so provided shall be free of charge, except where any provision of this Act expressly provides for the making and recovery of charges.

The minister was to provide hospital and other medical and nursing services throughout England and Wales

to such extent as he considers necessary to meet all reasonable requirements. (*Section 3*)

The Act vested in the minister a range of facilities and services which had previously been owned or provided by local health authorities, voluntary hospital authorities and other voluntary organisations, by the Government under the 1911 scheme, and by doctors practising privately.

The Act recognised the right of doctors to continue to practise privately, either full-time or in combination with certain types of NHS contract. They could admit patients to private beds in NHS hospitals.

The Act embodied the principle of the 1911 Act that medicines were normally to be dispensed at pharmacies and that normally doctors were not to dispense for their patients. Regulations could lay down the conditions for departing from this.

The 1946 Act set up a tripartite structure to administer the new arrangements. Different authorities controlled the hospitals, the primary care service and the mental hospitals.

The NHS took over control of 2688 hospitals from local authorities, charities and commercial bodies. The new structure consisted of 14 regional boards. Below them were 388 hospital management committees. The special position of teaching hospitals was recognised by the creation of 36 teaching hospital groups. Within each hospital the management was in the hands of an administrator, a matron and the senior doctor.

Local health authorities administered ambulance services, midwifery, home nursing and provision of care for the mentally ill.

The primary health care services were run by 134 executive councils. The health professionals – general practitioners, dentists, opticians and pharmacists – were (and remain) independent contractors. By contrast, staff in the hospital services were (and remain) employees.

This original structure has been changed over the years as the amending legislation reflected changes in both government and management theory.

The National Health Service Act 1977

This repealed the whole of the 1946 Act and consolidated a number of previous measures into one Act. It is now the principal Act dealing with the NHS. Since its introduction, the structure of the NHS has again been altered by both primary and secondary legislation. The 1977 Act, as amended, sets out the duties of government in the NHS, whilst the later Acts deal with the current structures of accountability and command, and with the more detailed arrangements for service delivery.

New Act to consolidate NHS law

The Government indicated at the beginning of 2006 that it would enact a new NHS Act to repeal the several previous laws and to consolidate the law into one Act.

General principles, scope and nature of the current NHS

Section 1 of the 1977 Act echoes the words of the 1946 Act by placing a duty on the S of S to

> continue the promotion in England and Wales of a comprehensive health service designed to secure improvement:
>
> (a)   in the physical and mental health of the people of those countries, and
> (b)   in the prevention, diagnosis and treatment of illness,
>
> and for that purpose to provide or secure the effective provision of services in accordance with this Act.

The key aims of the NHS today are

- to promote health and prevent ill health
- to diagnose and treat injury and disease
- to care for those with long-term illnesses and disability who require NHS services.

Actual care is provided by NHS staff in general practices, hospitals, treatment centres, pharmacies, NHS walk-in centres and in other community settings. The NHS employs around 1.3 million people, 633,000 of which are professionally qualified clinical staff. This includes 108,000 hospital doctors and general practitioners, 386,000 nursing, midwifery and health visiting staff, 122,000 scientific, therapeutic and technical staff and 15,000 ambulance staff who together diagnose, treat and support patients. These staff groups are supported by 360,000 other staff, such as nursery nurses and health care and nursing assistants. A further 199,000 people provide general infrastructure support in areas such as IT, catering, finance and management.

Free services

Section 1(2) of the 1977 Act states that

> the services so provided shall be free of charge except in so far as the making and recovery of charges is expressly provided for by or under any enactment, whenever passed.

In other words, the NHS shall be free except where a charge may lawfully be made. The NHS is funded through central taxation.

Other services

Section 2 gives power to the S of S to

> provide such services as he considers appropriate for the purpose of discharging his duties, and do anything else which is calculated to facilitate or be conducive or incidental to the discharge of his duties.

Besides the primary duty imposed by *Section 1* of the 1977 Act, *Sections 3, 4* and *5* impose further duties:
To the extent that he considers necessary, the S of S must provide

- hospital accommodation
- accommodation for other services
- medical, dental, nursing and ambulance services
- prenatal services and services for nursing mothers and young children
- services for the prevention of illness, care of the ill, and convalescence
- other services for diagnosis and treatment
- contraceptive services.

The services of "special hospitals" must also be provided for persons subject to detention under the Mental Health Act 1983 and who require treatment in high-security institutions.
The S of S also has power to provide

- invalid carriages
- treatment outside the United Kingdom for TB sufferers
- a microbiological service
- assistance for relevant research.

Income generation schemes

Section 7 of the Health and Medicines Act 1988 gives specific powers to the NHS to engage in "income generation schemes". In 2002 these powers were extended by Directions to include the use of companies. The schemes as such are not defined in the Act, which merely provides a framework for activities to take place. The Department of Health has issued guidance.

An "income generation scheme" is defined as one which seeks to provide a level of income which exceeds total costs, or at least provides an income contribution over and above the direct unit cost involved.

The S of S's power may only be exercised by bodies set up under the 1977 Act, i.e. NHS Trusts or Primary Care Trusts (PCTs). On 1 April 2005 the S of S issued Directions giving all Special Health Authorities income-generation powers, including the use of companies. The S of S must authorise each individual scheme.

Pharmaceutical services are arranged by PCTs, using contractors. Health Authorities cannot themselves be granted an NHS dispensing contract. They can lease their premises to a pharmacist or a company which can operate a pharmacy and be granted a contract.

The National Health Services and Community Care Act 1990

The majority of NHS hospital services are provided by NHS Trusts, which assumed responsibility for the ownership and management of hospitals or other establishments which were previously managed or provided by Regional, District or Special Health Authorities. Trusts may be either physical units, such as an acute hospital, or more nebulous institutions, such as an ambulance service.

Under the Act, NHS Trusts may make available facilities for private patients. Services provided by the NHS must still be provided free of charge. Non-NHS services should be charged for on a commercial basis. This includes the provision of private beds and the treatment of overseas visitors in hospitals.

The Health Act 1999

The Act:

(1) abolished fund-holding practices
(2) established PCTs
(3) allowed the making of Regulations to ensure practitioners (including pharmacists) are insured
(4) allowed the S of S to determine the remuneration for providing Part II services
(5) provided for a pharmaceutical price regulation scheme (PPRS) which may be voluntary or compulsory, and for powers to set prices charged to the NHS for medicines
(6) made it a criminal offence to evade paying NHS patient charges
(7) allowed for the pharmacy profession to be regulated by Orders
(8) set up the Commission for Health Improvement (ChImp) – now abolished by Health and Social Care (Community Health and Standards) Act 2003, and its functions transferred to the Commission for Healthcare Audit and Inspection.

The Act also repealed The Professions Supplementary to Medicine Act 1960, The Health Service Joint Consultative Committees (Access to Information) Act 1986 and The Nurses, Midwives and Health Visitors Act 1997.

The Health and Social Care Act 2001

This Act implements the NHS Plan 2000. The Act is in five parts:

- *Part 1* changes the way the NHS, including family health services, is run and funded in England and Wales.
- *Part 2* deals with pharmaceutical services in England and Wales and some aspects of such services in Scotland.
- *Part 3* provides for the establishment of Care Trusts and for the transfer of staff in connection with partnership arrangements.

- *Part 4* changes the way long-term care is funded and provided in England and Wales.
- *Part 5* deals with the control of patient information and the extension of prescribing rights as well as various miscellaneous and supplementary provisions.

Part 1 – changes the way the NHS is run

The following are of particular relevance to pharmacy:

Public–private partnerships

Section 4 inserts a new *Section 96C* into the 1977 Act. The S of S and the National Assembly for Wales (NAW), as well as Health Authorities, Special Health Authorities, Trusts and PCTs, may participate in public–private partnerships with companies that provide facilities or services to persons or bodies carrying out NHS functions.

The S of S may form or participate in forming companies to provide facilities, services, loans, guarantees or other financial provisions to the NHS.

Section 5 allows NHS bodies to form or invest in companies for income generation. Such activities must not interfere with any duties under the 1977 Act or operate to the disadvantage of patients. They are subject to any directions given by the S of S.

New arrangements for patient involvement

Sections 7–12 establish new arrangements for public and patient involvement in the NHS to run alongside the existing CHCS (more details later).

- Local authority overview and scrutiny committees (OSCs) will scrutinise the NHS and represent local views on the development of local health services.
- NHS organisations have a duty to involve patients and the public in decision making about the operation of the NHS.

Abolition of Medical Practices Committee

Sections 14 and *15* transfer arrangements for managing the numbers and distribution of General Practitioners (GPs) to Health Authorities (now PCTs).

Regulation of Health Service Practitioners

Sections 17–22 introduce new arrangements covering the regulation of family health service practitioners.

- Only practitioners, including deputies and locums, who are included in lists maintained by PCTs will be able to deliver family health services.
- Criteria to be admitted to (and to remain on) a list include probity and positive evidence of good professional behaviour and practice. This will involve a system of declarations, annual appraisal and participation in clinical audit.
- Primary Care Trusts may refuse to include a practitioner on the relevant medical, dental, ophthalmic or pharmaceutical list on the grounds of unsuitability.

Section 21 provides powers to make regulations providing for a person's inclusion in a PCT list to be subject to conditions.

    Section 24 provides for PCTs to keep supplementary lists of deputies and assistants who provide the various family health services (including GPs, dentists and people who provide pharmaceutical and optical services).

Financial interests and gifts

Section 23 requires practitioners to declare financial interests and the acceptance of gifts or other benefits.

Discipline arrangements

Section 25 provides for new arrangements for PCTs to suspend and remove practitioners from the relevant lists on the grounds of inefficiency, fraud or unsuitability.

    Section 27 created the Family Health Services Appeals Authority (FHSAA) as an independent body whose functions will include dealing with appeals by these practitioners against PCT decisions. The FHSAA is now part of the NHS Litigation Authority.

Abolition of NHS tribunal

Section 16 abolished the NHS Tribunal.

Part 2 – concerns pharmaceutical services

Chapter 1 provides for new arrangements under which community pharmacy and related services may be provided, initially on a pilot basis.

- These services are known as local pharmaceutical services (LPS).
- Primary Care Trusts may designate neighbourhoods or premises in connection with pilot schemes, and must conduct at least one review of each pilot scheme.
- Primary Care Trusts have power to vary or terminate pilot schemes.

New health service bodies

Section 33 allows potential providers of local pharmaceutical services to apply to the relevant authority to become health service bodies. One result will be that certain arrangements they make with other health service bodies will become NHS contracts.

Patient charges

Section 35 enables charges corresponding to those for pharmaceutical services under Part II of the 1977 Act to be levied for local pharmaceutical services, subject to exemptions.

Pilot schemes

Section 37 permits regulations to be made preventing the provision of pilot scheme services from the same premises as pharmaceutical services under Part II of the NHS Act 1977, except as provided in the regulations. It also permits regulations to make provision for the inclusion, re-inclusion, removal and modification of entries in pharmaceutical lists held under Part II of that Act.

Section 38 permits regulations to prescribe the extent to which pilot schemes are to be taken into account when considering applications for inclusion in those lists.

Section 40 deals with the provision of full-scale permanent LPSs (rather than under pilot schemes). The S of S or the NAW may bring this section into effect only if the results of pilot schemes show that the continued provision of LPSs would be in the interests of the NHS.

Chapter 2 introduces changes to the existing arrangements for the provision of pharmaceutical services.

Section 42 inserts a revised *Section 41* into the 1977 Act on the arrangements for pharmaceutical services. See Chapter 5 of this book.

Remote dispensing

Section 43 authorises arrangements made by Health Authorities for the provision of these pharmaceutical services by remote means.

The intention is to facilitate, and provide a means to control, the development of Internet and mail order, home delivery and other arrangements which may involve dispensing across PCT boundaries.

Part 3 – establishes Care Trusts

Grants new powers to establish Care Trusts to provide integrated care.

Part 4 – changes the way long-term care is funded and provided

Nursing care is excluded from community care services. Local authorities are responsible for meeting the care needs of people whose long-term care is funded through preserved rights to income support and jobseekers allowance.

Part 5 – patient information

Part 5 deals with the control of patient information and the extension of prescribing rights as well as various miscellaneous and supplementary provisions.

Use of NHS information

This has been dealt with in detail in Chapter 19.

Section 60 permits regulations to control the use of patient information.

The S of S may require or permit patient information to be shared for medical purposes where he or she considers that this is in the interests of improving patient care or in the public interest.

Section 61 establishes a Patient Information Advisory Group.

Extension of prescribing rights

Section 63 makes provision for the extension of prescribing rights to health professionals other than doctors, dentists and certain specified nurses, health visitors and midwives, who already have prescribing rights. This part also includes a number of supplementary provisions.

The Health and Social Care (Community Health and Standards) Act 2003

The HSC (CHS) received Royal Assent on 20 November 2003. The Act

- establishes NHS foundation trusts
- establishes a new health care inspectorate
- establishes a new inspectorate for social care
- provides for the recovery of NHS charges
- makes changes to the way in which primary dental and medical services are delivered and
- provides for a replacement of the Welfare Food Scheme and other miscellaneous matters.

Part 1 sets up Foundation trusts.

Section 1 sets out that an NHS foundation trust is a public benefit corporation which is authorised under this part to provide goods and services for the purposes of the "health service" in England. As this term is defined in *Section 128* of the National Health Service 1977 ("the 1977 Act") as being the health service that is provided by the S of S, the effect is that every NHS foundation trust has a primary purpose of providing health care under the NHS.

Subsection (2) makes it clear that a public benefit corporation is a body corporate. Each public benefit corporation must have a constitution that accords with *Schedule 1*.

Chapter 1 of *Part 2* establishes two new regulatory bodies – the Commission for Healthcare Audit and Inspection (the CHAI) and the Commission for Social Care Inspection (CSCI). Both inspectorates are established as executive non-departmental public bodies. Chapter 1 also abolished the National Care Standards Commission (the NCSC) and the Commission for Health Improvement (CHI). The majority of the NCSC's functions transferred to the CSCI, with the exception of those functions relating to the provision of independent healthcare, which transferred to the CHAI. All of the CHI's functions transferred to the CHAI.

Chapter 2 imposes a duty of quality on all NHS bodies that provide or commission health care, and provides for the standards.

Chapter 3 sets out the functions of the CHAI.

Chapter 5 sets out the functions of the CSCI, which is operational in England only.

Chapter 6 confers functions on the NAW ("the Assembly") in relation to social care similar to those conferred upon the CSCI.

Chapter 7 sets out the functions under Parts 1 and 2 of the Care Standards Act 2000 ("the CSA 2000") which have transferred to the CHAI and CSCI.

Chapter 8 provides for other functions of the CSCI.

Chapter 9 deals with the handling of complaints relating to the provision of NHS health care and local authority social services.

Finally, *Chapter 10* provides supplementary and general provisions in relation to the CHAI and CSCI, for example providing for joint working between both commissions.

Part 3 deals with the recovery of NHS charges. This part of the Act provides for the NHS to recover hospital treatment and/or ambulance costs where people receive compensation for injuries. This is an expansion of the current scheme for traffic accident cases as set out in the Road Traffic (NHS Charges) Act 1999. The costs would be recovered from the compensator and not the patient receiving the NHS treatment.

Part 4 of the Act makes provision for primary dental and medical services. For dentistry, the Act introduces a new duty on PCTs and Local Health Boards (LHBs) to provide or secure the provision of primary dental services. For medical services, the Act also introduces a new duty on PCTs and LHBs to provide or secure the provision of primary medical services.

Part 5 of the Act provides for the replacement of the Welfare Food Scheme, a scheme originally set up to provide milk and vitamins to mothers and children during a time of food rationing.

Advice from the health professions

Local Advisory Committees

At local level a system of Local Advisory Committees was set up to advise in both the primary and secondary care sectors.

For pharmacy, the primary care committees are the Local Pharmaceutical Committees (LPC). These consist of 9 or 15 members who provide pharmaceutical services as either contractors or employees. The PCT is obliged to consult them on certain matters, e.g. on applications for dispensing contracts. They must be consulted before local agreements for allocation of pharmacy monies are implemented. Health circular FHSL (96)9 – "Local pharmacy budgets, 1996/97" makes this clear. They may offer advice at any time.

Representative of contractors in the area
The LPCs are constituted under *Section 44* of the 1977 Act. This now states that where the PCT is satisfied that a committee formed for its area is representative of the persons providing pharmaceutical services in that area it may recognise that committee. *Section 43(6)* of the Health and Social Care Act 2001 amends *Section 44* to clarify that notwithstanding that people in the PCT's area may receive pharmaceutical services from people whose premises are outside that area, the LPC need only be representative of persons who are included in a PCT's own pharmaceutical list in order to be recognised by it.

Contractors in the area elect the LPCs. They adhere to the constitution adopted by the Pharmaceutical Services Negotiating Committee (PSNC), which represents contractor interests at national level.

Functions of the LPC
The functions are set out in *Section 45* of the Act. They are to be consulted about certain matters by the PCT, and may exercise any other functions which are given to them.

The expenses of an LPC may be met by a levy on local contractors. *Section 45(2)* allows PCTs to deduct sums from monies due to contractors. This is paid to the LPC. The S of S must approve the amounts.

Professional Advice to Primary Care Trusts

The Health Authorities Act 1995 amends the 1977 NHS Act at *Section 12(1)* to provide for professional advice to the authority.
Section 12(1) states

Every PCT shall make arrangements for seeing that they receive from

(a)   medical practitioners, registered nurses and midwives
(b)   other persons with professional expertise and experience of health care

advice appropriate for enabling the PCT effectively to exercise the functions conferred or imposed on them under or by virtue of this or any other Act

The Health Act 1999 inserts a new provision into the 1977 Act:

Advice for Primary Care Trusts. 16C.

Every PCT shall make arrangements with a view to securing that they receive advice appropriate for enabling them effectively to exercise the functions exercisable by them from persons with professional expertise relating to the physical or mental health of individuals.

Pharmaceutical Services Negotiating Committee

At a national level, the S of S has recognised the PSNC as a body "representative of the general body of chemists". Negotiations over pay for pharmaceutical services take place between PSNC and DH. PSNC are formally consulted on changes in the relevant Regulations, and Terms of Service.

Acts of Parliament mainly concerned with the NHS

The National Health Service Act 1946*
The National Health Service (Scotland) Act 1947
The National Health Service (Amendment) Act 1949
The National Health Service Act 1951*
The National Health Service Act 1952*
The National Health Service (Amendment) Act 1957*
The National Health Service Act 1961*
The National Health Service (Hospital Boards) Act 1964*
The National Health Service Act 1966
The National Health Service (Family Planning) Act 1967*
The Health Services and Public Health Act 1968
The National Health Service (Scotland) Act 1972
The National Health Service (Family Planning) Amendment Act 1972*

The National Health Service Reorganisation Act 1973* (repealed by HA Act 1995)
The Health Services Act 1976*
The National Health Service Act 1977
The National Health Service (Scotland) Act 1978
The Health Services Act 1980
The Health and Social Security Act 1984
The Health and Medicines Act 1988
The National Health Service and Community Care Act 1990
Health Authorities Act 1995
National Health Service (Amendment) Act 1995
Health Service Commissioners (Amendment) Act 1996
National Health Service (Private Finance) Act 1997
National Health Service (Primary Care) Act 1997
Audit Commission Act 1998
Health Act 1999
Health and Social Care Act 2001
NHS Reform & Health Care Professions Act 2002
Health and Social Care (Community Health and Standards) Act 2003

*Asterisked Acts have been totally repealed.

Chapter 2

Administration of the NHS

Administration

The Secretary of State for Health is the political head of the Department of Health (DOH) which sets overall health policy in England, including policy for the NHS. The S of S is assisted by a Minister of Health and a number of junior ministers. The S of S is responsible to Parliament for the operation of the NHS.

The Department's staff are civil servants. The most senior civil servant – the Permanent Secretary – is also the Chief Executive of the NHS. He is answerable to the S of S and Parliament for the way the Department is run, and provides strategic leadership to the NHS as its Chief Executive.

The DOH is managed by a board of directors. They support the Permanent Secretary to achieve the Department's objectives and ensure its work is conducted efficiently and effectively.

The DOH is organised into three business groups which focus on:

- developing effective DOH strategies and managing the Department's business
- improving the delivery of health and social care services
- setting, maintaining and monitoring standards and quality in the NHS and social care.

In relation to the NHS, the main functions of the DOH are to negotiate with the Treasury for funding, to set the policy framework and to monitor the performance of the NHS.

Chief professional officers, including a Chief Pharmaceutical Officer, provide expert knowledge in specialist health and social care disciplines.

NHS Executive

The NHS Executive (NHSE) manages the NHS directly through strategic health authorities and trusts. It is organised in two parts – a central unit (mainly located in the Department's Leeds office) and four regionally located Directorates of Health and Social Care.

There are four Directors of Health and Social Care (DsHSC), who are National Directors with seats on the Department Board. Their work has a territorial focus but they also have national responsibilities. The four Directorates cover London, South, North, and Midlands and East of England.

The Directors have small teams, some of whom work in government offices for the regions. The role of the DsHSC and teams can be summarised as follows:

Overseeing the development of the NHS and social care

This is a function of the whole Department, but the DsHSC have a key role. They will co-ordinate the Department's activities, liaising with the Modernisation Agency, finance colleagues and policy managers.

Assessing performance

The performance of the whole health and social care system, and in particular the new health authorities is assessed. The DsHSC can intervene where appropriate on issues of performance at a local level (e.g. poorly performing hospitals), though this intervention role will be increasingly at arm's length.

Managing senior NHS staff

This function includes the appointment and development of senior NHS staff.

Public health

Regional Directors of Public Health work as part of the DsHSC teams, with a responsibility for wide-scale factors affecting health and oversight of the local public health agenda.

Supporting Ministers and troubleshooting

The DsHSC support Ministers on issues relating to their regions or national responsibilities and "troubleshoot" where appropriate.

The NHSE sets a strategic framework for the NHS in accordance with the policy of the government. It manages the NHS to ensure that policy is implemented through the strategic health authorities and trusts. It gives out advice and information on good practice.

Strategic Health Authorities (SHAs)

In April 2002, 28 Strategic Health Authorities (SHAs) were set up to develop strategies for the NHS, and to monitor performance and standards. The NHS Reform and Health Care Professions Act 2002 changed the name from "Health Authorities" to SHAs. The Act has powers allowing the S of S to create or abolish authorities, or to vary the area for which they are established.

With the exception of NHSFTs they manage the NHS locally and are the key link between the DOH and the NHS. They also make sure that national priorities (such as improving cancer services) are integrated into local plans.

The S of S for Health delegates responsibility of the NHS to the Accounting Officer of the SHA who is accountable both to the S of S and directly to Parliament. A similar dual accountability role applies to chief executives of SHAs who are responsible both to their boards and, via the accounting officer, to Parliament. The Accounting Officer is responsible for the propriety and regularity of public finances in the NHS; for the keeping of proper accounts; for prudent and economical administration; for the avoidance of waste and extravagance; and the efficient and effective use of all the resources in his charge.

They are responsible for

- developing plans for improving health services in their local area
- making sure local health services are of a high quality and are performing well
- increasing the capacity of local health services, so they can provide more services
- making sure national priorities – for example, programmes for improving cancer services – are integrated into local health service plans.

The NHS Reform and Health Care Professions Act 2002 renamed Health Authorities (HAs) in England as Strategic Health Authorities and allowed for direct delegation of the S of S's functions to (PCTs).

The NHS (Functions of Strategic Health Authorities and primary care trusts and Administration Arrangements) (England) Regulations 2002, SI No. 2375, replaced the existing Regulations relating to the functions of HAs and PCTs in England.

Provision of NHS services

The majority of NHS services are provided by NHS trusts. Within each SHA, the NHS is split into various types of Trusts that take responsibility for running the different NHS services in your local area.

The different Trust types are:

- Acute Trusts
- Ambulance Trusts
- Care Trusts
- Mental Health Trusts
- Primary Care Trusts.

Acute Trusts

Hospitals are managed by NHS Trusts (also known as Acute Trusts).

Sections 5–11 of the NHS & CC Act 1990 deal with NHS Trusts, which according to *Section 5* are bodies established by the S of S to:

(a) assume responsibility for the ownership and management of hospitals or other establishments which were previously managed or provided by Regional, District or Special HAs; or

(b) provide and manage hospitals or other establishments or facilities.

From 1 April 1991, hospitals were gradually established as NHS Hospital Trusts. The Act allows that hospital trusts may be either physical units such as an acute hospital, or more nebulous institutions such as an ambulance service. The Act provides for statutory public consultation on the establishment of Trusts.

Establishment as a trust gives considerable freedom to manage affairs. The trust is run by a Board, which is able to employ its own staff, set rates of pay, borrow capital and dispose of assets. Such activities are severely restricted within the main NHS structure. Staff employed by Trusts are still considered as NHS staff. The property remains NHS property, although vested in the Trust.

The S of S retains certain powers over the Trusts. In particular, he is able to direct them as to the services which they must provide, and in this way he is able to ensure that essential services such as "Accident and Emergency" remain available locally. Each HA has a responsibility to ensure that certain core services are available locally.

The Powers of a Trust

The S of S may make an order to confer specific powers on a Trust in addition to those contained in Paragraphs 10–15 of Schedule 2 of the Act.

The specific powers are

(a)   to enter into NHS contracts as a provider
(b)   to undertake research
(c)   to train Trust staff and those likely to become employed by the Trust
(d)   to make facilities for training available to a university
(e)   to join with another body or individual to carry out its functions
(f)   to make charges for its services to private patients
(g)   to generate additional income using the powers in *Section 7(2)* of the Health and Medicines Act 1988.

There are some general powers:

(h)   to deal in land
(i)   to enter into legal contracts
(j)   to accept gifts of money, land or property
(k)   to employ staff
(l)   to do anything necessary or expedient to carry out its functions

Status

According to Schedule 2, Paragraph 18, a Trust shall not be regarded as the servant or agent of the Crown or except as provided by this Act, as enjoying any status, immunity or privilege of the Crown. An NHS Trust's property shall not be regarded as the property of, or property held on behalf of, the Crown.

Financial objectives of Trusts

Section 10 requires the NHS Trusts to break even, taking 1 year with another, and to achieve any financial objectives which are set.

Foundation Trusts

Foundation Trusts are a new type of NHS hospital run by local managers, staff and members of the public which are tailored to the needs of the local population. NHS foundation trusts are established in law as new legally independent organisations called Public Benefit Corporations. The primary purpose of NHS foundation trusts is to provide NHS services to NHS patients. These Trusts remain within the NHS.

Foundation Trusts have been given much more financial and operational freedom than other NHS Trusts. They have freedom to retain surpluses and to invest in delivery of new services, to manage and reward their staff flexibly and to access a wider range of options for capital funding. They are not allowed to sell off or mortgage NHS property or resources needed to provide key NHS services.

NHS foundation trusts are not subject to direction by the S of S. Instead, their performance will be monitored by an Independent Regulator. Each NHS foundation trust will have a Board of Governors responsible for representing the interests of the local community, staff and local partner organisations.

There are currently 37 NHS Foundation Trusts in existence.

Primary Care Trusts

There are 302 PCTs. They are local health organisations responsible for managing health services in their local area. On average they cover a population size of 150,000 – the smallest is approximately 90,000 and the largest approximately 300,000 They work with local authorities and other agencies that provide health and social care locally to make sure the community's needs are being met. They receive money directly from the DOH. They are responsible for 75% of NHS funds.

Amalgamation
It is expected that many PCTs will amalgamate with their neighbours to form larger administrative units.

Responsibility for planning secondary care
Despite the name they are also responsible for planning secondary care. They look at the health needs of the local community and develop plans to improve health and set priorities locally. They then decide which secondary care services to commission to meet people's needs. Therefore they work closely with the providers of the secondary care services that they commission to agree about delivering those services.

They are responsible for the provision of other health services including hospitals, dentists, mental health care, Walk-in Centres, NHS Direct, patient transport (including accident and emergency), population screening, pharmacies and opticians and for integrating health and social care so the two systems work together for patients.

Establishment

Primary care trusts were established by *Section 2* of the Health Act 1999, which inserted new provisions in the National Health Service Act 1977 – *Section 16A.* – (1) The S of S may establish bodies to be known as PCTs with a view, in particular, to:

(a)   providing or arranging for the provision of services under Part I of this Act,
(b)   exercising functions in relation to the provision of general medical services under Part II of this Act, and
(c)   providing services in accordance with *Section 28C* arrangements.

Each PCT shall be established by an order made by the S of S (referred to in this Act as a PCT order). A PCT shall be established for the area specified in its PCT order and shall exercise its functions in accordance with any prohibitions or restrictions in the order.

The creation of trusts began in April 2000.

Primary Care Trusts are allowed to commission and provide services, to employ staff and to own property. They are not prevented from setting up community pharmacies, although the S of S could give directions prohibiting this.

Boards of PCT

The board consists of five lay members, plus the Chief Executive, Finance Director and three professional members of the executive.

Funding

Primary Care Trusts are funded by the SHAs which make allocations to them. They receive a unified budget covering hospital and community services, GP prescription and the general practice infrastructure.

Each financial year is complete in itself, so funds (or arrears) cannot be carried over to subsequent years. PCTs are accountable to SHAs for outcomes. HA are required by the HA 1999 to pay to PCTs their share of Part II primary care expenditure.

Teaching PCT

Teaching PCTs have been established in a number of areas. A teaching PCT is a statutory NHS body based upon the existing PCT model. According to the DOH, all PCTs are expected to develop a learning culture and role within their organisation. A teaching PCT brings specific additional capacity into their locality to support all healthcare professionals and PCTs in the healthcare community.

Crime and Disorder Partnerships

From 30 April 2004, PCTs in England became responsible authorities within crime and disorder partnerships under *Section 5(1)* of the Crime and Disorder Act 1998, as amended by the Police Reform Act 2002. This status formalises the role PCTs have in participating in Crime and Disorder Reduction Partnerships (CDRP).

Care Trusts

Care Trusts are organisations that work in both health and social care. They may carry out a range of services, including social care, mental health services or primary care services.

They are set up when the NHS and Local Authorities agree to work closely together, usually where it is felt that a closer relationship between health and social care is needed or would benefit local care services.

Mental Health Trusts

Specialist mental health care is normally provided by mental health trusts or by local council social services departments.

Ambulance Trusts

There are 33 ambulance services covering England, which provide emergency access to health care. There are proposals to amalgamate these into 11 larger organisations.

NHS Walk-in Centres

NHS Walk-in Centres give you fast access to health advice and treatment. There are now 43 centres throughout England. Open 7 days a week, from early in the morning until late in the evening, they offer

- treatment for minor illnesses and injuries
- assessment by an experienced NHS nurse
- advice on how to stay healthy
- information on out-of-hours General Practitioner (GP) and dental services
- information on local pharmacy services
- information on other local health services.

NHS Direct

NHS Direct is a 24-hour phone line, staffed by nurses, which offers quick access to health care advice. NHS Direct was made a Special Health Authority in April 2004.

Special Health Authorities

These are health authorities which provide a health service to the whole of England. They were set up under *Section 11* of the NHS Act 1977. They are independent, but can be subject to ministerial direction like other NHS bodies.

Dental Vocational Training Authority – to be transferred to the Postgraduate Medical Education and Training Board.

Health and Social care Information Centre

Mental Health Act Commission

NHS Blood and Transplant Authority – replaced the National Blood Authority and UK Transplant on 1 October 2005.

NHS Business Services Authority – took over Dental Practice Board, NHS Counter Fraud and Security Management Service, NHS Pensions Agency and Prescriptions Pricing Authority from 1 October 2005.

National Institute For Health and Clinical Excellence

NHS Institute for Innovation and Improvement added July 05

National Patient Safety Agency
National Treatment Agency for Substance Misuse (NTA)
NHS Appointments Commission
NHS Direct
NHS Litigation Authority
NHS Logistics Authority
NHS Professionals

Prescription Pricing Authority

The Prescription Pricing Authority (PPA) is of special interest to pharmacists. It was created in 1978 as a Special Health Authority under provisions in the 1977 Act. It was reconstituted in 1990 by the Prescription Pricing Authority Constitution Order, SI 1990 No. 1718.

The Authority consists of eight members:

(1)   the chairman
(2)   a general medical practitioner
(3)   a pharmacist providing pharmaceutical services
(4)   a chief officer of a Family Health Service Authority (FHSA)
(5)   the chief officer of the PPA
(6)   three lay members, i.e. persons who are not and have never been a doctor, dentist, pharmacist, optician or nurse.

The appointment and tenure of office of the members is governed by the PPA Regulations, SI 1990 No. 1719.

Members are appointed, by the S of S, for a period not exceeding 3 years. The S of S also appoints the Chairman.

The functions of the PPA relate to the examining, checking and pricing of prescriptions for drugs, listed drugs, medicines and listed appliances supplied as part of pharmaceutical services. These functions are carried out on behalf of PCTs. In addition the S of S may direct the PPA to carry out other tasks.

Non-departmental public bodies (NDPB)

A number of bodies have been created to assist with the work of the NHS, but which are not part of the DOH:

Executive NDPB
Council for Healthcare Regulatory Excellence (CHRE)
Health Protection Agency which includes The National Radiological Protection Board and Public Health Laboratory Service
Human Tissue Authority
Health and social Care Information Centre
Agencies
MHRA
NHS Connecting for Health

Effects of devolution

The services are organised slightly differently in each of the countries of the United Kingdom. The regional tier is absent, and the functions are provided either by the local health authorities or at the national level.

Wales

During 1999 the National Assembly for Wales took on responsibility for the management and performance of the NHS in Wales. The NHS Directorate in Wales has a similar role to the NHSE. The Directorate is accountable to the Assembly.

In Wales there are currently 5 health authorities, 16 Trusts and 22 Local Health Groups (LHG) which are similar to the Primary Care Groups (PCGs) found in England. The HA's role includes quantifying the healthcare needs of their area and commissioning the necessary care accordingly, supporting the contractor professions, protecting public health and responding to the views of people and organisations in their area. NHS Trusts are charged with providing services and operating hospitals, community health service, ambulance services and other health facilities in accordance with contracts they have with HAs. In Wales the responsibility for producing health Improvement Programs lies with the LHGs. There are two special health authorities (the Welsh Common Services Authority and the Health Promotion Authority for Wales). Community health councils in Wales report to the Welsh Assembly.

The Health Promotion Authority for Wales and parts of the Welsh Health Common Services Authority will also become part of the Assembly.

Northern Ireland

In Northern Ireland the Department of Health and Social Services (DHSS) is required, under the provisions of the Health and Personal Social Services (Northern Ireland) (HSSE) Order 1972, to secure the provision of an integrated service designed to promote health and social welfare of the population.

Part of this provision is the Health Services in Northern Ireland which is managed by the HSSE.

The Health and Social Policy Group (HSPG) of the DHSS is responsible for promoting wider health and social gain. It sets the overall strategy for HPSS; promotes voluntary activity and community development in Northern Ireland; takes the lead in targeting health and social need; and is responsible for health promotion and protection, developing social policy and social legislation.

The strategy of the DHSS has three main aims:

(1) to promote health and social well-being
(2) to target health and social need
(3) to secure and improve the provision and delivery of health and social services.

Health and Social Services Executive

The HSSE is the Northern Ireland counterpart to the NHSE in England. Its primary purpose is to secure improvements to the health and social well-being of people in Northern Ireland. Its main functions are

- to provide leadership, direction and support to the HPSS in Northern Ireland;
- to set and ensure the achievement of specific objectives and targets for the HPSS in accordance with national and regional policies and priorities;
- to monitor the performance of HPSS in assessing need and improving health and social well-being of the population;
- to allocate resources and ensure that they are used effectively, efficiently and economically in accordance with the required standards of public accountability;
- to promote the managerial environment necessary to achieve these objectives;
- to provide advice, information and support to ministers relating to the management and performance of the HPSS.

The HSSE is headed by a Chief Executive who is supported by six directors.

Health and Social Services Boards

There are four Health and Social Services Boards in Northern Ireland. They act as agents of the DHSS in planning, commissioning and purchasing health and social services for residents in their areas – functioning in a similar role to HAs in England.

Each Board has a non-executive chairman, six executive and six non-executive members. The chairman and non-executive members are appointed by the minister with the approval of the S of S. By statute, two of the executive members are the chief executive/general manager and director of finance.

As commissioners and purchasers, Boards are required to plan, secure and pay for the services needed to meet the health and social care needs of their population. In deciding which services are needed, the Boards assess the population's health and social care needs by collecting information about patterns of death, illness and community care needs and by consulting local people. They also liaise with GPs and statutory and voluntary agencies to build up a picture of the health and social care needs of their residents.

Health and Social Services Trusts

The HSS Trusts are the providers of health and social services. They are responsible for the management of staff and services at hospitals and other establishments previously managed or provided by Boards. The Trusts control their own budgets and, although managerially independent of Boards, they are accountable to the HSSE.

There are 20 Trusts in Northern Ireland. It is the only part of the United Kingdom which, because of the integrated health and social services, has Trusts based solely on the delivery of community health and social services.

Each Trust is managed by a Board of Directors which contains up to five non-executive members and a non-executive chairman, who are appointed by the DHSS with the approval of the S of S and five executive members who are employees of the Trust.

Scotland

The Scottish Health Service is responsible to the Scottish Parliament. The Management Executive within the Scottish Office Department of Health is responsible for health service policy and central management. The Management Executive sets national objectives and priorities, agrees corporate contracts with area Health Boards and monitors their performance. Health Boards have a strategic management role and are responsible for planning and commissioning hospital and community health services for the people who live within their area. Health Boards are also responsible for the primary care services provided by GPs, dentists, community pharmacists and opticians, who are independent contractors. There are 15 Health Boards covering the whole of Scotland (12 mainland and 3 island Boards).

There are 46 NHS Trusts in Scotland responsible for providing hospital and/or community services in a particular area, under contract to Health Boards and others. Non-executive directors are referred to as trustees. All trust chairs are members of the appropriate health board. There is one national Trust responsible for the Scottish Ambulance Service. The Scottish Ambulance Service is a special Health Authority Board.

Health Boards, with the exception of the larger ones, have one acute and one PCT. There are 28 acute hospital trusts and 13 PCTs. PCTs are responsible for primary care, mental health, learning disabilities and community hospitals. Each Trust is accountable to the S of S via the Management Executive.

Each PCT operates through Local Health Care Co-operatives (LHCC) whose role is to plan and provide service delivery at a local level. There are 70 LHCCs. The PCT senior management team has representatives from each LHCC.

There are also a number of other national organisations responsible for associated services and include the Common Services Agency, the Health Education Board for Scotland, and the State Hospitals Board for Scotland. The patients' and public's interests in the NHS are represented by 16 Local Health Councils (one for each Health Board area except for the Western Isles which has two).

New proposals for the NHS in Scotland were set out in the Government's White Paper: *Designed to Care*. This announced that the 15 Health Boards would remain but that there would be a smaller number of Trusts of two types: acute hospital Trusts and primary care Trusts.

Chapter 3

The Supply of NHS Pharmaceutical Services

The PCT's duty

Primary Care Trusts are under a legal duty to arrange for the supply of pharmaceutical services to patients in their area.

According to *Section 41* of the NHS Act 1977 (as amended mainly by the 1980 and 1990 Acts), they must arrange for the supply of "proper and sufficient drugs and medicines and listed appliances" when they are ordered by a medical practitioner under the NHS. They must also make similar arrangements for the supply of the limited range of drugs and medicines which may be ordered by a dental practitioner, a nurse or other "prescribed person" under the NHS. The services which are so provided are known as "pharmaceutical services". The details of those arrangements are dealt with by Regulations.

The relevant section of the 1977 Act now reads:

Section 41 – *Arrangements for pharmaceutical services*

It is the duty of every Primary Care Trust, in accordance with regulations which shall be made for the purpose, to arrange as respects their area for the provision to persons who are in that locality of –

(a) proper and sufficient drugs and medicines and listed appliances which are ordered for those persons by a medical practitioner in pursuance of his functions in the health service, the Scottish health service, the Northern Ireland health service or the armed forces of the Crown

(b) proper and sufficient drugs and medicines which are ordered for those persons by a dental practitioner in pursuance of –

    (i) his functions in the health service, the Scottish health service or the Northern Ireland health service (other than functions exercised in pursuance of the provision of services mentioned in Paragraph (c); or

    (ii) his functions in the armed forces of the Crown;

(c) listed drugs and medicines which are ordered for those persons by a dental practitioner in pursuance of the provision of general dental services or equivalent services in the Scottish health services or the Northern Ireland health service;

(d) such drugs and medicines and such listed appliances as may be determined by the Secretary of State for the purposes of this paragraph which are ordered for those persons by a prescribed description of person in accordance with such conditions, if any as may be prescribed, in pursuance of functions in the health service, the Scottish health service, the Northern Ireland health service or the armed forces of the Crown; and

(e)   such other services as may be prescribed.

The persons referred to in (1)(d) may be PAMs, pharmacists, dental auxiliaries, ophthalmic opticians, osteopaths, chiropractors, nurses, midwives, health visitors, or any other health professionals the Secretary of State specifies.

The current Regulations are the NHS (Pharmaceutical Services) Regulations 2005, SI No. 641 (the Contract Regulations). A similar new set of regulations deal with general medical services – the NHS (General Medical Services) Regulations.

The NHS (Pharmaceutical Services) Regulations 2005 have already been amended by two sets of Amendment Regulations:

(1)   The (Pharmaceutical Services) (Amendment) Regulations 2005, SI No. 1015; and
(2)   The (Pharmaceutical Services) (Amendment No. 2) Regulations 2005, SI No. 1501.

Pharmaceutical services

According to the Definitions section of the Contract Regulations "pharmaceutical services" means pharmaceutical services other than directed services.

Pharmaceutical Services consist of:

(1)   the supply of drugs and medicines as above
(2)   the supply of appliances
(3)   the provision of certain "additional professional services"
(4)   the supply of contraceptive substances and appliances.

Pharmaceutical Services may be provided by:

(1)   pharmacists
(2)   pharmacy companies
(3)   appliance contractors.

Unless Regulations provide otherwise, arrangements for the dispensing of medicines may only be made with pharmacists or pharmacy companies (*Section 43*). The Regulations do not provide otherwise.

Dispensing is not defined in the NHS Act or in the Regulations. Since supply of medicines under the NHS is allowed by persons who are not pharmacists, it could be argued that the restriction referred to above in *Section 43b* refers only to the making up of medicines. Such an interpretation would however be at odds with the normal use of the term "dispensing" by the profession.

Unless Regulations provide otherwise, arrangements may not be made with a medical practitioner or dental practitioner under which he agrees to provide or is required to provide pharmaceutical services to any person to whom he is rendering General Medical Services (GMS) or General Dental Services (GDS).

Regulations do provide for General Medical Practitioners (GMPs) to provide Pharmaceutical Services (PS) to:

(1)   patients living in a rural area, more than 1.6 km from a pharmacy;
(2)   patients who have satisfied the PCT that they have serious difficulty in obtaining drugs or appliances from a pharmacy because of its distance or the poor communications.

The "contract" which governs the relationship between the PCT and the pharmacy is not contained in any single document, despite the size of the Contract Regulations, but consists of an amalgam of parts from various documents.

The nature of the arrangements between the PCT and those professionals providing the services to patients has been discussed by the courts. In 1968 the courts decided that the pharmacy had a contract with the Executive Council (a predecessor to the PCT) to provide services (*Appleby* v. *Sleep, 2 AER 265*). Other views have since been expressed that there is no contract as such, merely an administrative arrangement set out in regulations (*Roy* v. *Kensington and Chelsea FPC 1992 1AER 705 (HL)*).

Contractors obligations

Under the Contract Regulations 2005, there are three levels of service provision:

- Essential
- Advanced
- Enhanced.

Essential and Advanced services form part of a national contract. Essential services are obligatory for all contractors.

Components of essential service

Under their contract with a PCT, pharmacists are obliged to:

(a)   dispense all NHS prescriptions presented to them, within a reasonable time
(b)   maintain certain minimum hours of opening
(c)   provide on request an estimate of the time when the prescription will be ready
(d)   where required check evidence of entitlement to exemption or remission of charges
(e)   give advice to patients about the medicines
(f)   maintain patient medication records
(g)   dispose of unwanted drugs
(h)   promote healthy lifestyle messages to the public
(i)   provide information about other health and social care providers and support
(j)   provide advice and support to people caring for themselves or their families
(k)   allow certain persons to inspect the premises
(l)   participate in clinical governance.

Advanced services can be provided by all contractors, once they have met the accreditation requirements and after they have met the requirements of

Essential services. Advanced services are Medicines Use Review and prescription interventions.

Enhanced services are commissioned by PCTs according to their local needs. These include

- Minor ailments service
- Smoking cessation
- Supervised administration of medication
- Needle and syringe exchange schemes
- Anticoagulant monitoring
- Care home support
- Patient Group Direction services
- Clinical medication reviews.

Terms of service

When a contractor applies to be entered on the list of NHS pharmacies he agrees to the Terms of Service (TOS), which are contained in Schedule 1 of the NHS (PS) Regulations 2005.

The TOS incorporate

- The Drug Tariff (DT);
- The parts of the NHS (Service Committees & Tribunal) Regulations 1992 which concern the investigations of disputes between patients and pharmacists;
- The parts of the Patients' Forums (Functions) Regulation 2003 which concern entry and inspection of premises.

As a breach of any of these terms may result in a hearing by a discipline committee (discussed later), it is important that they be clearly understood. Each paragraph contains a number of requirements. Failure to comply with any one of them may give rise to a breach.

The requirements of these TOS are absolute. An error is just as much a breach as is a deliberate fraud. For instance, the supply of the wrong drug, in error, will constitute a breach. However, the TOS are not all-embracing. For instance, they do not cover errors on dispensing labels, although such an error might give rise to criminal proceedings under the Medicines Act.

Fundamental requirements of the terms of service

The fundamental requirement is to supply what is ordered.

> Paragraph 4
> A pharmacist shall, to the extent that Paragraphs 5–9 required in the manner described in those paragraphs, provide proper and sufficient drugs and appliances to persons presenting prescriptions for drugs and appliances by health care professionals in pursuance of their functions in the health service, the Scottish health service or the Northern Ireland health service.

Paragraph 5(1)

Where any person presents a non-electronic prescription form which contains:

(a)   an order for drugs, not being Scheduled drugs, or for appliances, not being restricted availability appliances; or

(b)   an order for a drug specified in Schedule 2 to the Prescription of Drugs Regulations, signed by a prescriber and including the reference "SLS"; or

(c)   an order for a restricted availability appliance, signed by a prescriber and including the reference "SLS"; or

a chemist shall, with reasonable promptness, provide the drugs so ordered, and such of the appliances so ordered as he supplies in the normal course of his business

"Signed" includes signature with a prescriber's advanced electronic signature. Paragraph 5 makes similar requirements for electronic prescriptions, and for repeatable prescriptions.

Promptness

A pharmacy must supply "with reasonable promptness".

In the past, Discipline Committees have generally taken the view that most medicines should be supplied either from stock in the pharmacy or from the next reasonable wholesaler delivery. They have also taken into account the nature of the condition being treated and the rarity or scarcity of the medicine. The situation which frequently causes problems is where the patient is repeatedly asked to return to the pharmacy to collect an item alleged to be on order but which has not been delivered. This may have resulted from failure to provide an effective system for passing on messages between members of staff, or to "progress chase" items on order. Breaches of the requirement to provide promptly have been found where a delay of several days occurred.

Paragraph 7(1) requires the pharmacy to give, on request, an estimate of the time when the completed prescription will be ready for collection. If the prescription is not ready at that estimated time, a revised estimate must then be given.

Refusal to provide drugs or appliances ordered

A pharmacy must supply any person who presents a valid form. However, Paragraph 9 sets out situations where the pharmacist may refuse supply. These are

- the pharmacist believes the form is stolen or a forgery
- there is an error on the form
- supply would be contrary to the pharmacist's clinical judgement
- there is a threat of violence
- the person presenting the form or someone accompanying him commits or threatens to commit a criminal offence
- there are technical reasons not to supply a repeatable prescription (discussed later)
- a review is required of the treatment ordered on a repeatable prescription.

In the last case the pharmacist must inform the prescriber.

Such drugs as may be so ordered

A pharmacy must supply any drugs ordered on a prescription form by a doctor except those covered by the Selected List rules. The requirement is to supply the drugs ordered on the form, not any similar drugs. This provision therefore prohibits the supply of generic equivalents. It also prohibits the supply of parallel imports where the name used on the product is different from that on the form. This provision has the somewhat unusual effect of occasionally requiring the pharmacist to supply an import where the doctor's poor spelling has unwittingly produced the foreign name.

Where the wrong drug is supplied in error it will constitute a breach of Paragraph 5(1).

There are additional rules governing the prescribing and supply of Schedule 2 drugs. These are dealt with later.

Dentists may only prescribe from the S of S's list which is in the DT. Although the list is in generic terms, it is accepted that proprietary products fitting those generic descriptions may be ordered and supplied.

Appliances

A pharmacy is only required to supply those appliances which he normally supplies in the course of his business.

Prescription forms

The expression "prescription form" means a form supplied by the PCT to enable persons to obtain pharmaceutical services as defined by the Act. All variations are included, e.g. FP10, FP10 (HP), FP14.

The term includes

> data that are created in an electronic form, signed with a prescriber's advanced electronic signature and transmitted as an electronic communication to a nominated dispensing contractor by the ETP service. (Regulation 2(1))

Signed

Paragraph 5(1) requires the prescriptions to be signed. The advent of electronic transmission of prescriptions meant that special provision had to be made for electronic signatures.

A "prescribers advanced electronic signature" is defined as an electronic signature which is

(a) uniquely linked to the signatory
(b) capable of identifying the signatory
(c) created using means that the signatory can maintain under his sole control and
(d) linked to the data to which it relates in such a manner that any subsequent change of data is detectable.

Services may only be provided on receipt of a signed form, except in emergency. Accordingly unless the form is signed no drugs can be supplied. It also follows that an amendment agreed over the phone with the prescribing doctor does not take effect until either the doctor requests an emergency supply, or he signs the original form again. In some circumstances pharmacists will have to balance the possibility of a service case against the need for the patient to have the medicine.

Supervision of dispensing

The dispensing of medicines must be by or under the direct supervision of a pharmacist. A company must undertake that all medicines supplied by them under the Act shall be dispensed by or under the direct supervision of a pharmacist (*Section 43* NHS 1977).

There are Medicines Act requirements with respect to supply, but they require only "supervision". "Direct supervision" is probably more onerous than "supervision". The courts have discussed this issue in cases brought under the Pharmacy and Poisons Act 1933, and supported the view that there is a distinction. It is difficult to find such a distinction in practice.

Paragraph 8(2) of the TOS states that

Drugs or appliances [so ordered] shall be provided by or under the direct supervision of a pharmacist; Where that pharmacist is an employee, he must not be

(a) someone who has been disqualified under *Section 46(2)(b)* of the Act, or
(b) someone who is suspended.

Section 46 deals with removal of a pharmacist from a list.

Forgeries

Paragraph 9 states that a pharmacist may refuse to dispense a form which he believes is stolen or a forgery.

Exemption declaration

Paragraph 7 requires the pharmacist to ask, in most cases, for evidence of entitlement to exemption.

Quality

Paragraph 8(5) of the TOS states that

Any drug which is provided as part of pharmaceutical services and included in the DT, BNF, DPF, EP or the BPC shall comply with the standard or formula specified therein.

The Drug Tariff helpfully adds that

> Any drugs which are not included in the DT [or the publications listed in Paragraph 8(5) of the Terms of Service] must be of a grade or quality not lower than that ordinarily used for medical purposes.

The DT contains a list of galenicals and generic medicines. If the pharmacist wishes the prescriber can specify a different standard, for example, by specifically referring to a foreign pharmacopoeia. Where a prescription calls for a generic drug which is included in a monograph in one of the listed publications the product supplied must comply with the relevant monograph and not just with the generic description.

Quantity

The quantity which is ordered should be supplied, unless the provisions of 3(3) apply. This sub-paragraph was originally inserted into the TOS in 1965 in order to allow for the change-over from the old apothecary system of measures to metric measurements. An agreed system of conversion allowed apothecary measures to be converted into an approximate metric equivalent, e.g. 12 fluid ounces into 300 ml.

In practice, flexibility is allowed for items which are supplied in special containers to protect the contents, and for creams supplied in tubes, etc.

The DT allows payment to be made on the basis that the total amount in the special container has been ordered, but such a supply is strictly outside the requirements of the Medicines Act 1968 (see section on patient packs).

Missing details on script

Paragraph 8(6) allows the pharmacist to fill in certain missing details of quantity, strength and dosage.

Where the prescription is for a drug other than a Controlled Drug (CD) in Schedule 4 or 5, and the quantity, strength or dose is missing, the pharmacist may use his judgement to decide the missing information. He may give up to 5-day treatment at the appropriate dose. Where the product is a liquid antibiotic, an oral contraceptive or a combination pack, he may give the smallest original pack even if that quantity is larger than a 5-day course.

Paragraph 8(6) states that

> If the order is an order for a drug; but is not an order for a controlled drug within the meaning of the Misuse of Drugs Act 1971, other than a drug which is for the time being specified in Schedule 4 or 5 to the Misuse of Drugs Regulations 2001, and does not prescribe its quantity, strength or dosage, a pharmacist may provide the drug in such strength and dosage as in the exercise of his professional skill, knowledge and care he considers to be appropriate and subject to sub-paragraph (7), in such quantity as he considers to be appropriate for a course of treatment for a period not exceeding five days.

Where the strength or dosage is missing the pharmacist has complete freedom to supply what is appropriate. Note that where the wrong strength is given the pharmacist is not authorised by the regulations to change it. The PPA interprets the regulations as requiring the doctor to initial any alteration to the prescription which alters the strength ordered.

Professional practice requires that where an overdose is inadvertently ordered the pharmacist should reduce the dose to a safe one, and discuss his action with the prescriber as soon as possible.

Paragraph 8(7)

Where an order to which sub-paragraph (6) applies is for:

(a) an oral contraceptive substance;
(b) a drug, which is available for supply as part of pharmaceutical services only together with one or more drugs; or
(c) an antibiotic in a liquid form for oral administration in respect of which pharmaceutical considerations require its provision in an unopened package, which is not available for supply as part of pharmaceutical services except in such packages that the minimum available package contains a quantity appropriate to a course of treatment for a patient for a period of more than 5 days, the chemist may provide that minimum available package.

Patient Packs

Although no provision is made for the adoption of Patient Pack (formerly described as Original Pack) dispensing as a normal procedure, the TOS make special provision for dealing with products which are difficult to dispense from bulk.

Paragraph 8(8)

Where any drug to which this paragraph applies (that is, a drug that is not one to which the Misuse of Drugs Act 1971 applies, unless it is a drug which is for the time being specified in Schedule 4 or 5 to the Misuse of Drugs Regulations 2001), ordered by a prescriber on a prescription form, is available for provision by a chemist in a pack in a quantity which is different to the quantity which has been so ordered, and that drug is

(a) sterile
(b) effervescent or hygroscopic
(c) a liquid preparation for addition to bath water
(d) a coal tar preparation
(e) a viscous preparation or
(f) packed at the time of its manufacture in a calendar pack or special container, the pharmacist shall, subject to sub-paragraph (9), provide the drug in the pack whose quantity is nearest to the quantity which has been so ordered.

Paragraph 8(9)

A chemist shall not provide, pursuant to sub-paragraph (8), a drug in a calendar pack where, in his opinion, it was the intention of the doctor, dentist or nurse prescriber who ordered the drug that it should be provided only in the exact quantity ordered.

Paragraph 8(10) provides two definitions as follows:

(1) "Calendar pack" means a blister or strip pack showing the days of the week or month against each of the several units in the pack.
(2) "Special container" means any container with an integral means of application or from which it is not practicable to dispense an exact quantity.

Emergency NHS supplies

Paragraph 6 deals with "urgent supply without a prescription". In an emergency, a pharmacy may supply a drug if the prescriber:

(1) is personally known to the pharmacist
(2) requests the supply
(3) undertakes to supply a signed form or transmit an electronic prescription to the ETP service within 72 hours and
(4) the drug is not a Scheduled drug
(5) if a CD the drug is in Schedule 4 or 5 to the Misuse of Drugs Regulations.

The pharmacist is enabled to supply before the form arrives. He is not obliged to do so. Prescriber means a doctor, dentist, independent nurse prescriber or a supplementary prescriber. The procedure does not apply to appliances.

Paragraph 6 states

Where in a case of urgency, a prescriber personally known to a pharmacist requests him to provide a drug, the pharmacist may provide that drug before receiving a prescription form or repeatable prescription, provided that–

(a) that drug is not a Scheduled drug; and
(b) that drug is not a controlled drug within the meaning of the Misuse of Drugs Act 1971, other than a drug which is for the time being specified in Schedule 4 or 5 to the Misuse of Drugs Regulations 2001; and
(c) the prescriber undertakes to

    (i) give the pharmacist a non-electronic prescription form or non-electronic repeatable prescription in respect of the drug within 72 hours, or
    (ii) transmit to the ETP service within 72 hours an electronic prescription.

Selected List

In 1985 the government introduced, by means of Regulations, the "Selected List Scheme". Doctors were prohibited from prescribing, and pharmacists from dispensing a number of medicines in various categories. The categories are

indigestion remedies
laxatives
analgesics for mild to moderate pain

bitters and tonics
vitamins
benzodiazepine tranquillisers and sedatives.

Most of the medicines in these categories were put on a Schedule to the Regulations. Medicines listed on the Schedule may not be prescribed or dispensed under the NHS. Generic products were unaffected.

In December 1992, the Department announced that the scheme would be extended to an additional 10 categories:

anti-diarrhoeal drugs
drugs for allergic disorders
hypnotics and anxiolytics
appetitite suppressants
drugs for vaginal and vulval conditions
contraceptives
drugs used in anaemia
topical antirheumatics
drugs acting on the ear and nose
drugs acting on the skin

The current list is in Schedule 2 to the NHS (General Medical Services Contracts) (Prescription of Drugs) Regulations 2004, SI No. 629. References in the TOS to "Scheduled drug" refer to medicines listed on that Schedule. The list of products is amended from time to time. An up-to-date list is included in the current DT.

Schedule 2 contains a list of medicines which can only be prescribed for certain listed conditions, and only if the prescription form is endorsed by the prescriber with the initials "SLS".

Paragraph 8(11)

Except as provided in sub-paragraph (12), a pharmacist shall not provide a Scheduled drug in response to an order by name, formula or other description on a prescription form or repeatable prescription.

Paragraph 8(12)

Where a drug has an appropriate non-proprietary name and it is ordered on a prescription form or repeatable prescription either by that name or by its formula, a pharmacist may supply a drug which has the same specification notwithstanding that it is a Scheduled drug, provided that where a Scheduled drug is a pack which consists of a drug in more than one strength, such provision does not involve the supply of part only of the pack.

Paragraph 8(12) is intended to restrict the supply of constituent parts of combination packs, which otherwise would not be caught by the rules.

Paragraph 8(13)

Where a drug which is ordered as specified in sub-paragraph (12) combines more than one drug, that paragraph shall apply only if the combination has an appropriate non-proprietary name, whether the individual drugs which it combines do so or not.

Paragraph 8(13) is similarly intended to catch certain products containing a number of constituent drugs.

Containers

Paragraph 8(14)

A pharmacist shall provide any drug which he is required to provide under Paragraph 5 in a suitable container. The DT expands this requirement.

Capsules, tablets, pills, pulvules, etc. shall be supplied in airtight containers of glass, aluminium or rigid plastics. Card containers may be used only for foil/strip packed tablets, etc.

Card containers shall not be used for ointments, creams or pastes.

Eye, ear and nasal drops shall be supplied in dropper bottles, or with a separate dropper where appropriate.

When an oral liquid medicine is dispensed, a 5 ml plastics spoon shall be supplied by the pharmacist unless the patient already has a spoon or the manufacturer's pack includes one.

Doses less than 5 ml

In 1992 the previous "dilution convention" agreed between the Royal Pharmaceutical Society of Great Britain (RPSGB) and the British Medical Association (BMA), under which doses of less than 5 ml were diluted, was abandoned. Under the new agreement, doses of less than 5 ml are to be measured by the patient using an oral syringe. The medicine is to be dispensed undiluted. The specification for the oral syringe is in the DT. Patients requiring an oral syringe are to be supplied with one, without charge.

Contraceptive services

The supply of contraceptive substances and appliances forms part of the "pharmaceutical services" to be provided. All contraceptive substances are available, but only those appliances included in the DT. For example, diaphragms are included in the DT, but condoms are not.

Under the provisions of SI 1975/719, a pharmacist could notify the FHSA that he wished to be excluded from the arrangements for the supply of contraceptive substances. It was intended to take account of religious or moral objections to contraception. The provision disappeared from the regulations in 1987, when an amendment (SI 1987/401) replaced the existing Regulation 26 with a new version which omitted the "conscience clause". It is also missing from the current Contract Regulations. When applying for a contract the pharmacist can specify the services he intends to provide. This would seem to be an opportunity to indicate any religious or moral restrictions on the service.

Contractors are only required to supply such appliances as they normally stock, so no problem arises with contraceptive appliances.

Opening hours

Part 3 of Schedule 1 of the Contract Regulations deals with opening hours.

Except where the pharmacist has agreed to open for not less than 100 hours, pharmaceutical services shall be provided at the premises for not less than 40 hours each week.

The PCT can direct a pharmacy to open for more than 40 hours, or it can allow less hours. Where the PCT allows a variation from 40 hours it may set the times and days of opening.

When doing this the PCT must seek to ensure that the hours of opening are such as to ensure that services are provided on such days and at such times as are necessary to meet the needs of people in the neighbourhood or other likely users of the pharmacy.

Each pharmacy must provide the PCT with opening hours and a list of services. Any change must also be notified to the PCT.

Notices

Paragraph 22(2)

Each pharmacy, except a mail order or Internet pharmacy, must display

(a)   a notice which shows the opening hours, and
(b)   when the pharmacy is closed, a notice which indicates the addresses of other pharmacies nearby and their opening hours
(c)   when the pharmacy is closed, a notice which indicates the addresses of LPS pharmacies nearby, their services and their opening hours.

Illness of pharmacist

Paragraph 22(6)

> Where a chemist is prevented by illness or other reasonable cause from complying with his obligations under paragraph 22(1), he shall, where practicable, make arrangements with one or more pharmacists or LPS pharmacists whose premises are situated in the neighbourhood for the provision of pharmaceutical services or LPS during that time.

The obligation to make alternative arrangements is with the affected pharmacy, but only when "practicable". The provision applies to illness or "other reasonable cause".

When alternative arrangements cannot be made, there is no breach of the TOS if there is a temporary suspension of services, provided:

● the PCT is notified as soon as practical
● all reasonable endeavours are used to resume service as soon as possible (Paragraph 22(9)).

The TOS explicitly state in Paragraph 22(10) that "planned refurbishment' of a pharmacy is neither a 'reasonable cause' for the purposes of sub-paragraph (7) nor a 'reason beyond the control of the pharmacist' for the purposes of sub-paragraph (9)".

Changes to hours made by PCT

Paragraph 24 deals with review of hours by the PCT, in cases where it appears to the PCT that the needs of the neighbourhood are not being met. The LPC must be consulted. The changes must be notified to the pharmacy. There is an appeal process.

Variation of hours instigated by the pharmacy

Paragraph 25 deals with applications to vary the previous hours.

Supervision

Paragraph 8(2) requires the provision of drugs or appliances to be under the direct supervision of a pharmacist.

A pharmacist shall make all the necessary arrangements for measuring patients, and for fitting, when the appliance which is ordered requires this. (Paragraph 8(4))

Provision of advice to patients

The pharmacist must provide appropriate advice to patients:

- about any drug or appliance provided to them
- about the safekeeping of the products
- about returning unwanted products to the pharmacy.

The advice is to enable patients to utilise the products appropriately, and also to meet their "reasonable needs" for general information.

The pharmacist must also:

- advise patients to only request repeats which are needed
- provide owing slips and estimates when the product will be available
- keep patient medication records, including in appropriate cases, of advice given and interventions made. (Paragraph 10)

Disposal of unwanted drugs

Where the PCT has made suitable arrangements, the pharmacist must accept and dispose of unwanted drugs from:

- a private household
- a residential care home.

The pharmacist must carry out a risk assessment and train staff, on the handling of waste drugs, and have protective equipment available. (Paragraph 14)

Healthy lifestyle messages

Where it appears to the pharmacist that a patient:

- has diabetes
- is at risk of CHD, especially with high blood pressure
- smokes or is overweight

then the pharmacist must, where appropriate, provide that person with advice aimed at increasing his knowledge and understanding of the relevant health issues.

In addition to the advice, the pharmacist may refer the patient elsewhere, and/or give written material. (Paragraph 16)

Where appropriate, records must be kept.

When requested by the PCT the pharmacy must participate in up to six public health campaigns each year. (Paragraph 17)

Signposting

Pharmacists must provide contact information to users of the pharmacy when it appears that they require advice, treatment or support that the pharmacist cannot provide, but which is available elsewhere in the health or social services. (Paragraphs 18 and 19)

Records must be kept when appropriate.

Support for self-care

A pharmacist must provide advice and support to people caring for themselves or their family:

- on treatment options and use of over-the-counter (OTC) medicines
- on lifestyle changes. (Paragraphs 20 and 21)

Records must be kept when appropriate.

Information to be provided to PCT

Certain information about the pharmacist or the superintendent and directors of a company must be provided to the PCT, such as:

- information about criminal convictions, binding over, cautions, etc.
- investigations into professional conduct by licensing, regulatory or other bodies
- investigations by the NHS Counter Fraud and Security Management Service in relation to fraud
- investigations by another PCT or equivalent body
- removal or suspension on fitness to practise grounds from any equivalent list. (Paragraphs 29 and 30)

A company need only provide this information to its "Home PCT" provided it has informed that PCT of all other PCTs won whose lists it is included. (Paragraph 31 as amended)

A pharmacist shall tell the PCT of any change in the information recorded about him, including any change of private address, change in registered office of a company and any change affecting his inclusion in the EDP list.

Particulars of qualified staff

Paragraph 34

The PCT can require the name of any registered pharmacist employed in the dispensing of a particular prescription. (Paragraph 34(2))

Charges

Paragraph 36 states that subject to Regulations made under *Section 77* of the Act, all drugs, containers and appliances are to be supplied free.

The NHS (Charges for Drugs and Appliances) Regulations 2000, SI No. 620 are the ones made under *Section 77*. They are updated each year and contain the charges to be made for the supply of medicines and appliances.

Availability of records

Paragraph 37 allows the PCT to inspect the pharmacy:

- to satisfy itself that the pharmacy is complying with the TOS
- to monitor and audit the provision for patient care
- to monitor and audit the management of the services.

There must be reasonable notice of entry, and the LPC should be invited to be present. Residential parts of the premises may only be inspected with permission.

Inducements

Paragraph 28 states that

> A pharmacist or his staff shall not give, promise or offer to any person any gift or reward (whether by way of a share of or dividend on the profits of the business or by way of discount or rebate or otherwise) as an inducement to or in consideration of his presenting an order for drugs or appliances on a prescription form or for nominating he pharmacist as his dispensing contractor in his NHS Care Record.

This does not prohibit the supply of free controlled dosage systems to users of the pharmacy, nor the availability of collection and delivery systems, etc.

Professional standards

Requirements as to professional standards were first inserted in 1996.

Paragraph 27 now reads:

> A pharmacist shall provide pharmaceutical services and exercise any professional judgement in connection with the provision of such services in conformity with the standards generally accepted in the pharmaceutical profession.

The requirement refers to the "generally accepted" standards. Although it does not specifically refer to the RPSGB Code of Ethics, it is that document which will in most cases set out the generally accepted standards.

Withdrawal from the pharmaceutical lists

A pharmacy may give 3-month notice to the PCT requesting removal from the lists, if practicable.

Pharmacies which work 100 hours a week must give 6-month notice, if practicable. (Paragraph 35)

Complaints procedure

National Health Service pharmacies are required to have in place a system for dealing with expressions of dissatisfaction by users of pharmaceutical services. The system should be essentially the same as that set out in Part II of the NHS (Complaints) Regulations 2004, SI No. 1768.

See also Chapter 9.

Remuneration

Part 4 of the Regulations sets out how the PCT must pay the pharmacist.

Paragraph 56(1) requires the PCT to pay according to the DT. Where this is not possible the PCT may determine a fee where appropriate, with consultation of the LPC. This facilitates a degree of locally determined remuneration.

Payments must be made to suspended pharmacists, according to a determination made by the S of S.

Electronic transmission of prescriptions (ETP)

The Contract Regulations are worded on the assumption that ETP becomes commonplace.

The PCT must keep a separate list of pharmacists who participate in ETP. (Regulation 72)

There is provision for electronic signatures, which are tightly defined.

Prescription form includes electronic forms.

Chapter 4

The Drug Tariff

Form and Content of the Drug Tariff

Every month the S of S approves and the PPA publishes the "Drug Tariff" (DT). It contains a list of drug prices; detailed information on appliances; sets the standards of and payments for drugs and appliances; and details what can and cannot be prescribed on NHS prescriptions and by which class of practitioner (that is doctor, dentist or nurse). Separate Tariffs are produced for England and Wales, Scotland and Northern Ireland.

Regulation 56(1) of the NHS (PS) Regulations 2005 states,

For the purpose of enabling arrangements to be made for the provision of pharmaceutical services, the S of S shall compile and publish a statement (in these regulations referred to as "the Drug Tariff") which he may amend from time to time and which (subject to Paragraph (2) shall include . . .

(a)   the list of appliances for the time being approved by the S of S for the purposes of *Section 41* of the Act and, in the case of a restricted availability appliance, the categories of person for whom or purposes for which the appliance is approved

(b)   the list of chemical reagents for the time being approved by the S of S for the purposes of *Section 41* of the Act

(c)   the list of drugs for the time being approved by the S of S for the purposes of *Section 41* of the Act

(d)   the prices on the basis of which the payment for drugs and appliances ordinarily supplied is to be calculated

(e)   the method of calculating the payment for drugs not mentioned in the DT

(f)   the method of calculating the payment for containers and medicine measures

(g)   the dispensing or other fees or allowances payable in respect of the provision of pharmaceutical services or directed services

(h)   the dispensing or other fees or allowances payable in respect of the temporary provision of pharmaceutical services or directed services under Regulation 54

(i)   arrangements for claiming fees, allowances and other remuneration for the provision of pharmaceutical services or directed services, and

(j)   the method by which a claim may be made for compensation for financial loss in respect of oxygen equipment specified in the DT.

Regulation 56(2) states that

The DT may state in respect of any specified fee falling within Paragraph (1)(g) or (h), or any other specified fee, allowance or other remuneration in respect of the provision of pharmaceutical services by chemists included in the pharmaceutical list of a PCT, that the determining authority for that fee, allowance or other remuneration for those chemists is the PCT, and in such a case Paragraphs (5) and (6) shall apply.

Regulation 56(3) states that

The prices referred to in Paragraph 1(d) may be fixed prices or may be subject to monthly or other periodic variations to be determined by reference to fluctuations in the cost of drugs and appliances.

Besides the list included in the Regulations the DT also contains many other items of information useful to pharmacists and prescribers.

By virtue of Paragraph 1 of Schedule 2 of the NHS (PS) Regulations 2005, the DT lists of drugs and appliances are incorporated into the TOS. In other words, whatever is in the DT about prices to be paid for drugs and appliances is considered to be something which is agreed to by the pharmacist on taking up the contract.

The DT is produced on a monthly basis and the amendments for the month are listed in the preface. The preface bears the words "Pursuant to Reg 56(1) of the NHS (PS) Regs 2005 the Secretary of State for Health as respects England and pursuant to the National Health Service (PS) (Amendment) (Wales) Regulations 2005 has amended the Drug Tariff with effect from [date]".

Amendments, including prices, come into effect on the date specified, regardless of whether the DT has been received by the pharmacist and regardless of whether the particular amendment has actually been printed in the DT.

Part I – Requirements for the supply of drugs, appliances and chemical reagents

The DT sets out much of the arrangement for prescribing and dispensing for NHS patients. The basic principles of prescribing under the NHS are that

(1) Doctors may prescribe any medicine, unless its use at NHS expense is specifically prohibited by the S of S, or its use is restricted to specified circumstances.
(2) Doctors may prescribe an appliance or chemical reagent, only if its use at NHS expense is approved by the S of S, and only in the circumstances specified.
(3) Doctors may prescribe a "borderline substance" only if its use at NHS expense is approved by the S of S, and only in the circumstances specified.

Clause 1 requires that any drugs supplied must comply with the standard specified in the DT (if any such standard is included). Otherwise the drug must comply with the relevant standard in the BNF, DPF, EP, BP or BPC. The prescriber may indicate that he requires some other standard. If the prescriber has not indicated the standard, and the drug does not appear in one of the relevant publications then the grade or quality must be no lower than that ordinarily used for medicinal purposes.

Clause 2 states that only the appliances listed in the DT may be supplied, and that they must comply with the specifications listed in the DT. Certain items in Part IXA are not prescrible on forms FP10 (CN) or FP10 (PN) and these are marked.

In practice the "Technical Specifications" of the DT were last issued as a separate document in 1981, although they are available on request from the PPA. However many of the individual entries contain details which in effect are specifications, e.g. the size of a bandage. Dressings are included in the category "appliances". Neither the NHS Act nor the Regulations refer to dressings as such except to define them as appliances.

Since June 1998, "medical devices" (as defined in the Medical Devices Regulation 1994) which are supplied on prescription have been required to bear a CE mark.

Clause 3 states that only the chemical reagents listed may be supplied.

Pharmacists are not required to ascertain the purpose for which prescribed items are to be used. All drugs may be supplied except those on Schedule 1. Pure chemical compounds, organic or inorganic may be supplied as drugs. Chemical reagents other than those listed could therefore be supplied, and the pharmacist would be paid for their supply. If they were prescribed as reagents the doctor would be liable to pay the cost if action were brought under the NHS (General Medical Services) Regulations.

Clause 4 states that the requirements for the Domiciliary Oxygen Theraphy Service (DOTS) are in Part X of the DT. However the supply of oxygen by community pharmacies was discontinued by the DOH in 2005.

Clause 5 deals with claims for payment. Forms must be endorsed, sorted and despatched as PCTs (or local health boards in Wales) direct. The DT contains a number of rules about how prescription forms are to be handled in order for the correct payments to be made.

Where contractors have failed to despatch the forms on time, PCTs have held this to be a breach of the TOS. Occasional lateness is not considered to be a problem, but persistent and serious lateness is. The late submission of forms to the PPA causes extra costs and disrupts the PPA system.

Clause 5A deals with the handling of forms for repeat dispensing services.

Part 2 – Requirements enabling payments to be made

Clause 6 contains a very brief description of the payment systems.

Calculating payments

Clause 7 contains a more detailed description of the way payments are calculated for drugs. There is also a statement that if, after being requested to properly endorse a form the contractor fails to do so, then the S of S may decide the price.

Clause 7D is unusual in nature. It is a deeming provision. If the contractor's overall use of a particular product would seem to justify the use of a larger pack size than that endorsed, then the endorsement will be ignored and the price paid will be based on the appropriate larger size. The actual words refer to "that normally required pursuant to orders on prescription forms" – a remarkably unclear phrase. Further there is no indication of what constitutes the criteria for determining that a larger size ought to have been used.

Clause 8 states that the basic price for drugs, appliances and chemical reagents listed in Parts VIII and IX of the Drug Tariff is the price in the DT. For other generic and branded drugs it is the manufacturers list price.

The PPA may, under specified circumstances, accept an endorsement that a price higher than the "statutory maximum price" has been paid.

Endorsement

The forms must be endorsed as required. The intention of endorsement is to ensure that the Pricing Authority has sufficient information to price accurately. The principle is that as far as possible the actual price paid by the pharmacist is paid by the NHS. Account is taken of the discounts obtained on purchases by averaging them and deducting an average discount from the totals of list prices. Additional rules for endorsement are found in Clauses 9–13, the remainder of Part II, in Part III, and in the Notes to Part VIII.

Clause 9 contains the main endorsement requirements. No endorsement is needed except for "broken bulk" or where the quantity supplied differs from the order, for

(a)   generic drugs listed in Part VIII
(b)   appliances listed in Part IX
(c)   chemical reagents listed in Part IX.

The pack size and name of maker or wholesaler is needed for orders for generic drugs not in the DT.
   Where no product is available to contractors at the Part VIII price, the prescription may be specially endorsed. This concession is only allowed when the Secretary of State has agreed that the product is not available. The contractor must have made all reasonable efforts to obtain the product at the DT price. The endorsement must include the brand name or manufacturer or wholesaler of the product, the pack size, the phrase "no cheaper stock obtainable" (or "NCSO") and be signed and dated on behalf of the contractor.
   The PPA may request additional information in order to price the prescription.

Clause 10 allows what is supplied to deviate from the exact quantity ordered only in specified circumstances. These are where it is particularly difficult to open the container and dispense a part of its contents.

Broken bulk

Clause 11 sets out the rules whereby a contractor may be paid for the whole amount of a drug when less has been supplied. The rules appear to set out an objective test – that the remainder cannot readily be disposed of – whereas in practice a subjective test is used. The contractor may claim if he believes he will not readily dispose of the remainder. Subsequent supplies are deemed to have been made from the remainder for the next six months, or until the remainder would in any event have been used up.
   The PPA interpret the "broken bulk" facility by using a "two-thirds" rule. If a contractor receives two or more prescriptions in the same calendar month, totalling more than 2/3 of a pack, the PPA assume that this establishes usage and so considers the broken bulk claims as invalid.
   In a service case where a contractor made a large number of broken bulk claims which were unjustified, the FHSA decided that constituted a breach of the TOS and recommended a very large withholding. The conduct was also regarded as fraud by the Crown Court, resulting in a heavy fine.

Miscellaneous matters

Clause 12 Out-of-pocket expenses over 10p may be claimed in certain circumstances.

Clause 13 extends the broken bulk rules in Clause 11 to allow for payment of the full cost of using reconstituted products with a short life.

What may be supplied?

Pharmacists will be paid for any medicines (including OTC medicines, homoeopathic preparations and herbal products) provided the item does not appear in Schedule 1 of the NHS (GMS Contracts) (Prescription of Drugs, etc.) Regulations 2004, which is reproduced in the DT as Part XVIIIA.

(1) Quantity. Clause 10 allows what is supplied to deviate from the exact quantity ordered only in specified circumstances. These are where it is particularly difficult to open the container and dispense a part of its contents.

(2) Quality. Drugs and medicines supplied must comply with the standards in the appropriate book: BNF, DPF, EP, BP, BPC or the DT itself. Where a drug or medicine does not appear in one of those then the grade or quality supplied should be the ordinary medicinal grade.

For appliances, the quality will be determined either by an official standard referred to in the name, e.g. absorbent lint BPC, or by a specification in the DT itself. DT Technical Specifications are obtainable on request from the PPA.

(3) Type. Any drug or medicine which is ordered may be supplied provided it is not included in Schedule 1 (printed as Part XVIIIA of the DT).

Drugs or medicines included in Schedule 2 may only be supplied when the prescription bears the endorsement "SLS" inserted by the prescriber. Additionally the conditions referred to in the Schedule must be complied with, although the pharmacist is under no obligation to verify these.

There is no requirement that the drugs or medicines supplied shall be licensed medicinal products (licensed under the Medicines Act 1968).

Only the appliances listed in Part IXA, B and C may be supplied.

The only chemical reagents which may be supplied are those listed in Part IXR.

Some diagnostic reagents are regarded as drugs. Neither the 1977 NHS Act nor the NHS (PS) Regulations 2005 refer specifically to diagnostic reagents. The effect of *Section 41* and *Section 128* of the Act together with Regulation 56 is that the DT can make provision for diagnostic reagents only if they are drugs, chemical reagents, medicines or appliances. Since it is difficult to regard something used for determining whether an illness exists to be the means of treating that illness, diagnostic reagents might not be regarded as medicines. The definition of a medicinal product in the Medicines Act specifically includes a substance used in "diagnosing disease or ascertaining the existence, degree or extent of a physiological condition".

For NHS purposes, however, the matter was clarified by a notice, ECL 80/1953 (ECN 132), which states that the Minister is prepared to regard certain diagnostic reagents as drugs for the purposes of the NHS (GMPS) Regulations. The list comprises

Dick Test
Protein Sensitisation Test Solution
Schick Test
Tuberculin Tests:
    Koch Test
    Mantoux Test
    Patch Test
    Diagnostic Jelly

How are payments made?

The DT lays down the basic rules which will be followed by the PPA when calculating the payments to be made in respect of the drugs, etc. supplied on Forms FP10 and variants.

Basically, payment is made for the quantity supplied on the script. The price paid is calculated from the normal wholesale price of the product for supply to community pharmacists. This price is normally set out by the manufacturer in price lists.

A discount is deducted from the total due to each contractor for each months dispensing. The discount is calculated according to the total amount due, on a sliding scale constructed to reflect the discounts generally achieved by contractors in their purchasing.

Zero discount

The DT contains two "Zero Discount" (ZD) lists. These lists contain both individual brand names (e.g. Eprex Injection) and descriptions of product groups (e.g. Alternative Medicines). Products on List A will not have discount deducted from the DT price. No endorsement is necessary.

Products on List B will not have discount deducted if the contractor received no discount from the supplier, and the prescription is endorsed ZD.

How must the forms be endorsed?

Rules for endorsing the forms are found in Clauses 9, 10 and 11, Part III and the Notes to Part VIII.

At the end of each calendar month the contractor must sort the prescription forms in a manner directed by the FHSA. They must then be despatched, together with the appropriate claim form, not later than the fifth day of the next month.

The claim form is standard, and also contains instructions for sorting.

Containers

Part IV specifies that card containers may only be used to dispense foil or strip packed tablets, capsules, etc. All other medicines, including creams and ointments must be supplied in airtight containers of glass, aluminium or rigid plastic. Where appropriate, a dropper bottle or separate dropper shall be used.

Appliances and dressings

Part IX of the DT lists the appliances and dressings which may be supplied. The list is very specific, in some instances only certain sizes may be supplied although others are made. For example, only 10 cm Non-Sterile Gauze Swabs, packed in 100s may be supplied.

In some entries, where a general specification is given, any make which meets the specification may be supplied e.g. WOW bandage BP. In others only the specified makes may be supplied. This is particularly noticeable where items for incontinence are concerned, where the detail extends to the model number.

Borderline substances

Under the NHS a general medical practitioner may prescribe (and the NHS may pay for) only drugs, medicines and certain appliances. Drugs and medicines are not clearly defined, but the category does not include food or cosmetics. Hospitals are not restricted in the same way and are able to provide anything needed for the care of the patient.

Note that the NHS Acts use the terms "drugs" and "medicines" whereas the Medicines Act 1968 uses the term "medicinal product". The two terms "medicine" and "medicinal product" are not synonymous. "Medicinal product" is defined in the Medicines Act as a substance which is made or sold for use in treating, diagnosing or preventing disease or otherwise altering the normal physiological state.

"Drug" is a wider term which includes pure chemicals which are not produced for any particular purpose, e.g. glucose, but which are used in therapeutics. "Medicines" refers to the product ready for administration, e.g. tablet.

There are circumstances where a patient will benefit from the prescribing of food or cosmetics. Certain metabolic disorders are best treated by the supply of special foods which do not contain a particular amino acid. Photosensitivity reactions caused by drugs can be minimised by the use of sunscreens.

Prescribers are requested to endorse prescriptions for borderline substances which are written in accordance with the advice of the Committee with the letters ACBS.

Prescriptions are monitored by the Prescription Pricing Authority, which may refer them to PCTs. Where an PCT receives a prescription for a product which it does not believe is a drug it may refer the matter to the local LMC under procedures provided by Regulation 20 of the NHS (Service Committees & Tribunal) Regulations 1974.

Advisory Committee or Borderline Substances (ACBD)

The Advisory Committee on Borderline Substances exists to provide the S of S for Health with expert independent medical advice on those substances which, although not drugs or medicines, are used in a similar manner. The Committee advises on the classification and on whether or not they should be prescribed by GPs at NHS expense or prescribed only for patients with specified medical conditions.

The Terms of Reference which were announced in December 1992 are

> To advise UK Health Ministers as to whether particular substances, preparations or items should not be treated as drugs for the purpose of the GMS Regulations; and to advise on appropriate amendments to Schedules 10 and 11 to the NHS (GMS) Regulations 1992 and the corresponding schedules in the regulations in Scotland and Northern Ireland accordingly.

In considering whether a particular substance, preparation or item should be included in such schedules, the Committee will have regard to the need to ensure that substances which have therapeutic use in the treatment of disease in the community can be provided as economically as possible under the NHS.

The Committee itself contains experts from many disciplines and is advised by medical and pharmaceutical assessors within the DOH. The members are appointed by the S of S for Health in England, and the S of S for Scotland and Wales, after consultation with professional bodies. Members are appointed for a period of three years.

The Committee is a non-statutory body. Its existence has no basis in law and depends only upon the need for advice from an authoritative independent body.

Requests for consideration

It is open to doctors, manufacturers or the Health Departments to request the Committee to consider any substance or product of a borderline nature. The manufacturers are asked to provide the following information about the product:

(1) the indications for use
(2) details of formulation
(3) relevant clinical trials
(4) promotional policy
(5) confirmation that the product will be available for dispensing by community pharmacies
(6) applicability of the Medicines Act (e.g. exemption under the Food and Cosmetics Order)
(7) descriptive literature, samples, packaging.

The ACBS advises manufacturers in writing of the proposed unfavourable recommendations, giving them at least 30 days in which to make representations. An oral hearing may be granted if the case is complex. The manufacturer may be represented at the oral hearing, either legally or by other experts.

The Committee considers all relevant information provided by the manufacturer of the substance concerned.

If the S of S accepts the decision of the Committee that a product should not be regarded as drug, he may place the product on Schedule 10 to the NHS (GMS) Regulations. This is the list of products which may not be prescribed by GPs.

Medical Foods Regulations

The Medical Food Regulations (England) 2000, SI No. 845, implement European Commission Directive 99/21/EC, which was developed to meet the Commission's requirement under framework Directive 89/398/EC to introduce specific rules for dietary foods for special medical purposes.

Corresponding regulations have been introduced in Wales, Northern Ireland and Scotland.

Medical foods are a unique group of foods used in the dietary management of specific diseases or medical conditions. The government considered that the population group for whom these products are intended is particularly vulnerable, and therefore specific controls, in addition to the general provisions of the Food Safety Act, are appropriate.

The Regulations define foodstuffs which may be sold as "Food(s) for Special Medical Purposes" (FSMPs); lay down specific compositional and labelling requirements for them; and introduce a notification system to facilitate efficient monitoring of new products.

Maximum and minimum vitamin, mineral and trace element levels for specific categories of FSMPs are set by the Regulations.

The labelling requirements supplement those required by the Food Labeling Regulations 1996 (as amended) and are intended to provide sufficient nutritional and other information to health professionals and consumers to ensure the appropriate and effective use of these products under medical supervision.

The Regulations introduce a formal obligation to notify new products when first placed on the market.

Statutory procedure for classifying borderline substances

The Medicines for Human Use (Marketing Authorisations, etc.) Amendment Regulations, SI No. 2000/292 amend the 1994 marketing Authorisations Regulations to give power to stop a company selling a product, which the licensing authority believes is a medicine, without a marketing authority. The licensing authority must explain why they consider the product to be a medicine. There is an appeal to a review panel.

Maximum price legislation

The basic price for a generic medicine listed in Parts VIII and IX of the DT is the price stated in the DT.

However, maximum prices are set by the DOH. The list is available on a website www.doh.gov.uk/generic.

An exemption allows contractors to claim a higher price in certain circumstances as set out in Clause 8.

The prices of medicines supplied for NHS use are controlled in a number of ways.

Pharmaceutical Price Regulation Scheme

First, the majority of branded medicine manufacturers belong to a voluntary price regulation scheme. The current scheme, called the Pharmaceutical Price Regulation Scheme (PPRS) was agreed between the DOH and the Association of the British Pharmaceutical Industry (the trade organisation for the pharmaceutical industry). It came into effect on 1 January 2005 and is scheduled to run for 5 years. It covers those medicines which are manufactured by scheme members and which:

(a) have EC or UK marketing authorisations
(b) are sold as branded products and
(c) are supplied to the NHS.

The scheme includes branded medicines regardless of whether patent protection is in force, and medicines supplied on tender or on contract. OTC medicines dispensed against an NHS prescription are included. Generic medicines, "standard" branded generics and OTC medicines sold directly to the public are not included. A "standard" branded generic is defined as an out-of-patent product to which the manufacturer/supplier, who is not the originator company, has applied a brand name and that is directly comparable to a true generic, that is readily available.

Under this scheme prices are controlled indirectly. The control is exerted by limiting the profits made by manufacturers. Target profits are set as a percentage of capital invested. If the figure is exceeded the company is required to reduce its prices or to make a repayment to the DOH. However, prices may only be raised with the approval of DOH. A company has freedom to set the price for new products within the constraint of the profit target.

Statutory control of prices

Membership of the PPRS is voluntary. Companies that choose not to become members of the 2005 PPRS are subject to the statutory price control under *Section 34* of the Health Act 1999.

Control of branded medicine prices

The Health Service Medicines (Control of Prices of Branded Medicines) Regulations 2000, SI No. 123, came into force on 14 February 2000.

The Regulations, which apply to the United Kingdom, control the price of branded medicines sold for NHS purposes. They apply only to medicines which:

(a) have EC or UK marketing authorisations
(b) are sold as branded products and
(c) are supplied to the NHS and
(d) are supplied by companies which are not scheme members within the meaning of *Section 33(4)* of the Health Act 1999.

Under the Regulations, the maximum price which may be charged for the supply for health service purposes of a branded health service medicine of a particular presentation shall not exceed 95.5% of the 1999 price and for newer products the initial price. Financial information must be provided to the DH. There are penalties for failing to supply information, and for supplying above the specified price.

Control of generic medicine prices

The Health Service Medicines (Control of Prices of Specified Generic Medicines) Regulations, 2000 SI No. 1763, came into effect on 3 August 2000.

These Regulations allow the DOH to control the prices of generic medicines which are sold "for the purposes of the national health services in England and Wales, Scotland and Northern Ireland".

Under the Regulations, the maximum price which is charged by a manufacturer or supplier for the supply of a specified generic medicine for health service use shall not exceed the "specified price".

"Supply" means supply by way of sale to a person lawfully conducting a retail pharmacy business or to a registered medical practitioner, in order to enable that person or practitioner (as the case may be) to provide pharmaceutical services within the meaning of –

(a) *Section 41* of the National Health Service Act 1977 in England or Wales;
(b) *Section 27* of the National Health Service (Scotland) Act 1978 in Scotland; and
(c) Article 63 of the Health and Personal Social Services (Northern Ireland) Order 1972 in Northern Ireland.

The "specified price" is the price specified in the list. Provision is made for the maximum price to be increased.

The Regulations apply only to the medicines specified in the list of controlled prices, which is published on the website at the address http://www.doh.gov.uk/generics. Printed copies of the list are available from the DOH.

They apply only to medicines that have marketing authorisations.

The manufacturers and wholesalers must provide sales information to the S of S. There are penalties for failing to supply information, and for supplying above the specified price.

Appeals

A manufacturer or supplier affected by price controls made under the statutory provisions has a right of appeal in accordance with The Health Service Medicines (Price Control Appeals) Regulations 2000, SI No. 124.

Control of OTC prices

Following a decision of the Restrictive Practices Court on 15 May 2001, there are no longer any controls on the prices of OTC medicines sold to the public.

Chapter 5

Applications to Dispense NHS Prescriptions

This chapter is concerned mainly with the provisions governing the opening of a pharmacy, and the application for an NHS contract in an urban area. The rural dispensing arrangements are dealt with in Chapter 4.

Neither this chapter nor the one on rural dispensing arrangements is intended to give a step-by-step set of instructions on how applications should be made or how they are processed. Instead we aim only to outline the procedures.

The opening of a new pharmacy is subject to a number of controls. One set of controls relate to professional matters. They derive from the Medicines Act 1968 and from the law governing the profession of pharmacy. These are dealt with in Chapter 9. The other set of controls relate to the granting of an NHS contract. A pharmacy may open without an NHS contract although such pharmacies are few in number.

Applications for NHS contract

Until 1983 an application to dispense NHS prescriptions in a pharmacy was automatically granted. Since 1983 there have been a number of restrictive measures.

In 1987, amending regulations introduced a system of control to link the number of persons included in a pharmaceutical list as closely as possible to the need of the local population for reasonable access to the full range of NHS pharmaceutical services. At the same time they were intended to take account of the cost to the taxpayer of providing pharmaceutical services. A new contract was only to be granted if it was "necessary or desirable" to secure adequate provision in the neighbourhood.

In 2003 the Office of Fair Trading published a report "The Control of entry regulations and retail pharmacy services in the UK" which recommended abolition of the statutory controls on entry in order to increase competition.

The government decided not to implement the proposals in full, but introduced a package of changes designed to increase competition whilst retaining controls on entry.

A new contract for NHS community pharmacies was introduced at the same time.

The main law is now found in the NHS (PS) Regulations 2005, SI No. 641 (the "Contract Regulations"). The Regulations have already been amended twice, by the NHS (Pharmaceutical Services) Amendment Regulations 2005, SI No. 1015, and the NHS (PS) (Amendment No. 2) Regulations 2005, SI No. 1501.

A guide to the Control of Entry parts of these Regulations has been issued by the DOH as "Information for PCTs (Control of Entry)."

Since 1992 there have been a number of court decisions which have attempted to clarify the previous Regulations and many of these decisions will be applicable to the new Regulations.

Duty of the PCT

Section 41 of the NHS Act 1977 states,

> it is the duty of every PCT, in accordance with regulations, to arrange as respects their area for the provision to persons who are in the area of pharmaceutical services.

The pharmaceutical list

The PCT has a duty to keep "pharmaceutical lists" of persons who undertake to provide pharmaceutical services. The lists are of:

(a)   those who provide drugs (pharmacies)
(b)   those who provide appliances.

Each list contains the name and address of the contractor, and the hours at which the service is provided. The list of pharmacies must also indicate whether or not the pharmacy has undertaken to provide "directed services". (Regulation 4)

Pharmaceutical services are the provision of:

(a)   proper and sufficient drugs, medicines and appliances ordered by doctors and dentists; and
(b)   such other services as may be prescribed in the regulations (*Section 41* NHS Act 1977).

   Section 42 allows regulations to be made to ensure the effective provision of those services.
   Section 42 also introduces a test for granting applications – the "necessary or desirable" test.

Application to PCT

Anyone who wishes to operate an NHS pharmacy in a PCT area, to open additional or new premises, or to change the services which are provided must apply to the PCT.
   Some applications are automatically granted. Others are subject to the "necessary or desirable" test.
   Any application must contain the information which is set out in Schedule 4 of the Contract Regulations.

Who may apply for a contract?

Section 43 of the NHS Act 1977 limits the classes of persons who may provide pharmaceutical services.

> No arrangements shall be made by an HA (except as may be provided by regulations) with a medical practitioner or dental practitioner under which he is required

or agrees to provide pharmaceutical services to any person to whom he is rendering general medical services or general dental services. (Section 43(1))

No arrangements for the dispensing of medicines shall be made (except as may be provided in regulations) with persons other than persons who are registered pharmacists, or are persons lawfully conducting a retail pharmacy business in accordance with section 69 of the Medicines Act 1968 and who undertake that all medicines supplied by them under the arrangements made under this part of this Act shall be dispensed either by or under the direct supervision of a registered pharmacist. (Section 43(2))

Primary Care Trusts have been advised by the DOH to summarily reject applications to dispense medicines which are from persons who are not entitled to conduct a retail pharmacy business. The Guidance states that all applications for inclusion in the pharmaceutical list must be rejected if they are not from pharmacists, partnerships of pharmacists or from companies.

The procedures which the PCT must follow are set out in the Regulations. There is an appeal procedure to the FHS Appeals Unit.

Exemptions from the Control of entry test

The Contract Regulations introduce automatic exemptions from the control of entry tests for:

- pharmacies located in large out-of-town shopping centres
- pharmacies that intend to open for more than 100 hours a week
- consortia establishing new One-Stop Primary Care centres
- pharmacies which only provide mail order or Internet services
- minor relocations
- change of ownership of pharmacy.

Provided the conditions set out in the Regulations are met, the application is automatically granted.

Pharmacies located in large out-of-town shopping centres

The development must approved by the S of S for the purpose of these regulations. It must be of 15,000 square metres gross lettable floor space and considered out of town. The criteria are set out in Regulation 15. A list is published of the developments which meet the criteria.

Pharmacies that intend to open for more than 100 hours a week

The willingness to keep open for more than 100 hours becomes a condition of the grant. The PCT may not vary or remove the condition. If the condition is breached the premises may be removed from the list if:

- the person has repeatedly breached the condition without good cause or
- the breach is serious and the safety of a patient has been or may be put at serious risk.

Consortia establishing new one stop primary care centres

The premises must be a "one-stop primary care centre", which is defined in Regulation 16.

The premises must be under the management of a consortium – an association of persons with a formal structure, which is committed to running the centre and which is also defined in Regulation 16.

Pharmacies which only provide mail order or Internet services

These are defined in Regulation 13(1)(d) as:

> premises at which essential services are to be provided but the means of providing those services are such that all persons receiving them do so otherwise than at those premises.

Applications for a minor relocation

A person who is on the pharmaceutical list may apply to change the address from which he provides services. If the PCT is satisfied that the change is a minor relocation, and other conditions are satisfied, then the application must be granted.

The other conditions are that

- the same services are being provided
- the provision of services has not been interrupted unless allowed by the PCT.

This applies even if the move is from one PCT to another adjoining PCT.

What is a minor relocation?

A "minor relocation" is not defined in Regulations, but the Court of Appeal gave guidance in 1995. A relocation is minor if

- it is within the same neighbourhood
- the move is over a short distance
- there is no significant change to the population served.

Minor relocations of up to 500 metres

Where

> the relocation is to premises which are less than 500 metres by the most practicable route by foot from the applicant's existing premises.

The application may be granted by the PCT without formal notification to the persons set out in Regulation 23, and without hearing representations (Regulation 6(3)).

The "necessary or desirable" test

The "necessary or desirable" test is used to determine applications which do not fall into the categories set out above.

> An application shall be granted only if the PCT is satisfied . . . that it is necessary or desirable to grant it in order to secure, in the neighbourhood in which the premises are located, the adequate provision, by persons included in the list of the services, or some of the services specified in the application.

The test can be met in either of two possible ways. The application may be "necessary" or it may be "desirable". The two words are not mutually exclusive, so presumably an application may also be "necessary and desirable".

Regulation 12(2) sets out the matters which the PCT must consider when determining the application:

- whether any of the proposed services are already being provided
- whether people in the neighbourhood already have a reasonable choice services or providers
- any other information the PCT considers is relevant
- any representations received.

The PCT is to disregard any services in the neighbourhood provided by a wholly mail order or Internet pharmacy.

Regulation 24 allows PCTs generally to "determine an application in such manner as it thinks fit". It may determine an application without hearing any representations.

Applications for change of ownership

A person taking over the ownership of an NHS pharmacy must apply to the HA to provide NHS pharmaceutical services. The application must be granted by the HA provided

- when the application is made a person on the list is providing services from the premises specified
- the same services will be provided from those premises
- the provision of services will not be interrupted
- the new owner does not fall into the "European diploma" category
- fitness to practise requirements are met (Regulation 8).

Preliminary consent

Prior to 1983 there was no control of entry to the pharmaceutical list, and an application to go on the list was automatically granted.

Preliminary consent was originally introduced into the 1983 Regulations to allow a likely contractor to "test the water" without committing himself. It was not necessary to specify the exact location of premises in an application for preliminary consent, so the applicant was able to maintain some degree of commercial confidentiality. An applicant who was granted "preliminary consent" was automatically granted admission to the pharmaceutical list on subsequent application. This dual system caused some problems when the test of "necessary or desirable" was introduced.

The Contract Regulations now provide that an application for preliminary consent shall be subject to the same test as a full application. The procedures remain slightly different, however.

An application for preliminary consent may be made regardless of whether the premises are situated in a rural area or in an urban area.

Making an application for preliminary consent

Applications for preliminary consent are dealt with in Regulations 40 and 41.

Applications must be in writing

The application must be in writing (Regulation 40(2)). No form is prescribed in the Regulations. The application must specify the premises or state the location of the premises. "Location" is not the same as address and is less specific, although it must in each case be sufficiently precise to enable the "necessary or desirable" test to be applied.

The application must set out the services to be provided and provide the information which Schedule 4 requires.

The application is subject to the same test as a full application (Regulation 40(3)).

Effect of the grant of preliminary consent

Once a person has been finally granted preliminary consent then the PCT must grant any full application made during the net 6 months, provided the premises are in the same location and the same services are to be provided.

European diplomas

The Regulations place certain restrictions on pharmacists who hold diplomas in pharmacy granted by universities in other EU countries. Such pharmacists are required to satisfy the PCT as to their knowledge of English before an application can be granted (Regulation 11).

Guidance from the Courts

"Necessary or desirable"

The Court of Appeal gave guidance on the "necessary or desirable" test in *Ex parte Lowe* No. 2, 2001.

The Court said that

- An application can only be granted for the purpose of securing the adequate provision of pharmaceutical services by pharmacists.
- Adequacy is a question of degree. A spectrum of adequacy runs from "wholly adequate" to "wholly inadequate".

- The real issue is where on that spectrum of adequacy does a particular case belong.
- That question has a variety of answers, which include
  - Wholly adequate: There is no doubt that the existing provision is sufficient and hence it would be neither necessary nor desirable to grant the application.
  - Wholly inadequate: There is no doubt that the existing provision is insufficient and hence it would be both necessary and desirable to grant the application.
  - Marginal: Some point between the two answers above, where it is not necessary to grant the application, but it might be desirable to do so in order to secure the adequate provision of services.
  - Decisions must be pragmatic because there are spaces on the spectrum between marginal and wholly adequate or wholly inadequate.

"Persons on the pharmaceutical list"

The test refers to persons on the pharmaceutical list. This formulation excludes dispensing doctors. Thus services provided by dispensing doctors are excluded when consideration is given to the need or desirability, in the locality, of services provided by pharmacists.

What is a "neighbourhood"

In a Northern Ireland case (Re: An application by Boots, 1994), Lord Justice Murray in the NI High Court said people must "live in some proximity" to be neighbours.

The High Court ruled in 1966 that absence of a resident population did not prevent a shopping centre from being a "neighbourhood". Mr Justice Tucker said:

> I have reached a clear finding that shopping centres can indeed constitute neighbourhoods.

He also said that when assessing the adequacy of existing pharmacy provision the authority should pay regard to the needs of everyone who might be expected to be in, but not necessarily resident in, the neighbourhood at any time and for any purpose. (*Ex parte Boots the Chemists Ltd* – the "Cribbs Causeway"case)

In another High Court case in 1996, it was suggested

> There must be some communality for a neighbourhood.
>
> (*Ex parte Baker*)

In 1999 Mr Justice Kay, again in the High Court (*Ex parte Tesco*) ruled that a superstore was not a neighbourhood in its own right, but was part of a neighbourhood which included local villages. He rejected an argument that it was irrelevant to consider whether or not an area had a resident population.

"Minor relocation" has been judicially considered [*R v. Cumbria FPC, ex parte Boots the Chemists Ltd*] and the relevant portion of the judgment reads,

We have been asked to give guidance on the meaning of "minor relocation". We do so with hesitation; it is a matter of fact and degree. The primary consideration is geography, whether the move is over a short distance. But what is a short distance depends on the circumstances. In a densely populated town a move of a few hundred yards might not be minor. In the depths of the country a move of several miles might be.

Second, the FHSA must consider if the population served in the new premises will be the same as the old. It might be that the distance is small, but a physical barrier – a river, a motorway – would mean that the new premises would be difficult to reach by the population served by the old premises. The HA is entitled to take account of this, and of the availability of public transport and whether the population is pedestrian or car-borne, bearing in mind that major users are elderly. . . .

The Court of Appeal gave judgments in two cases in 1995 on the interpretation of various phrases relating to applications for minor relocation.

The facts in *R* v. *Yorkshire Regional Health Authority ex parte Gompels* were as follows.

The doctor's surgery in a small town decided to move from the High Street to purpose-built premises nearby. Two of the pharmacies in the town applied to relocate their premises from the High Street to near the new surgery. Another High Street pharmacy opposed the minor relocation applications on the grounds *inter alia* that the relocations could not be minor if the redistribution of prescriptions would threaten the viability of that pharmacy.

The Court of Appeal held that the continuing viability of adversely affected pharmacies was irrelevant. The application has to be granted if "within the neighbourhood . . . the HA is satisfied that the change is a minor relocation".

As to what constitutes a "minor relocation" the Court of Appeal was divided. One judge said that the essential question was one of geography and topography. He said "The words 'minor relocation' are plain English words which mean no less and no more than they say".

The other two judges disagreed. One said that the SHA must also consider the significance and consequence of the move as they affect users of the service. He thought the word "minor" was synonymous with "unimportant".

The other referred to the 1988 case above and suggested that it would be a minor relocation if the new location is substantially as convenient to the population served as the old location.

Removal from pharmaceutical list

The PCT has the power to remove a contractor from the list in a number of circumstances.

The PCT must remove a name from the list where it determines that

(a) the contractor has died (Regulation 45(2)a)
(b) is no longer a pharmacist or RPB (Regulation 45(2)b).

There are provisions in the MA 1968 for an RPB to be carried on by "representatives" where a pharmacist has died or been declared legally incompetent, e.g.

because of mental illness. The representative "stands in the shoes of" the pharmacist and the business remains on the list. The main requirement for the carrying on of the business by representatives is that a pharmacist be employed to handle professional matters (see Chapter 10 under the heading "Representatives").

Regulation 45(4) enables the representatives to continue on the list.

The PCT must remove a name from the list where it determines that the contractor has breached one of the conditions set out in Regulation 13(2)(a) or Regulation 13(4), which relate to either providing 100 hours service a week, or being a wholly mail order or Internet pharmacy.

The PCT may remove a name from the list where it determines that the contractor has not provided services for 6 months.

In the above two cases the PCT is required to follow a procedure:

- The contractor must be given 28 days' notice of the intention to make a determination.
- He must be given an opportunity to make representations.
- The PCT must consult the LPC.

The PCT may remove a name from the list where a contractor has failed to comply with a condition imposed under Regulations 21, 30, 42 or 43 (Regulation 44).

The PCT may remove a name from the list on "fitness to practise" grounds (Regulation 47).

Applications from appliance contractors

Applications from appliance contractors, or from those who wish to provide only appliances are dealt with in a broadly similar way. However, there is no requirement that the applicant be a pharmacist. The necessary or desirable test applies. The rules relating to controlled localities have no application for appliance contractors. The availability of appliances from pharmacies in the locality is a factor to be considered when determining whether the existing service is adequate.

Planning law

The planning regulations which affect pharmacies are found in the Town and Country Planning (Use Classes) Order 1987. This lists the various classes of activity for which planning permission may be granted.

An explanatory note attached to the order says that "dispensaries" will fall into Class A1. This is the class for shops. If the "dispensary" is ancillary to a hospital then it may fall into Class C2 (residential institutions).

Under a previous order it was possible for pharmacies which were "dispensing-only" to fall into a category of professional use of residential premises, thereby avoiding planning restrictions applicable to shops.

It is not necessary for the relevant planning permission to have been granted prior to the granting of an application for minor relocation or for a new contract.

Chapter 6

Rural Dispensing

History

Doctors and pharmacists have argued over who should dispense for patients in rural areas since the advent of the NHS. In 1975 the two professions agreed a voluntary standstill on changes in dispensing arrangements while they engaged in discussions. Following these discussions a number of actions occurred:

1977 – "Report of the National Joint Committee of the medical and pharmaceutical professions on the dispensing of NHS prescriptions in rural areas" – commonly known as the "Clothier Report"

1983 – The Rural Dispensing Committee was to determine applications for dispensing in rural areas, and to determine the "rurality" of an area

1990 – RDC abolished and decisions made by FHSAs (now PCTs)

2001 – The professions reach agreement on further reform

2004 – Advisory Group on Reform of the NHS Regulations 1992 propose introduction of more competition and choice

2005 – Proposals implemented in NHS (PS) Regulations 2005.

The current rules

The NHS Act 1977 made it clear that doctors would only be allowed to dispense drugs in exceptional circumstances and that the prime suppliers of medicines would be pharmacists. Exceptions were made in rural areas where there was no pharmacy and where patients would have extreme difficulty in getting to a pharmacy (Lord Justice Schieman in *R* v. *North Staffs HA, ex parte Worthington* 1996).

Controlled locality

The current rural dispensing rules apply to areas termed "controlled localities". A controlled locality is an area which has been determined by the PCT to be "rural in character". The PCT is required to delineate the boundaries of the controlled areas on a map. Where a previous determination of rurality has been made under earlier regulations then that area continues as a controlled locality.

The PCT may at any time determine whether an area is rural. The PCT must determine rurality if requested in writing by the LPC or LMC (Regulation 31(3)).

What does "rural" mean?

The DOH has issued guidance in the document "Information for Primary Care Trusts (Control of Entry)". This states that factors which might be taken into account include

- environmental – balance of land use
- employment patterns
- size of communities
- distance between settlements
- overall population density
- public transport arrangements
- level of local services.

The guidance document suggests that the decisions are ones of common sense rather than ones made by the application of rigid criteria.

Areas which have not been classed as "controlled" are not necessarily urban.

The "five-year rule"

Regulation 31(10) states that where a PCT has decided whether or not an area is rural, the question may not generally be considered again in the next 5 years. The exception is where the PCT is satisfied that there has been a "substantial change of circumstances" in relation to the area, or to a part of it, since the matter was last determined.

Meaning of "substantial change"

No definition is given in the Regulations. The guidance document states that each case should be considered on its merits. Examples are given such as changes in the size of the population, changes in transport facilities, changes in levels of services.

Appeals

Dispensing doctors and pharmacy contractors affected by the decision may appeal against a rurality decision, as may the relevant LMCs and LPCs.

Applications by pharmacists to dispense in rural areas

Applications are made in a similar manner to those relating to non-controlled areas. They are subject to special procedures set down in Regulations. The Regulations lay down a timetable, and indicate which other persons or bodies should be consulted before a decision is taken.

Stage 1

The PCT must first of all determine whether to grant the application would preju-dice the proper provision of general medical services or pharmaceutical services in an area.

The PCT must refuse an application if granting the application would prejudice the proper provision in the locality of:

- primary medical services
- dispensing services
- Local Pharmaceutical Services
- pharmaceutical services.

Regulation 18(2) states

> The PCT
>
> (a)   shall refuse an application to the extent that it is of the opinion that to grant it would prejudice the proper provision of primary dispensing services, local pharmaceutical services or pharmaceutical services in any locality.

The application may not be granted if there would be prejudice to either medical or pharmaceutical services. Thus an application from a pharmacy to dispense may not be granted if to do so would prejudice the proper provision of pharmaceutical services – for example those provided by the doctor.

Location

At this stage an application is not required to give the exact address of the proposed pharmacy, but the location must be given sufficiently clearly for the test to be applied. In practice that seems to mean that it must be possible to look at the population within a 1.6 km radius of the proposed site, so as to determine how they are affected.

What is meant by "proper provision"

Proper provision means provision of the service to the standard which the contractor is obliged to provide in order to comply with the TOS.

What is meant by "prejudice"?

The services will be prejudiced if the contractor would be unable to comply with the TOS. A reduction in the standard of service will not, in itself, constitute prejudice to the proper provision. This interpretation has been approved by the S of S in a number of decisions and it is also given in the guidance document.

Stage 2

If the PCT finds that there is no prejudice it must then determine, as a separate decision, whether the application is "necessary or desirable". The two stages are distinct and separate, and must be done in the correct order. The same people, at the same meeting, may make the decisions.

The "necessary and desirable" stage for pharmacists is the same as that which governs the applications for dispensing in urban areas. See Chapter 5.

The PCT may make its determination in such manner as it thinks fit. It may dispense with an oral hearing if it wishes.

The PCT must consider whether it should impose any conditions under Regulation 20.

Applications for minor relocation within a controlled area

If the PCT decides that granting the application would not result in a significant change in the arrangements for the provision of pharmaceutical services in any part of the controlled locality, then the application may be dealt with as a minor relocation under Regulation 6 or 7.

The guidance document suggests that the following should be considered in deciding on "significant change":

- impact on population served
- accessibility of premises

When processing an application the PCT should consider whether the application relates to premises in a reserved location.

Reserved locations

The 2005 Contract Regulations introduce a new concept of "reserved location".

According to Regulation 35(2)(a), a "reserved location" is an area within 1.6 km of the proposed location where the patient population is less than 2750.

If a PCT determines that an area is a reserved location it must delineate this on a map, and publish the map (Regulation 35(9)).

If an area is a reserved location then:

- The "prejudice" test does not apply.
- Patients within that area may continue to have their prescriptions dispensed by a dispensing doctor.

Applications by doctors

Existing dispensing practices were required to register their premises with the PCT by 30 April 2005 (Regulation 68(2)).

The dispensing doctor list includes

- the premises where the doctor has premises approval
- whether the premises approval is granted, temporary or residual
- the date on which premises approval took effect or where it has not taken effect, the date when it was finally granted
- the area where the doctor has outline consent and premises approval
- premises, identified separately, where the doctor has outstanding applications for premises approval (Regulation 68(4)).

New applications to dispense by GPs are not granted if there is a pharmacy within 1.6 km radius of the premises from which the medical practice wishes to start dispensing (Regulation 18(2)).

Otherwise doctors may apply for "outline consent" to dispense for those of their patients who live more than one mile from a pharmacy (Regulation 61). The same test is used – whether to grant the application would prejudice the proper provision of general medical or pharmaceutical services.

The application must specify the area for which the grant of "outline consent" is sought. The application must be in writing, but no particular form is specified.

The effect of a grant is that the doctor may then dispense to any of his patients residing in the specified area, who request him to dispense, and who live more than 1.6 km from an NHS pharmacy.

In certain circumstances, doctors are enabled to dispense for patients without making an application as outlined above.

The "serious difficulty" rule

Regulation 60 states that

> Where a patient satisfies a PCT that he would have serious difficulty in obtaining any necessary drugs or appliances from a pharmacy by reason of distance or inadequacy of means of communication he may at any time request in writing the doctor on whose list he is included to provide him with pharmaceutical service

This provision applies to any patient, including those resident in urban areas.

In considering whether the patient has a serious difficulty, the PCT is expected to consider:

- personal circumstances of the patient
- local arrangements for medical and pharmaceutical services
- transport
- any collection and delivery services
- availability of telephones
- any other relevant factors.

There is no appeal procedure from a decision of the PCT that the patient does not have any serious difficulty.

Temporary Residents

Doctors who provide pharmaceutical services to at least some of the patients on their list may also dispense to any temporary residents which they accept.

Appeal procedure

An appeal may be made to the FHS Appeals Unit on the issue of rurality, and on decisions to grant a contract. The Appeals Unit may, but is not required to, hold an oral hearing.

An appeal against a decision made under the Regulation 12 procedure may be summarily dismissed by the unit if it decides the appeal is frivolous, vexatious or discloses no reasonable grounds of appeal.

Chapter 7

Prescription Charges

The basic principle expressed in the National Health Act 1977 is that services are to be free unless there is some statement to the contrary.

Section 1(2) of the 1977 Act states

> The services so provided shall be free of charge except in so far as the making and recovery of charges is expressly provided for by or under any enactment, whenever passed.

Section 77 of the 1977 Act provides the power for making charges for pharmaceutical services:

> Regulations may provide for the making and recovery in such manner as may be prescribed of such charges as may be prescribed in respect of:
>
> (a)   the supply under this Act (otherwise than under Part II) of drugs, medicines or appliances (including the replacement and repair of those appliances); and
> (b)   such of the pharmaceutical services referred to in Part II as may be prescribed.

The effect of *Section 77* is that charges may be made for the supply both in the hospital and in the community, of medicines and appliances.

The Regulations

The current Regulations are the NHS (Charges for Drugs and Appliances) Regulations 2000, SI No. 620. These substantive Regulations are amended each year as new charges are announced.

Charges for drugs

The Regulations require that, subject to the exemptions, a pharmacist must make and recover from a patient the specified charge in respect of the supply of "each quantity of a drug". The term "drug" includes "medicine". The interpretations given in the Drug Tariff are, for example:

(1)   The supply of Water for Injection with an antibiotic, or in accordance with the BNF, is not charged.
(2)   The supply of different strengths of the same tablet results in only one charge.
(3)   The supply of both tablets and capsules of the same strength of the same drug would be two charges.

Definitions

The 2000 Regulations include a number of definitions which are specific to the Charges Regulations and important to their meaning. In the 2000 regulations:

(1) "Appliance" means a "listed appliance", but excludes contraceptive appliances.
(2) "Chemist" means any person who provides pharmaceutical services or LPS (other than a doctor).
(3) "Drugs" includes medicines, but do not include contraceptive substances.
(4) "Elastic hosiery" means anklet, legging, kneecap, above-knee, below-knee or thigh stocking.

Who is a patient?

"Patient" means

- any person for whose treatment a doctor is responsible under his TOS; *or*
- any person who applies to a chemist for the provision of pharmaceutical services including a person who applies on behalf of another person; *or*
- a person who pays or undertakes to pay on behalf of another person a charge for which these regulations provide; *or*
- any person who seeks information or treatment from a walk-in-centre, i.e. a centre at which information and treatment for minor conditions is provided to the public under arrangements made by or on behalf of the S of S.

This last definition is added by the NHS (Charges for Drugs and Appliances) Amendment Regulations 2000, SI No. 122, which has the effect of making prescription charges applicable to supplies of drugs and appliances made from walk-in-centres.

When the regulations refer to a "patient" the word also includes someone acting on behalf of the patient, such as a parent and also, say, someone collecting the prescription for a neighbour. That parent or neighbour must pay the charge on demand. Pharmacists are under no obligation to dispense a prescription until after the appropriate charges have been paid. They are entitled to collect the charge when the prescription is handed over for dispensing.

Out-of-hours providers

The introduction of new arrangements for out-of-hours provision of medical services has required a further amendment, in the 2005 Amendment Regulations, to cover the situation where an out-of-hours provider supplies medicine or appliances. Thus an amended Regulation 4A allows a provider of out-of-hours services to make and recover the usual charges from a patient, except for medicines for immediate treatment or where they are personally administered by the provider.

How many charges?

Provided the order is on one form, the supply of the same medicine in more than one container (whether ordered by the prescriber in that way or not) is treated as the supply of one quantity.

Guidance on what constitutes "each quantity of a drug" is found in the DT.

Elastic hosiery and tights

Each piece of hosiery, e.g. a stocking, is treated as one appliance and attracts a separate charge.

Appliances

There is only one charge payable for the supply of two or more appliances of the same type (excluding elastic hosiery). The supply of two or more component parts of the same appliance also attracts only one charge.

Prescription form

"Prescription form" means a form provided by an NHS Trust, and NHS Foundation Trust or a PCT and issued by a prescriber, or data that are created in an electronic form, signed with a prescribers advanced electronic signature and transmitted as an electronic communication to the ETP service, to enable a person to obtain pharmaceutical services or local pharmaceutical services and does not include a repeatable prescription.

This definition includes all variants of the forms including those issued by a hospital for dispensing at community pharmacies.

The 2005 Amendment Regulations (SI No. 578) altered the definitions to reflect the advent of ETP.

A "repeatable prescription" means a prescription which

(a)   either

　　　(i)   is contained in a form provided by a PCT and issued by a repeatable prescriber which is in the format specified in Part I of Schedule 1 to the GMS Contract Regulations and which is generated by a computer and signed in ink by a repeatable prescriber; or

　　　(ii) is data that are created in an electronic form, signed with a repeatable prescriber's advanced electronic signature and transmitted as an electronic communication to the ETP service;

(b)   is issued or created to enable a person to obtain pharmaceutical services or local pharmaceutical services; and

(c)   indicates that the drugs or appliances ordered on that prescription may be provided more than once and specifies the number of occasions on which they may be provided.

Hospital patients

The general rule is that treatment in hospital is free. Hospitals can only charge for medicines which are provided to a patient for administration outside of the hospital. That means that medicines for the following are free:

- inpatients
- day patients whose medicines are administered to them whilst they are in the hospital
- patients attending A & E departments whose medicines are administered whilst they are in the hospital.

Charges are made for any medicines which are to be administered outside of the hospital.

Charges for medicines and appliances are the same as in community pharmacies, except for certain appliances which are only supplied under the NHS by hospitals. These appliances are surgical brassières, abdominal or spinal supports, and wigs.

Prisoners

No charges are payable by "prisoners", i.e. those detained in prisons.

Instalment prescribing

Where a medicine is ordered on a single prescription form, and it is supplied in instalments, the standard charge is payable when the first instalment is supplied. Only one charge is made, regardless of the number of instalments.

Receipts

Patients are entitled to a receipt if they ask for one. This must be on the form provided by the PCT.

Exemptions

The following persons are exempt from charges:

(1) persons under 16 years
(2) persons under 19 years in full-time education
(3) a person aged 60 years or over
(4) a woman holding a maternity exemption certificate (expectant women and those who have given birth within the last 12 months)
(5) a person holding a medical exemption certificate
(6) a person holding a prescription prepayment certificate
(7) a person holding a War Pension exemption certificate (exemption only for prescriptions to treat their accepted disabilities)

(8)   a person named on a current HC2 charges certificate (low income)
(9)   a person receiving free-of-charge contraceptives
(10) a person who is, or whose partner is, receiving various Social Security and similar allowances and payments.

These are

- Income Support
- Income-based Jobseekers Allowance
- Pension Credit Guarantee Credit
- Working Tax Credit
- Child Tax Credit.

Exemption certificates

Exemption certificates are supplied to the patient by the PPA. They are valid for 5 years.

The following medical conditions entitle the person to exemption:

- a permanent fistula requiring continuous dressing or an appliance (Fistula includes caecostomy, colostomy, laryngostomy and ileostoma)
- epilepsy requiring continuous anti-convulsive therapy
- diabetes mellitus except where treatment is by diet alone
- myxodema or other conditions which require supplemental thyroid hormone
- hypoparathyroidism
- diabetes insipidus and other forms of hypopituitarism
- forms of hypoadrenalism (including Addison's disease) for which specific substitution therapy is essential
- myasthenia gravis
- a continuing physical disability which prevents the patient leaving his residence without the help of another person.

Prepayment certificates

Prepayment certificates are available. The regulations state the amount to be paid for the 4-month and the 12-month certificate.

All exemptions, and the prepayment certificate, apply to all drugs and appliances provided to that patient. The exemption is not limited to treatment specifically for the condition for which exemption was granted.

Accuracy of exemption statement

Paragraph 7(3) of the TOS requires the pharmacist to ask any person who fills in the exemption section on the back of the prescription form for evidence of entitlement to exemption. The question need not be asked if the exemption is claimed by virtue of sub-Paragraphs a, c, e, f or g of Regulation 7(1) of the Charges Regulations and at the time the pharmacist had such evidence available to him.

If no satisfactory evidence is produced the pharmacist must endorse the form to that effect.

No exemption declaration need be made where the exemption is on age grounds and the age is computer generated on the prescription form. (Regulation 11 of 2005 Amendment Regulations)

Declaration on prescription form

The declaration of entitlement to exemption or remission which appears on the prescription form must be duly completed, by or on behalf of the patient, in order for the exemption to be valid.

The amended Regulations require that where a person pays a prescription charge he shall sign the declaration on the prescription form that the relevant charge has been paid.

Penalty charges

The NHS (Penalty Charge) Regulations 1999 came into force on 1 November 1999. They provide that a penalty notice may be served on any person who fails to pay a required prescription charge (or a charge for dental treatment and appliances, optical services or any other appliances).

A penalty notice requires payment of the amount that the person has failed to pay plus an additional penalty charge calculated according to the Regulations.

Where the amount required to be paid under the penalty notice is not paid within 28 days, a further sum by way of penalty ("a surcharge" equal to 50% of the penalty charge) must be paid.

A person is not liable to a penalty charge, or a surcharge, if he shows that he did not act wrongfully, or with any lack of care, in respect of the original charge.

These Regulations are administered by a section of the PPA.

Additionally a person who fails to pay a charge when not exempt *may* be prosecuted for the new criminal offence of evading a prescription charge. (Guidance issued by the DOH restricts this to repeat offenders. The Guidance also indicates that either a penalty charge or a prosecution may be appropriate but not both.)

A patient's representative is jointly and severally liable with the patient for unpaid charges in a manner specific to this Act and *may* be issued with a penalty charge notice. The Guidance states that where a representative has signed the declaration of exemption, they are to be the initial recipient of any penalty notice and debt recovery action with the patient only being joined in that action if the representative enters a defence or otherwise fails to pay.

County Court judges should be asked to apportion liability between patients and representatives. (There is some debate as to how likely it is that a Judge will be prepared to do this.)

Bulk prescriptions

No charges are payable for "Bulk prescriptions". A bulk prescription is an order for two or more patients bearing the name of a school or institution in which at least 20 persons normally reside, and a particular doctor is responsible for the treatment of at least 10 of those persons.

The order must be for non-POM medicines or for prescribable dressings which do not contain POM products.

Bulk prescribing is only allowed on NHS forms FP10NC and FP10C.

Contraceptives

There are no charges for contraceptive substances, or for those contraceptive appliances which are listed in the DT. *Section 77* gives Ministers power to charge for the supply of contraceptive substances and appliances, although the Regulations themselves specifically exclude contraceptive substances and appliances from charges.

Treatment of Sexually transmitted diseases

Prescriptions issued by hospital or PCT clinics for the treatment of sexually transmitted diseases are free.

Dispensing doctors

Dispensing doctors must charge patients for medicines and appliances in exactly the same way as pharmacists. They have similar obligations in respect of the evidence of exemption.

No charges are payable where the medicine or appliance is supplied for immediate treatment, and no order is written on a prescription form.

Similarly no charge is payable for items administered or applied to the patient by the doctor personally. Although the Regulations state "personally", it also applies when the nurse acts on behalf of the doctor.

Prescription charge refunds

The TOS in the NHS (Pharmaceutical Services) Regulations 2005 state, "Where any person who is entitled to a repayment of any charge paid under the Charges Regulations presents a pharmacist with a valid claim for the repayment within 3 months of the date on which the charge was paid, the pharmacist shall make the repayment".

Reward scheme

A reward scheme, set up under Regulation 59 of the NHS (PS) Regulations 2005, allows pharmacists to claim a financial reward when they have identified fraudulent prescription forms and thereby prevented fraud. Participation is voluntary. It is not a requirement of the Terms of Service.

The Basic Reward is £70. It is payable when a fraudulent prescription form is identified and reported, regardless of whether or not the items have been dispensed.

A Bonus Reward may be payable when the identification of a fraudulent form contributes to the detection and prevention of a fraud, or the recovery for the NHS of sums lost through fraud, regardless of whether items have been dispensed. It is

5% of the total savings resulting from the information provided, up to a maximum of £10,000. It is administered by the NHS Business Authority.

A similar scheme operates in Wales, though the details are different.

Wales

The NHS (Charges for Drugs and Appliances) (Wales) (Amendment No. 2) Regulations 2005, SI No. 1915, came into effect on 1 August 2005.

The standard £4 (reducing to £3 from April 2006) charge in Wales is only applicable to scripts written on a form supplied by a Welsh Local Health Board or NHS Trust. Forms from the rest of the United Kingdom are subject to the normal English charge (currently £6.50).

Prescriptions for under 25-year-old patients are exempt from any prescription charge if dispensed in Wales even if the prescription is not a Welsh one.

Chapter 8

The Interests of the Public

The NHS Plan set out plans to establish a new system of patient and public involvement (PPI), replacing Community Health Councils in England, as part of the modernisation programme. The system was also designed to respond to the Bristol Royal Inquiry report, which recommended representation of patient interests "on the inside" of the NHS and at every level.

New arrangements for patient involvement

Sections 7–12 of the Health and Social Care (HSC) Act 2001 establish new arrangements for public and patient involvement in the NHS.

- Local Authority overview and scrutiny committees (OSCs) scrutinise the NHS and represent local views on the development of local health services.
- NHS organisations have a duty to involve patients and the public in decision making about the operation of the NHS.

Local Authority overview

Section 7 of the HSC Act 2001 amended *Section 21* of the Local Government Act 2000 to require local authorities with social services responsibilities to ensure that their overview and scrutiny committee or committees had the power to scrutinise the planning, provision and operation of health services.

The Local Government Act 2000 (Constitutions) (England) Direction 2000 stated that scrutiny arrangements should be set out in local authority constitutions.

Overview and scrutiny committees are sub-committees of Local Authorities, set up under the Local Authority (Overview and Scrutiny Committees Health Scrutiny Functions) Regulations 2002.

Directions to local authorities set out the powers of the OSCs. They can review and scrutinise health service matters, and make reports and recommendations.

The role includes

- being consulted by the NHS where there are to be major changes to health services;
- scrutinising ongoing operation and planning of services;
- referring contested service changes to the S of S;
- calling NHS managers to give information about services and decisions;
- reporting their recommendations locally.

Duty to involve patients

Section 11 of the HSC Act 2001 confers on PCTs and NHS Trusts a new statutory duty to involve patients and the public in the planning and decision-making processes of that body. This covers both the hospital and the community health services for which they are responsible and the family health services provided by practitioners in their area.

Independent Complaints Advocacy Services (ICAS)

Section 12 of the HSC Act 2001 places a statutory responsibility on the S of S for Health to make appropriate arrangements for the delivery of independent advocacy services to support people in making complaints about the NHS.

The DOH set up the ICAS on 1 September 2003. The service may be provided by the local authority or by other persons or bodies. ICAS is provided on a regional contract basis, managed by the DOH. The independent providers are

- Citizens Advice Bureaux
- Carer's Federation
- POhWER
- South East Advocacy Projects (SEAP).

What does ICAS do?

Independent Complaints Advocacy Services provides information, support and guidance to help complainants articulate their concerns and navigate the complaints system. This may include assistance with constructing a complaints letter, drafting or attendance at meetings.

Patient Advocacy and Liaison Services (PALS)

The new arrangements are complemented by a non-statutory arrangement, Patient Advocacy and Liaison Services (PALS). PALS are trust-based services able to assist and support patients. They provide information and resolve problems and difficulties. They act on behalf of their service users when handling patient and family concerns.

It is intended that they will be situated in or near main reception areas of hospitals and act as a welcoming point for patients and carers.

The PALS will also advise patients on how to access independent advocacy to support their complaints.

The service provide

- confidential advice and support to patients, families and their carers
- information on the NHS and health-related matters
- confidential assistance in resolving problems and concerns quickly
- explanations of NHS complaints procedures and contact details
- information on the NHS locally
- a focal point for feedback from patients to inform service developments
- an early warning system for NHS Trusts, PCTs and PPI Forums by monitoring trends and gaps in services and reporting these to the trust management for action.

Patient and Public Involvement Forums

Patient and Public Involvement Forums (PPI Forums) were set up by the Patients' Forums (Membership and Procedure) Regulations 2003, SI No. 2123, and their functions are set out in the Patients' Forums (Functions) Regulations 2003, SI No. 2124.

They exist in NHS trusts (including foundation trusts) and PCTs. They represent the views of local communities about the quality and configuration of health services to PCTs and trusts.

The NHS Reform and Health Care Professions Act 2002 provides patients' forums with the power to refer issues to overview and scrutiny committees as appropriate.

The Appointments Commission has the responsibility to appoint members to forums. Their functions include

- monitoring and reviewing the services arranged and or provided by the trust from the perspective of the patient – this includes both the range and operation of services;
- seeking the views of patients receiving services;
- inspecting premises where NHS services are delivered;
- making reports and recommendations. Trusts will be required to respond to these reports;
- referring matters of concern to OSCs and the CPPIH, SHAs, the Healthcare Commission and the National Patient Safety Agency, etc. – and to any other person or body the forums deem appropriate, including the media;
- promote the involvement of the public in decisions and consultations on matters generally affecting health;
- provide training and support to empower local communities;
- identify trends and concerns resulting from PPI activity and make reports;
- work with the other trust forums in their areas to ensure a strategic and cohesive view;
- provide a one-stop shop service by providing advice and information to the public about public involvement and information and support about complaints;
- monitor and review how well the NHS is meeting its duty to involve and consult the public.

The DOH has given Directions to PCTs. These require that contracts to provide health services, which are placed with independent providers after 1 December 2003, must include provisions that

- require those providers to allow entry to Patients' Forums to enter and inspect premises where those services are provided; and
- require those providers to give information in relation to those services to Patients' Forums when requested.

The Freedom of Information Act 2000, which came fully into effect 1 January 2005, replaced the previous NHS Guidance on Openness.

The Act gives a general right of access to all types of recorded information held by public authorities. The Information Commissioner oversees the operation of the Act (discussed later).

New monitoring arrangements for healthcare quality

The HSC (Community Health and Standards) Act 2003 contains a number of provisions designed to improve quality of the NHS.

Chapter 1 established two new regulatory bodies – the Commission for Healthcare Audit and Inspection (CHAI) and the Commission for Social Care Inspection (CSCI). Both inspectorates were established as executive non-departmental public bodies.

Chapter 2 of imposes a duty of quality on all NHS bodies that provide or commission health care, and provides for the standards.

Chapter 3 sets out the functions of the CHAI.

Chapter 5 sets out the functions of the CSCI which is an England only body.

In Chapter 6, the Act confers functions on the NAW ("the Assembly") in relation to social care similar to those conferred upon the CSCI.

Chapter 7 sets out the functions under Parts 1 and 2 of the Care Standards Act 2000 ("the CSA 2000") which have transferred to the CHAI and CSCI.

Chapter 8 provides for other functions of the CSCI.

Chapter 9 deals with the handling of complaints relating to the provision of NHS health care and local authority social services.

Finally, Chapter 10 provides supplementary and general provisions in relation to the CHAI and CSCI, for example providing for joint working between both Commissions.

In April 2004, the Commission for Healthcare Audit and Inspection became known as the Healthcare Commission. Its legal name remains unchanged.

The Healthcare Commission

The Healthcare Commission is an independent body, set up to promote and drive improvement in the quality of healthcare and public health. It replaces the work of the Commission for Health Improvement. It also took over some responsibilities from other Commissions. Its main statutory duties in England are to:

- assess the management, provision and quality of NHS healthcare and public health services;
- review the performance of each NHS trust and award an annual performance rating;
- regulate the independent healthcare sector through registration, annual inspection, monitoring complaints and enforcement;
- publish information about the state of healthcare;
- consider complaints about NHS organisations that the organisations themselves have not resolved;
- promote the co-ordination of reviews and assessments carried out by ourselves and others; and
- carry out investigations of serious failures in the provision of healthcare.

In carrying out those duties, the Commission is required to pay particular attention to:

- the availability of, access to, quality and effectiveness of healthcare
- the economy and efficiency of the provision of healthcare

- the availability and quality of information provided to the public about healthcare
- the need to safeguard and promote the rights and welfare of children and the effectiveness of measures taken to do so.

The Healthcare Commission:

- takes over the private and voluntary healthcare functions of the National Care Standards Commission; and
- covers the elements of the Audit Commission's work which relate to efficiency, effectiveness and economy of healthcare.

The Healthcare Commission also has certain duties in respect to Wales, mainly relating to national reviews and an annual "State of Healthcare" report.

However, local inspection and investigation of NHS bodies in Wales rests with the Healthcare Inspectorate Wales, while the Care Standards Inspectorate Wales inspects those organisations providing independent healthcare.

Under the Government's review of legislation on mental health, it is expected that most of the functions of the Mental Health Act Commission (MHAC) will transfer to the Healthcare Commission and that MHAC will be abolished, though not before April 2007.

Access to meetings

NHS trusts and authorities are subject to the Public Bodies (Admission to Meetings) Act 1960. This states that generally the public have access to any formal meeting of the trust. An exception may be made where the trust resolves to exclude the public because of the confidential nature of the business to be discussed.

The DOH has issued guidance indicating that trusts are expected to conduct their business in as open a manner as possible.

Non-executive members are appointed for their personal skills and experience, and not as representatives of any particular professional group. They are expected to have links with the local community. The DOH advise that those working in provider units managed by the trust, or in units which have a contract with the trust should not be appointed. This is to avoid a conflict of interest.

The Health Service Commissioner for England

The 1973 Act provided for the creation of the post of Health Service Commissioner. His function is to investigate and report and make recommendations on complaints about the activities of health authorities and those for whom they are responsible.

Separate Commissioners were created for England and for Wales. The NHS (Scotland) Act 1972 similarly created the post for Scotland. The provisions of the 1973 Act were repeated in the consolidating Act of 1977.

How to complain

The Commissioner acts only on a written complaint, received within a year of the event. The complaint must be made by the person who has suffered the injustice (unless he is unable to act for himself).

Jurisdiction

The commissioner investigates complaints that a person has suffered injustice or hardship because of a failure by a health authority to provide services properly, or as a result of maladministration.

From 1 April 1996, Health Service Commissioner (Amendment) Act 1996 extended the jurisdiction of the commissioner.

Section 1 adds family health service providers and independent providers to the list of those about whom the commissioner may investigate complaints.

Section 6 removes a statutory bar on the commissioner investigating matters of clinical judgement.

Section 7 allows the commissioner to investigate complaints about family health services.

Audit Commission

The Audit Commission covers NHS bodies. The Audit Commission is an independent body responsible for ensuring that public money is used economically, efficiently and effectively. Its function is the audit of local authority and NHS bodies. It is responsible for appointing external auditors to audit financial statements and to carry out reviews of governance arrangements and performance in all local authorities, strategic health authorities, trusts and other public bodies such as the police and fire authorities. In the course of producing its national studies it may send out questionnaires to collect data and visit a sample of NHS trusts.

The Health Act 1999 established that the Audit Commission may work with the Commission for Health Improvement (CHI) to support it to undertake a number of its functions.

Public Health Observatories

There are eight regional Public Health Observatories (PHOs) in England, together with ones in Scotland, Wales and Northern Ireland.

They were established as part of the implementation of the White Paper "Saving Lives: Our Healthier Nation".

Their role is to:

- monitor the health of the population and the underlying causes of this
- highlight future health problems
- assess the health impact of potential and past policies
- work in partnership with regional and local health policy makers, the NHS and the public health community and those interested in the health of the population.

The Health Protection Agency

The Health Protection Agency was created on 1 April 2003 to cover England and Wales.

It provides an integrated approach to health protection in order to reduce the impact of infectious diseases, poisons, chemicals, biological and radiation hazards.

It provides

- information and advice to professionals and the public, and
- independent advice to the Government on public health protection policies and programmes.

It integrates expertise that was previously distributed between a number of organisations, including:

- The Public Health Laboratory Service (PHLS), including the Communicable Disease Surveillance Centre and Central Public Health Laboratory
- The Centre for Applied Microbiology and Research
- The national focus for chemical incidents
- The regional service provider units that support the management of chemical incidents
- The National Poisons Information Service
- NHS public health staff responsible for infectious disease control, emergency planning and other protection support.

It works in partnership with the National Radiological Protection Board (NRPB). (Primary legislation is planned to transfer functions from the NRPB to the Health Protection Agency.)

Independent Regulator of Foundation Trusts – Monitor

Monitor is a non-departmental public body established under the HSC (Community Health and Standards) Act 2003. It is responsible for authorising, monitoring and regulating NHS Foundation Trusts. It monitors their activities to ensure that they comply with the requirements of their terms of authorisation. It has powers to intervene in the running of a foundation trust in the event of failings in its healthcare standards or other aspects of its activities, which amount to a significant breach in the terms of its authorisation.

Chapter 9

Complaints and Discipline in the NHS

Complaints and breaches of the terms of service

Primary Care Trusts will start to monitor contractors' compliance with the terms of the new contract from October 2005.

Under the provisions of the NHS (PS) Regulations 2005, pharmacy contractors are required to have in place arrangements, for the handling and consideration of complaints about any matter connected with its provision of pharmaceutical services, which are essentially the same as those set out in Part II of the NHS (Complaints) Regulations 2004. The regulations also impose a duty on PCTs to ensure that pharmacy contractors have those arrangements in place.

According to Paragraph 32 of Schedule 1 to the Contract Regulations

> a pharmacist shall have in place arrangements for the handling and consideration of complaints about any matter connected with his provision of pharmaceutical services which are essentially the same as those set out in Part II of the NHS (Complaints) Regulations 2004 SI No 1768.

The complaints procedure is intended only to resolve complaints. It does not investigate disciplinary matters or apportion blame.

The arrangements for handling complaints must be in writing and a copy must be given, free of charge, to any person who makes a request for one.

The pharmacy contractor is responsible for compliance with the regulations and must designate a "complaints manager", to manage the procedures for handling and considering complaints.

A deputy complaints manager may also be authorised in the absence of the complaints manager.

The Complaints Regulations derive from powers given to the S of S for Health in the NHS (Community Health and Standards) Act 2003 to make provision for the handling and consideration of complaints by NHS bodies in England (or a cross-border Special Health Authority). Chapter 9, Regulations 113–119, deals with complaints about health and social care.

Although the intention had been to implement the Complaints Regulations in full from June 2004, Ministers decided on a phased implementation following an approach from the Shipman Inquiry. Amended Complaints Regulations will be issued in 2005 once the Department has been able to give proper consideration to any recommendations made by the Shipman Inquiry, which published its 5th report on 9 December 2004.

Therefore, the Local Resolution stage of the complaints procedure remains broadly unchanged across all services. The Complaints Regulations consolidate and rationalise the statutory requirements set out in the various Directions referred to in Regulation 24 for Local Resolution by NHS bodies and introduce the reformed independent review stage carried out by the Healthcare Commission.

The Complaints procedure has three stages:

- Local Resolution
- Independent review
- Referral to an Ombudsman.

First stage – local resolution

The first stage of the procedure is to make a complaint to the practitioner concerned. The PCT may have an informal scheme for resolution of disputes with service providers. This stage is intended to give the contractor an opportunity of responding and if possible resolving the complaint.

Some complaints are excluded, such as:

- employee/employer matters;
- complaints being investigated by the Ombudsman;
- complaints where the complainant has given written warning that he intends to take legal proceedings;
- complaints raising Data Protection or Freedom of Information issues.

Complaints may be brought by the patient or by a representative of that patient. The complaint may be made orally or in writing. Written records must be made about the complaint. The complaint should be made within 6 months.

The response must be sent within 20 working days or as soon after as is practicable.

Second stage – Independent review

If the complainant is not satisfied with the response at the local level the matter may be taken to the next stage. In England, independent reviews are carried out by the Healthcare Commission.

In Northern Ireland, independent reviews are carried out by health boards.

Usually complaints must be made either within 6 months of the event or within 6 months of realising that there are grounds for complaint.

Healthcare Commission

The Healthcare Commission is responsible for reviewing complaints about the NHS or independent healthcare in England that have not been resolved locally.

Procedure on receipt of complaint

The Commission acknowledges the complaint and then ensures that it has all of the information needed to carry out an initial review to determine whether or not it is possible or appropriate for the complaint to be looked at further by the Commission. The complaint may then go to an investigation or a panel.

The initial decision will be based on:

- the request for a review
- the necessary consent forms
- the case file from the original investigation of the complaint
- relevant medical records.

At the initial review stage the Healthcare Commission may decide

- that the complaint is not eligible because it does not meet the Healthcare Commission's criteria;
- to take no further action;
- to refer the complaint back to the healthcare provider or NHS body for further action;
- to refer the complaint to another body for further action or investigation, e.g. the General Medical Council or the Health Service Ombudsman;
- to refer the complaint for action by another section of the Healthcare Commission;
- to carry out a full investigation of the complaint; and
- to refer the complaint for a panel hearing.

Appeal from decision at initial review stage

If a complainant is unhappy with the outcome of the initial review they will be able to complain to the Health Service Ombudsman.

Reference back

A reference back may be accompanied by a recommendation from the Healthcare Commission that the healthcare provider or NHS body do a certain number of things to resolve the complaint including

- giving more information to the complainant
- carrying out further investigation
- taking remedial action, e.g. offering treatment that may rectify a problem, improving procedures, following disciplinary procedures, arranging for an independent person to mediate between the complainant and the healthcare provider.

Healthcare Commission investigation

If the Healthcare Commission makes the decision to investigate then terms of reference are agreed with both parties.

Independent expert advice may be sought, e.g. medical or legal advice or advice from a patient or public interest perspective.

People connected with the complaint, including witnesses, may be interviewed.

When the investigation is completed, a draft report will be prepared and sent out for comment on factual accuracy. The report will summarise the investigation and make recommendations. The report will then be finalised and distributed to following parties:

- the complainant
- the patient if different from the complainant
- the person complained against
- the Chief Executive of the relevant NHS organisation
- any experts consulted
- the strategic health authority.

Recommendations as a result of an investigation

Similar recommendations to those available at initial review stage can be made.

An investigation will normally be completed within 6 months.

Panel investigation

Complaints may be investigated by a panel of three people – a chair and two panel members. The terms of reference will be agreed following comments from the parties involved. All parties will have a chance to check the draft report for factual accuracy before it is finalised and distributed. The recommendations made by a panel will be similar to those possible at the end of initial review.

The panel process will normally be completed within 4 months of the date of the request.

Third stage – Ombudsman

If the independent review does not resolve the complaint then it may be referred to the Health Service Ombudsman.

New arrangements for dealing with serious allegations

Fitness to practice procedures

The Department of Health issued guidance to PCTs on the Fitness to Practise procedures in July 2005. [Delivering quality in primary care: PCT management of Primary Care Practitioners' Lists – community chemist contractors/bodies corporate.]

The Fitness to Practise provisions permit a PCT to defer or reject an application for inclusion in the pharmaceutical list, and also provide the power to remove a pharmacy contractor from the pharmaceutical list.

PCT lists of practitioners

The HSC Act 2001 introduced new arrangements covering the regulation of family health service practitioners. The details are set out in the Contract Regulations 2005.

Primary Care Trusts are required to maintain lists of all practitioners, who undertake to provide services in their area. This list system was extended by the HSC Act 2001 to cover those who assist in the provision of primary care services (e.g. deputies or locums).

Declaration of convictions

The intention is that persons have to declare any criminal convictions, bindings-over following a criminal conviction and cautions in order to be admitted to a list or remain in it. PCTs will verify the information that they are given, using the Criminal Records Bureau.

This requirement extends to:

- Pharmacist owners
- Partnerships
- Limited companies.

All directors and superintendents of limited companies must provide the information. Limited companies with pharmacies in more than one PCT only have to make a declaration to the PCT where the head office is situated. They must give that PCT details of all other locations.

Grounds for refusal to admit to list

Primary Care Trusts may refuse a practitioner admission to the appropriate list on the grounds of unsuitability, prejudice to efficiency or because of previous fraudulent behaviour. Regulations allow the PCT to set conditions for inclusion in a list.

Under the new system:

- Only practitioners, including deputies and locums, who are included in lists maintained by PCTs are able to deliver family health services.
- Criteria to be admitted to (and to remain on) a list include probity and positive evidence of good professional behaviour and practice. This involves a system of declarations, annual appraisal and participation in clinical audit.
- PCTs may refuse to include a practitioner on the relevant medical, dental, ophthalmic or pharmaceutical list on the grounds of unsuitability, prejudice to efficiency or because of previous fraudulent behaviour.

Mandatory refusal

Regulation 19 sets out circumstances where a PCT must refuse to grant an application on fitness grounds.

These are

(a)   where the applicant, a director or a superintendent:

- has been convicted of murder in the United Kingdom
- has been sentenced to a term of imprisonment of over 6 months for an offence committed after 1 April 2005;

(b)   where the applicant:

- is subject to national disqualification
- has not updated his application following an investigation or hearing set out in Regulation 26(4).

Discretionary refusal

Primary Care Trusts have discretion to refuse applications on grounds of suitability, fraud or efficiency.

Primary Care Trusts should take into account issues such as:

- nature of offence or incident
- timescale
- number of offences or incidents
- any action taken or penalties imposed
- relevance to provision of NHS pharmaceutical services
- whether any offence was a "sexual offence"
- decisions of other PCTs.

Removal or suspension of practitioners

Primary Care Trusts may suspend and remove practitioners from the relevant lists on the grounds of inefficiency, fraud or unsuitability. They may also impose conditions on continued presence on the list.

The criteria are similar to those relevant to decisions on applications.

Where a director or superintendent of a limited company has been convicted of murder or has been sentenced to more than 6 months imprisonment, the limited company has 28 days to remove that person from office, or the entire limited company will be removed from the list.

Contingent removals

The PCT may impose conditions on persons on the list to prevent:

- any prejudice to the efficiency of the service
- any continuation of fraud.

If the conditions are not agreed then the PCT may remove that person from the list. Conditions must be reviewed on receipt of a written request.

Conditions cannot be imposed in "suitability" cases. The guidance states that "a chemist is either suitable or unsuitable. There are no degrees of suitability". Therefore the PCT must remove the contractor form the list if it decides he is unsuitable.

Suspension

The PCT may suspend a contractor if the action is necessary to protect the public (*Section 49I* of the NHS Act 1977).

A suspended contractor may appoint a "temporary chemist" to provide services on his behalf.

Suspension may only be for 6 months unless:

- the FHSAA agrees otherwise;
- the PCT is awaiting the outcome of regulatory body or criminal investigations;
- the PCT has decided to remove, or contingently remove a contractor from the list and it has imposed a suspension until the appeal process has been completed.

Suspended contractors are paid according to Directions from the DOH, which take account of previous levels of payment.

Hearings

The regulations include provision for a practitioner to be given notice of any allegations against him; for him to put his case at a hearing before a PCT makes a decision; and for him to be informed of a PCT's decision, the reasons for it and his right of appeal. The hearings are in private. Legal representation is not allowed, although parties may have legally qualified persons to assist and provide advice.

Appeals

The Act sets up a right of appeal to the FHSAA against a PCT's decision to impose conditions, to vary a condition, to vary terms of service or to remove a person from a list for a breach of a condition. The regulations provide for a decision not to have effect until the FHSAA has determined the appeal (and must do so in relation to a decision to remove the person from a list).

If a PCT suspends a practitioner, it must specify the period of suspension unless the Regulations provide otherwise.

National disqualification

A Health Authority may apply to the FHSAA for the national disqualification of a practitioner that it has removed from one of its lists.

Referral to Royal Pharmaceutical Society

The Regulations allow a PCT or the S of S to bring a matter to the attention of the Royal Pharmaceutical Society. Any relevant documents may be passed to the RPSGB.

Chapter 10

Retail Pharmacy

The nature of the control

The operation of a pharmacy is subject to a number of laws, which deal with ownership and with the activities carried on in the premises. In excess of 200 different pieces of legislation exist. This chapter deals only with those directly relevant to the establishment of the professional practice.

History

The Pharmacy Act 1852 established a system of control over the practice of pharmacy by requiring registration as a "chemist and druggist" or a "pharmaceutical chemist". Passing an exam entitled the person to registration and to the right to sell poisons.

The Pharmacy and Poisons Act 1933 compelled all pharmacists to become members of the then PSGB. The Statutory Committee system was established to disqualify persons from membership and hence from being an "authorised seller of poisons".

The Pharmacy Act 1954 removed the connection between poisons and pharmacy (which had been present since the Arsenic Act 1851) and dealt only with the profession of pharmacy. The 1954 Act is still extant, covering the registration process applicable to individual pharmacists.

The current legislation dealing with premises is the Medicines Act (MA) 1968. Subject to certain exceptions, the MA 1968 requires that the sale of medicinal products to the public takes place in registered premises and that the sale is by or under the supervision of a pharmacist.

Retail pharmacy business

The MA does not use the term "pharmacy" but "retail pharmacy business" (RPB). This is defined as:

> a business (not being a professional practice carried on by a practitioner) which consists of or includes the retail sale of medicinal products other than medicinal products on a general sale list (whether medicinal products on such a list are sold in the course of that business or not).

In other words, a business is a "retail pharmacy business" if it is:

- a business which consists of the retail sale of POM or P medicines
- a business which includes the retail sale of POM or P medicines, and
- not part of the professional practice of a practitioner, which in this instance means a doctor, dentist or vet.

The words in brackets at the end of the definition do not appear to add anything at all to the meaning.

Registered pharmacy

Section 74(1) defines a "registered pharmacy" as the premises where a person is lawfully conducting a RPB. The Registrar of RPSGB is required to keep a register of premises where a person is "lawfully conducting a retail pharmacy business" *(Section 75)*.

Applications to enter premises in the register of premises are made in writing to the Registrar. The RPSGB provides a printed form for convenience, but its use is not mandatory provided the specified details are given. According to the Medicines (Pharmacies) (Applications for Registration and Fees) Regulations 1973, SI No. 1822, all applications must be accompanied by a plan of the premises. The fees were set out in the same Regulations, but are amended each year.

The phrase "registered pharmacy" refers to the premises, and the phrase "retail pharmacy business" refers to the professional practice of a pharmacist who sells medicines and dispenses prescriptions.

Who may own a pharmacy?

The MA 1968 lists the persons who can operate a pharmacy.
A RPB may be lawfully carried on by:

(a) a pharmacist
(b) a partnership of pharmacists
(c) a "body corporate"
(d) a "representative" of a pharmacist.

There are a number of additional conditions for each circumstance outlined above.

Pharmacist
The part of the RPB which concerns the retail sale of medicines (whether or not they are General Sale List (GSL)) must be under the personal control of the pharmacist owner or of another pharmacist. The meaning of "personal control" is dealt with in Chapter 12.

Partnerships
In England, Wales and Northern Ireland, partnerships can only carry on a pharmacy if all the partners are registered pharmacists. In Scotland, the partnership running

the pharmacy must have one partner who is a pharmacist, but the rest need not be qualified as pharmacists.

The part of the business concerned with the sale or supply of P and POM medicines, and the dispensing of medicines must be under the personal control of one of the partners who is a pharmacist, or under the personal control of another pharmacist.

The Limited Liability Partnership Act 2000 came into force on 6 April 2001. The limited liability partnership is a hybrid of partnerships and companies. Limited liability partnerships are treated by the Medicines Act as companies rather than partnerships and therefore they may include non-pharmacist members. They need to appoint a superintendent pharmacist.

The general law relating to partnerships is discussed in Chapter 29.

Body corporate

This is a term applied to any association of individuals which is so constituted as to acquire a collective legal personality. The law recognises that some groups of people ought to be treated as a single individual, which is a separate "legal entity" from those who make up the group.

There are two types of "body corporate":

(1) A "corporation sole". The Crown, Ministers and an archbishop are examples. The idea of a "body corporate" enables the post to be sued instead of the person who holds the post for the time being.
(2) A "corporation aggregate". There are various types, including

   public corporations such as the Post Office
   co-operative societies
   mutual building societies
   private and public limited companies.

The most important, and numerous, are private limited companies. Generally speaking, where the term "body corporate" is used the term "company" can replace it.

The business of keeping, preparing and dispensing P and POM medicines must be under the management of a superintendent pharmacist.

The sale or supply of P and POM medicines by retail or as dispensed medicines must be:

(a) under the personal control of the superintendent *or*
(b) under the personal control of another pharmacist who is subject to direction by the superintendent.

Superintendent

(1) The superintendent must be a pharmacist.
(2) He must not act in a similar capacity for any other body corporate.
(3) He must send a statement to the registrar stating whether or not he is a member of the board of the body corporate.
(4) The statement must be in writing, signed by him and signed on behalf of the body corporate.

Representative

A representative of a pharmacist may carry on the pharmacy in certain circumstances (*Section 72*). These are

(a)   where the pharmacist has died
(b)   where he has become bankrupt
(c)   where he has become mentally unfit and a receiver has been appointed under
      the Mental Health Act 1983.

The representative is

(a)   the executor or administrator of a deceased pharmacist. For the first 3 months
      after the death any person beneficially interested in the estate may carry on the
      business;
(b)   the trustee in bankruptcy (or similar);
(c)   the receiver (or similar) of a mentally unfit pharmacist.

The representative may carry on business for a period of 5 years after the death of
a pharmacist, or for 3 years in any other case.

The name and address must be notified to the Registrar of the RPSGB. At all
premises where the retail sale or supply of P and POM medicines occurs, the sale of
all medicines must be under the personal control of a pharmacist.

Retail sale

Section 131 of the MA 1869 defines "retail sale" as the sale of a substance or article to
a person who buys it other than to sell it, supply it, administer it or cause it to be
administered in the course of business.

Supply in circumstances corresponding to retail sale

Section 131 defines this as a supply *otherwise than a sale* of a substance or article to a
person who buys it other than to sell it, supply it, administer it or cause it to be
administered in the course of business.

Between them these definitions cover almost all possible kinds of transactions.
One kind remains – a supply, without being a sale, which is for the same purpose as
a wholesale transaction. Such a supply does not seem to have been envisaged by the
Act and no provisions are made to control the transaction.

Supply of NHS Medicines

Legally, the supply of medicines on a NHS prescription is not a sale.

This has been considered by the courts on two occasions. In 1965, the House of
Lords considered whether the Minister of Health could import medicines for which
Pfizer Corporation held patents in this country. In dealing with this, they decided
that there was no sale of medicines by a hospital to a patient (*Pfizer Corporation v.
Minister of Health [1965] 1 AER, 450*).

In 1968 a court had to deal with contaminated medicine supplied to a patient. The
case was brought under the Food and Drugs Act, which required that the medicine

had been sold to the complainant. The court decided that the pharmacy had a contract with the then Executive Council for the supply of services. The pharmacy was paid remuneration for the services, and there was not a sale of medicine to the Executive Council (*Appleby* v. *Sleep, 2 AER 265*).

Dispensing only pharmacies

The definition of an RPB, taken from *Section 132* of the Act, suggests that a business where no retail sales took place (that is which only dispensed NHS scripts) would not be a RPB. But *Section 52* also restricts supply in "circumstances corresponding to retail sale" to an RPB in a registered pharmacy. This clumsy phrase "supply in circumstances corresponding to retail sale" covers the supply of dispensed medicines in the NHS. Therefore even dispensing-only pharmacies have to be registered, because the operation of such pharmacies can only be as part of a "retail pharmacy business". The Act does not envisage a pharmacy where no retail sales occur.

Wholesale dealing

This is a sale to a person who buys the substance in order to sell it, supply it, administer it or cause it to be administered in the course of business.

Register of Pharmaceutical Chemists

A pharmacist is a person whose name is entered in the Register of Pharmaceutical Chemists. This was established originally by the Pharmacy Act 1852, but now exists, in England, Wales and Scotland, as a result of *Section 2(1)* of the Pharmacy Act 1954. For Northern Ireland, the Register is maintained under a requirement in *Section 9* of the Pharmacy and Poisons Act (Northern Ireland) 1925. The register is computer-based and is kept by the Registrar of RPSGB (and the Registrar of PSNI). A printed version is produced every year for reference, but the definitive version is the updated computerised list.

Restricted titles

The use of some professional titles is restricted to a pharmacist. Only pharmacists may "take or use" any of the following titles:

pharmacist
pharmaceutical chemist
pharmaceutist
member of the Royal Pharmaceutical Society
fellow of the Royal Pharmaceutical Society.

Unqualified persons may not use the above titles. The abbreviations MRPharmS and FRPharmS are the approved abbreviations indicating membership and fellowship of the Society. The older forms MPS and FPS are still used occasionally.

Additionally, the MA specifies that no one may use any of those titles in connection with a retail business (or a business which consists of or includes a supply in circumstances corresponding to retail sale) unless the premises are a registered pharmacy or a hospital.

Pharmacy

The use of the term "pharmacy" is restricted to a registered pharmacy or the pharmacy department of a hospital.

Its use in circumstances which cannot be confused with the operation of a pharmacy, for instance a restaurant is still unclear. In 1998 the Society considered whether or not to instigate proceedings against a restaurant called "Pharmacy", but it did not take any action in court. The restaurant subsequently closed.

Use of title by companies

Companies operating an RPB may use the title "pharmacy" in connection with the premises.

Companies may also use the following titles:

chemist and druggist
druggist
dispensing chemist
dispensing druggist.

A body corporate may only use the title "chemist" if the superintendent is a member of the board. It may use "pharmacy" even though the superintendent is not on the board.

Representatives may use any title which the pharmacist was entitled to use.

European Union Nationals

Article 7 of the EC Directive 85/433 (which deals with the mutual recognition of the qualifications of EC pharmacists) allows nationals of Member States of the EC to use the lawful academic titles of their home state. They may do this if they are registered with the RPSGB.

Display of certificate of registration

The certificate of registration of the pharmacist in personal control at each premises must be "conspicuously exhibited" [*Sections 70* and *71 MA 68*].

Staffing

With effect from 1 January 2005, pharmacists have a professional obligation to ensure that pharmacy support staff are competent in the areas in which they are working to a minimum standard equivalent to the new Pharmacy Services S/NVQ level 2 qualification. Anyone not up to the required standards must be undertaking training. This requirement applies to all staff involved in the assembly of a prescription, including stock ordering, receiving and storing, and includes the following activities:

- sale of OTC medicines and the provision of information to customers on symptoms and products
- prescription receipt and collection
- the assembly of prescribed items (including the generation of labels)
- ordering, receiving and storing pharmaceutical stock
- the supply of pharmaceutical stock
- preparation for the manufacture of pharmaceutical products (including aseptic products)
- manufacture and assembly of medicinal products (including aseptic products).

Counter assistants

Since 1996 it has been a professional requirement of the RPSGB that any assistant who is given delegated authority to sell medicines under a protocol should have undertaken, or be undertaking an accredited course relevant to their duties. The Society's requirement is that courses should cover the knowledge and understanding associated with units 2.04 and 2.05 of the Pharmacy Services S/NVQ level 2, entitled Assist in the Sale of OTC medicines and provide information to customers on symptoms and products and Assist in the supply of prescribed items (taking in a prescription and issuing prescribed items).

Standard Operating Procedures (SOPs)

Since 1 January 2005 it has been a RPSGB requirement for pharmacies to have SOPs in place for the dispensing process, including the transfer of prescribed items to patients.

The requirement applies to both the hospital and community sectors and covers all of the activities which occur from the time that prescriptions are received in the pharmacy or by a pharmacist until medicines or other prescribed items have been collected or transferred to the patient.

Chapter 11

Manufacture and Licensing of Medicinal Products

The Medicines Act 1968 and other controls

In this chapter we deal with the licensing of the product, its manufacture and distribution.

Although there were some controls on poisons in the 19th century, and on biological products in the early 20th century, the current legislative framework for medicines production and supply dates from the Medicines Act 1968.

European Directives

Since 1968 the EU has issued several Directives which establish a community-wide system of control on medicines. The guiding principle of European and UK medicines legislation is to ensure the quality, safety and efficacy of medicinal products, with the overall aim of safeguarding public health.

A number of Directives cover the licensing of medicines.

The main European medicines legislation is Directive 2001/83/EC, *on the Community code relating to medicinal products for human use*, which repealed and re-enacted the original Directive 65/65/EEC and many subsequent directives on related subjects, with the aim of simplifying the European regulatory structure.

It requires that medicines placed on the market must have a licence (known as a marketing authorisation). This is based on showing that the product meets standards of safety, quality and efficacy.

From 1 January 1994 the licensing system consists of a centralised system and a decentralised or national (European member state) system. The centralised licensing system is administered by the European Medicines Evaluation Agency (EMEA) and enables the granting of an EC-wide marketing authorisation.

The decentralised system is under the control of member states and provides for the granting of marketing authorisations which may be recognised in other member states. In the United Kingdom this system is administered by the MHRA on behalf of the government.

The Medicines Act 1968

The MA 1968, together with the Medicines for Human Use (Marketing Authorisations, etc.) Regulations 1994, lays down a general framework for controlling dealings in medicinal products by way of a licensing system. This requires persons responsible for the composition of a product to hold a licence. Licences are also required by wholesale dealers and by manufacturers. It is unlawful for the products concerned to be manufactured, sold or supplied in, or imported into, the United Kingdom (and certain biological products may not be exported) except with the appropriate licences, certificates or exemptions.

A number of general remarks about the Act are appropriate at this point. The MA 1968 was produced in response to two main factors: the Thalidomide tragedy in the early 1960s, and the Directives issued by the European Economic Community (as it was then called). Although the United Kingdom did not join until 1973, the intention to do so was well known. In many ways the MA 1968 was a consumer safety act, concerned with protecting the public from faulty products by introducing a licensing system.

The opportunity was taken to include controls on the operation of pharmacies.

The MA 1968 is written in a difficult style. It starts off by prohibiting almost all dealings with medicines – referred to as "medicinal products". It continues by setting out a number of exemptions to the general rules, thereby allowing, for instance, the sale and manufacture of medicines. The first set of exemptions relate to licences. The second set refers to various activities done by professionals – practitioners. The third set removes some types of products from some controls, e.g. GSL.

In order to discover the rules governing an activity it is usually necessary to read a number of inter-related sections of the Act. For example, *Section 8* prohibits the manufacture of any medicinal product except in accordance with a licence. *Section 10* exempts pharmacists from the provisions of *Section 8*, but only for certain activities done in certain places, in certain ways.

Also the Medicines Act often sets out very general law, and the detail is found in Regulations. An example is the POM Order, which sets out in detail how prescription medicines are to be treated.

The Act allows for secondary legislation (Orders or Regulations), which can (and do) very considerably modify the provisions of the Act itself. In this way the later requirements of the EU Directives have been incorporated into the existing framework.

The basic framework of medicines control was set out in the MA 1968. Subsequently EC legislation has become dominant in this area, and UK legislation now reflects EC law. However, instead of producing a new Medicines Act, the changes are set out in various Regulations.

Medicines for Human use (Marketing Authorisations, etc.) Regulations 1994

The United Kingdom set out the new provisions of the EC Directive in the Medicines for Human use (Marketing Authorisations, etc.) Regulations 1994, SI No. 3144 (MAR 1994). These replace the provisions of the Medicines Act 1968 which deal with the licensing of medicines and their labelling. They also replace a mass of subordinate legislation which previously covered the same areas. They follow the same style as the main Act, but refer to "relevant Community provisions" in an attempt to avoid duplication.

Since the 1994 Regulations were introduced the original EC Directive has also been replaced, and a further set of UK Regulations, The Medicines (Codification

Amendments, etc.) Regulations 2002, SI No. 236, brings the terminology in the MAR Regulations up to date.

The UK Licensing Authority

Licences are issued by the "Licensing Authority" which for human medicines consists of the Health and Agriculture Ministers of the United Kingdom.

In practice, the licensing of human medicines is handled by the Medicines and Healthcare products Regulatory Agency (MHRA) of the DOH.

The licensing of veterinary products is generally dealt with by the Veterinary Medicines Agency, an Executive Agency of the Department for Environment, Food and Rural Affairs.

Medicinal products

A medicinal product is defined by Directive 2001/83/EC as:

(1) any substance or combination of substances presented for treating or preventing disease in human beings or animals;
(2) any substance or combination of substances which may be administered to human beings or animals with a view to making a medical diagnosis or to restoring, correcting or modifying physiological functions in human beings or animals is likewise considered a medicinal product.

Certain products used outside the human body, such as preservation agents for transplant organs are also included.

Relevant medicinal products

The MAR 1994 regulations apply to all medicinal products to which Directive 2001/83/EC applies, which are described in the Regulations as "relevant medicinal products".

"Relevant medicinal products" are all medicinal products for human use, except

(a) those prepared on the basis of a magistral or officinal formula
(b) medicinal products intended for research
(c) intermediate products intended for further processing by an authorised manufacturer.

Magistral refers to a medicine made in a pharmacy in accordance with a prescription for an individual patient.

Officinal formula refers to a medicine made in a pharmacy to a pharmacopoeial formula for direct supply to patients.

In practice most medicines which are sold or supplied in the United Kingdom are covered by the EC Directive definition.

Persons who are responsible for the composition of a product must hold a licence, termed a "marketing authorisation". In order to get an MA, a company must demonstrate the efficacy, safety and quality of its proposed medicine.

The MRHA acts as the government's licensing body. Medicines are considered for approval after laboratory screening, animal testing and closely monitored trials on healthy volunteers and patients.

The potential new medicine goes through four phases of clinical assessment in humans. In phase one a small number of healthy volunteers receive it; in phase two, 2–400 patients receive it; in phase three, 3000 patients receive it. If the results are satisfactory, the data (which will consist of many thousands of pages) are presented to the MRHA, which will refer the evidence to an advisory committee – the Commission on Human Medicines (CHM). The CHM may then recommend that the MHRA should grant a marketing authorisation.

After the drug has gone into general use, phase four studies are done on many thousands of patients. Doctors assist companies in post-marketing surveillance by reporting back on new products and any adverse reactions are reported to the CHM using the Yellow Card System.

Medicinal claims

The MHRA will generally regard a product as a medicinal product if medicinal claims are made for it. Medicinal claims are claims to treat or prevent disease, or to interfere with normal operation of a physiological function of the human body.

Medicines Act definition

Section 130 of the MA 1968 defines a "medicinal product" as any substance or article which is manufactured, sold, supplied, imported or exported for use wholly or mainly as something which is administered, or is an ingredient of something which is administered, for a medicinal purpose.

Medicinal purpose

A "medicinal purpose" is

- treating disease
- preventing disease
- diagnosing disease
- ascertaining the existence, degree or extent of a physiological condition
- contraception
- anesthesia
- preventing or interfering with the normal operation of a physiological function in any other way.

Administration

Administer means to give to someone as a medicine. This may be done orally, by injection, by introduction into the body in any other way, and by external application.

There may be direct contact with the body, e.g. a cream, or indirect, e.g. inhalation.

Marketing Authorisation (MA)

The MAR 1994 Regulations prohibit the placing on the market of most medicinal products unless they have an EU or UK marketing authorisation.
   According to Regulation 3(1) of MAR 1994:

> except in accordance with any exception or exemption set out in the relevant Community provisions and subject to Paragraphs 1 and 3 of Schedule 1:
>
> (a)   no relevant medicinal product shall be placed on the market; and
> (b)   no such product shall be distributed by way of wholesale dealing,
>
> unless a marketing authorisation is respect of that product has been granted . . . and is in force . . .

In effect a marketing authorisation is required by the person responsible for the composition of the product, i.e. either the manufacturer or the person to whose order the product is manufactured.
   Prior to 1994 the marketing authorisation was termed a "product licence". These were designated on the product label with the initials PL and a number. This "PL" designation is still used for marketing authorisations.

Placed on the market

A product is placed on the market when it is first made available in return for payment or charge with a view to distribution, use or both on the Community market.
   The term "made available" means the transfer of the ownership of the product, or the passing of the product to the final consumer or user in a commercial transaction. It may be for payment or free of charge. The legal instrument by which the transfer is achieved, e.g. sale, loan, lease, gift, etc. is irrelevant.
   A product is not placed on the market if it is made in a hospital pharmacy and then used elsewhere in the same hospital to treat patients.

Exemption in Section 7 of MA 1968

Section 7 of the MA 1968 only applies to products which are not covered by the MAR 1994 regulations.
   Section 7 of the Act states that, except where exempted by provisions in the Act or Regulations, a "marketing authorisation" is required by any person who in the course of his business sells, supplies, exports, imports or procures the sale, supply, export, manufacture or assembly of a medicinal product. It is an offence to carry out these activities without a marketing authorisation.

Conditions for granting a "marketing authorisation"

Applications must be in writing, comply with relevant EU provisions and be accompanied by the correct fee. Details of the necessary accompanying material are set out in EC Directive 2001/83/EC.

The licensing authority has to be satisfied as to the safety, quality and efficacy of a product before it may grant an MA. The appropriate committee (CSM, VPC or ACRHP) must be consulted where the authority intends to refuse a licence.

Safety includes consideration of the extent to which the product:

(a)   if used without proper safeguards, is capable of causing danger to the health of the community; or

(b)   may interfere with the treatment, prevention or diagnosis of disease; or may be harmful to the person administering it (*Section 132*, MA 1968).

Twenty-six copies of the application and accompanying material are required for a new application.

The application must be accompanied by a statement indicating whether the product should be a POM, P or GSL medicine.

There must be a Summary of Product Characteristics (SPC) which contains certain required information about the therapeutic indications, contra-indications and side-effects of the product. Other information includes dosage, method and route of administration, shelf life, storage precautions and the results of clinical trials and tests.

Section 28 states the grounds for suspending, revoking or varying a licence. The most important is the availability of new factual information relevant to the licence. Other reasons include failure to keep to conditions in the licence, e.g. standards of quality.

Licences are also required by wholesale dealers and by manufacturers. It is unlawful for the products concerned to be manufactured, sold or supplied in, or imported into, the United Kingdom (and certain biological products may not be exported) except with the appropriate licences, certificates or exemptions.

Provision of safety information

Article 8 of Directive 2001/83/EC introduced an obligation on applicants for authorisation to provide all information relevant to the evaluation of quality, safety and efficacy of a product.

This obligation is set out in the Medicines (Provision of False or Misleading Information and Miscellaneous Amendments) Regulations 2005, SI No. 1710, which came into effect on 1 August 2005.

Regulation 3 amends the MAR 1994. It creates new criminal offences for failures to provide information relevant to the evaluation of safety, quality or efficacy of a medicinal product for human use and for the provision of information to the licensing authority which is relevant to an evaluation of the safety, quality or efficacy of medicinal products for human use but which is false or misleading in a material particular.

Manufacturer's Licence (ML)

Section 8 of the MA 1968 provides that subject to exceptions, every person who makes or packs a medicinal product in the course of business must have a manufacturer's licence (ML).

Specials licence

A pharmacist or a doctor may ask a pharmaceutical manufacturer to prepare a medicinal product for him. No product licence is necessary provided the manufacturer holds a manufacturer's licence specifically authorising him to produce "specials". The manufacturer is prohibited from advertising the products or from soliciting the orders (SI 1994 No. 3144).

Assembly

This term is used to include various packaging activities:

enclosing the product in a container, which is then labelled before sale or supply,

labelling the container of medicine.

A container is the box, bottle or carton, etc. in which the product is contained. It does not mean the capsule in which the product is to be administered.

The assembly of a medicine is an activity which requires a manufacturer's licence, or an exemption.

Wholesale

Section 8 also requires that everyone who wholesales or offers for sale by wholesale a medicinal product must hold a "wholesale dealer's licence". Persons holding a manufacturer's licence do not need a separate licence for the wholesale supply of the products they manufacture. Pharmacies are also exempt, provided the volume of wholesaling is insignificant (less than 5% of turnover is used by the MHRA).

Appeal process

An aggrieved applicant for a licence may first take his case to the CSM, VPC or ACRHP. He may then appeal to the Medicines Commission (MC). The final appeal is to an independent person appointed by the licensing authority.

The European Medicines Evaluation Agency

The European Medicines Agency (formerly the European Medicines Evaluation Agency) is a part of the EU bureaucracy. It is established by Article 55 of the EC Regulation No. 726/2004. Its function is to handle the EC centralised procedure, which is used for new active substances and certain high-technology and biotechnology products. The EMEA is advised by the Committee for Proprietary Medicinal Products (CPMP) whose members are drawn from the member states of the EU. Where the centralised procedure is used, companies submit one single marketing authorisation application to the EMEA. A single evaluation is carried out through CHMP or through the Committee for Medicinal Products for Veterinary Use (CVMP). If the relevant Committee concludes that quality, safety and efficacy of the medicinal product is sufficiently proven, it adopts a positive opinion. This is sent to the Commission to be transformed into a single market authorisation valid for the whole of the European Union.

The Advisory Machinery

A number of committees of experts are established under the Act, to advise Ministers about the matters dealt with by the Medicines Act.

The Commission for Human Medicines

The Medicines Commission, established by *Section 2* of the Act, was abolished in 2005 by The Medicines (Advisory Bodies) Regulations 2005, SI No. 1094, and replaced with CHM. The former Committee on Safety of Medicines was also abolished and replaced by the CHM.

The functions of the CHM are set out in a new *Section 4* of the Act:

(1)   The Commission shall give to any one or more of the Ministers specified in Paragraphs (a) and (b) of *Section 1(1)* of this Act advice on matters:

    (a)   relating to the execution of this Act
    (b)   relating to the exercise of any power conferred by this Act
    (c)   relating to the execution of the Marketing Authorisation Regulations or the Clinical Trials Regulations
    (d)   relating to the exercise of any power conferred by those regulations or
    (e)   otherwise relating to medicinal products

where either the Commission consider it expedient, or they are requested by the Minister or Ministers in question to do so.

(2)   Without prejudice to the preceding subsection, and to any other duties or powers imposed or conferred on the Commission by or under this Act, the Marketing Authorisation Regulations or the Clinical Trials Regulations, it shall be the duty of the Commission:

    (a)   to

        (i)   give advice with respect to safety, quality or efficacy in relation to medicinal products,
        (ii)   promote the collection and investigation of information relating to adverse reactions, for the purposes of enabling such advice to be given, and
        (iii) undertake the functions mentioned in *Section 4(4)* of this Act,

    except in so far as those functions are for the time being assigned to a committee established under *Section 4* of this Act; and [a]
    (b)   to advise the licensing authority in cases where the authority

        (i)   are required by the provisions of Part 2 of this Act, or by the provisions of the Marketing Authorisation Regulations or the Clinical Trial Regulations, to consult the Commission with respect to any matter arising under those provisions, or
        (ii)   without being required to do so, elect to consult the Commission with respect to any matter arising under any of those provisions.

(c)   to give advice on general matters of policy relating to medicines control. In certain circumstances it also considers applications for licences. It reports to the licensing authority which must take account of its report in determining an application.

Composition

The Commission has at least eight members, who are appointed by Ministers. The Ministers shall appoint the members of the Commission. Chairmen of the Expert Advisory Groups are automatically appointed as members of the Commission.
The Expert Advisory Groups include

Biologicals Expert Advisory Group, to advise on safety, quality and efficacy of medicinal products of biological or bio-technological origin, including vaccines;
Chemistry, Pharmacy and Standards Expert Advisory Group, to advise on the quality, and quality in relation to safety and efficacy, of medicinal products which are the subject of an application for a marketing authorization, or a request for authorisation pursuant to Regulation 17 of the Clinical Trials Regulations;
Pharmacovigilance Expert Advisory Group, to advise on pharmacovigilance and other issues relating to the safety of medicinal products; and
"such other Expert Advisory Groups as it considers appropriate".

Veterinary Products Committee

This advises DEFRA on veterinary products.

British Pharmacopoeia Commission

The British Pharmacopoeia (BP) Commission is responsible for preparing the BP, which contains standards for human medicines. It is also responsible for selecting non-proprietary names for medicinal substances.

Advisory Committee on the Registration of Homoeopathic Products

The Advisory Board on the Registration of Homoeopathic Products (ABRHP) was established in 1994 to give advice on the safety and quality of a homoeopathic product for human and veterinary use, for which a certificate of registration could be granted. It is governed by the Registration of Homoeopathic Products Order 1994 (SI 1994/102) as amended by the Medicines (Advisory Board on the Registration of Homoeopathic Products Order 1995 (SI 1995/309).

Statutory procedure for classifying borderline substances

The Medicines for Human Use (Marketing Authorisations, etc.) Amendment Regulations, SI No. 2000/292 amend the MAR 1994 Regulations to give power to stop a company selling a product, which the licensing authority believes is a medicine, without a marketing authority. The licensing authority must explain why they consider the product to be a medicine. There is an appeal to a review panel.

Medical Foods Regulations

The Medical Food Regulations 2000, SI No. 845 implement Directive 99/21/EC which introduced specific rules for foods used for the dietary management of specific diseases or medical conditions. Maximum and minimum vitamin, mineral and trace element levels for specific categories of FSMPs are set by the Regulations. There is an obligation to notify new products when first placed on the market.

Medical devices

Prior to 1994 many medical devices were controlled under the MA 1968. They are now controlled under consumer safety legislation, specifically The Medical Devices Regulations 1994, SI No. 3017.

A medical device is

an instrument, apparatus, appliance, material or other article, whether used alone or in combination, together with any software necessary for its proper application which

(1) is intended by the manufacturer to be used for human beings for the purpose of:

    (a) diagnosis, prevention, monitoring, treatment or alleviation of disease;

    (b) diagnosis, prevention, monitoring, treatment or alleviation of or compensation for an injury or handicap;

    (c) investigation, replacement or modification of the anatomy or of any physiological process; *or*

    (d) control of contraception; *and*

(2) does not achieve its principal intended action in or on the human body by pharmacological, immunological or metabolic means, even if it is assisted in its function by such means.

The definition includes devices which are intended to administer a medicinal product or which incorporate a substance which would be a medicinal product if used on its own. Such devices include intra-uterine devices, diaphragms, dental fillings, contact lens care products, non-medicated dressings, sutures and ligatures. Medical devices must comply with the regulations and with the "essential requirements" set out in Directive 93/42/EEC. There are specific labelling requirements. The MHRA administers the legislation.

Exemptions from the need to hold licences

Pharmacists
Section 10 provides that no licence is required for the normal activities of a pharmacist. Some activities are covered simply because they are done by a pharmacist, whereas others are covered only if the activities take place in a registered pharmacy.

Doctors, dentists, vets

Section 9 exempts doctors, dentist and vets from the need to have PLs and MLs. They may prepare, import, order the preparation or importation, manufacture, assemble, sell, supply or procure the manufacture, sale or supply of a medicinal product for administration to a patient.

What can a pharmacist do?

The Act allows certain activities to be done by pharmacists which would otherwise require the holding of a licence.

(1) All pharmacists are allowed to procure the assembly of a medicinal product. The activity may also be done under the supervision of a pharmacist (*Section 10*).
(2) Where the activity takes place in a registered pharmacy, a hospital or a health centre a pharmacist may assemble a medicinal product (*Section 10*).
(3) Where the activity takes place in a registered pharmacy, a hospital or a health centre, *and* it is done in accordance with a prescription given by a practitioner, a pharmacist may prepare or dispense a medicinal product (*Section 10*).

The terms "prepare" and "dispense" are not defined in the Act, and therefore take their normal meaning. However, *Section 10* provides exemptions from *Sections 7* and *8*, which although they do not refer to preparation or dispensing, do refer to manufacturing. *Section 10* does not use "manufacturing", leading to the conclusion that preparation and dispensing are activities which are similar to but less than manufacture.

In 2005 the MHRA issued Guidance Note No. 14 stating that "The supply of unlicensed relevant medicinal products for individual patients" – which indicates how in practice MHRA will determine whether an activity is "preparation" or "manufacture". Criteria include location of the process, nature of the activity and scale of the activity.

(4) Where all the following conditions apply, a pharmacist may prepare or dispense a medicinal product.
    It must be done:

    - in a registered pharmacy
    - by or under the supervision of a pharmacist
    - in accordance with a specification furnished by the person to whom the product is or is to be sold or supplied
    - the person is going to administer the product to himself or to someone under his care (*Section 10*).

(5) A pharmacist may prepare a stock of medicinal products in a hospital or health centre ready for dispensing them in accordance with a prescription given by a practitioner (*Section 10*).
(6) A pharmacist may prepare or dispense a medicinal product in a registered pharmacy, if the following conditions are satisfied:

    - the product is for administration to a person
    - the pharmacist was requested by or on behalf of that person to exercise his judgement as to the treatment required
    - the person was present in the pharmacy at the time of the request (*Section 10*).

(7)   A pharmacist can prepare a stock of medicinal products in a registered pharmacy:

- with a view to dispensing them in accordance with a prescription given by a practitioner *or*
- with a view to dispensing them in accordance with a specification from a person who is going to administer them to himself or to someone under his care.

SPC and PILs

The EC Directive 92/37/EEC required all medicines to be supplied with a "patient information leaflet" (PIL). The information is directed at patients and the leaflet must be understandable. The contents are approved by the MHRA. The official implementation date of the Directive was 1 January 1999. Continental Europe has adopted patient packs, so it is easy for manufacturers and pharmacists to comply with the Directive. In the United Kingdom products are still dispensed from bulk, or patient packs are opened and split. The RPSGB announced in December 1998 that pharmacists should continue to dispense products whether or not they come with approved PILs. The current Professional Standards Directorate FactSheet is more equivocal and suggests pharmacists discuss the matter with their legal advisors.

Directive 2001/82/EC as amended by Directive 2003/63/EC and Directive 2004/27/EC also deals with PILs.

Under The Medicines (Marketing Authorisations and Miscellaneous Amendments) Regulations 2004, SI No. 3224, effective from 1 January 2005, PILs must be drawn up in accordance with new clear and easy to use reflect the results of consultations with target patient groups.

It is a requirement of the licensing process that there must be a Summary of Product Characteristics (SPC) which contains certain required information about the therapeutic indications, contra-indications and side-effects of the product. Other information includes dosage, method and route of administration, shelf life, storage precautions and the results of clinical trials and tests.

Chapter 12

Control on Sales of Medicines

Various parts of the MA 1968 place restrictions on the supply of medicines by restricting who may sell medicines and where they may be sold.

Control of retail sales

The underlying principle of MA 1968 control on the retail sales of medicines is that they should normally be supplied through pharmacies. There are three main exceptions to that.

First, certain medicines are designated by Statutory Instruments as ones which may be sold to the public by an ordinary shop.

Secondly, medicines may be sold by a hospital or health centre even where there is no pharmacy if the products are sold or supplied in the course of the business of the hospital or health centre *and* they are for the purpose of being administered in accordance with the directions of a doctor or dentist.

It does not matter whether they are to be administered in the hospital, or health centre or elsewhere. The doctor or dentist is not required to be an employee of the hospital, or to be associated with it in any way.

The "directions of a doctor" need not comply with the requirements for a prescription set out in SI 1983 No. 1212.

Thirdly, Patient Group Directions may empower certain health professionals to supply medicines to the public in accordance with protocols. This supply may take place anywhere.

Legal categories of medicines

The EC Directive on Legal Classification (92/26/EC) came into effect on 1 January 1993. This Directive has now been superceded by Directive 2001/82/EC, which consolidated a number of earlier directives. This Directive requires Member States to classify medicines into those which may only be sold or supplied on prescription, and those which may be obtained without a prescription.

The Directive lays down the criteria which must be used to determine whether a product should be subject to prescription control. These criteria have been incorporated into the Medicines Act by the Medicines Act 1968 (Amendment) (No. 2) Regulations 1992, SI 1992 No. 3271. This introduced a new *Section 58A* into the Act.

Marketing authorisation

Regulation 4 of the MAR 1994 Regulations requires each application for the grant of the MA 1968 to indicate whether the product is one that could be available:

(a)   only on prescription
(b)   only from a pharmacy
(c)   on general sale.

The application must also indicate whether the authorisation should include any other restrictions on the sale or supply of the product, for example a restriction on promotion.

Where the community marketing authorisation contains such restrictions, Ministers are required to include the product in the POM Order.

General Sale List

This is a list of medicines which can be sold, with reasonable safety, without the supervision of a pharmacist. The sales have to take place from proper shops, i.e. ones which can be closed so as to exclude the public. This prohibits sales being made from vans or other vehicles, or from open market stalls.

There is a separate list of products which may be sold from automatic vending machines.

To sum up, GSL medicines may be sold:

● without the supervision of a pharmacist
● from any ordinary shop (not a pharmacy)
● shop must be one which can be closed up
● not from a vehicle or market stall.

Pharmacy medicines

Pharmacy (P) medicines may be sold only in a registered pharmacy by or under the supervision of a pharmacist. This is the default category, into which all medicines fall unless placed by legislation into either of the other two categories.

Pharmacy medicines may only be sold:

● in a registered pharmacy
● by or under the supervision of a pharmacist

Prescription Only Medicines

POM medicines may only be sold or supplied in a registered pharmacy, by or under the supervision of a pharmacist, in accordance with the prescription of a doctor, dentist or veterinary practitioner. A nurse prescriber can write prescriptions for the POM Medicines listed in the Nurse Prescribers' Formulary.

Section 58A requires that a product is to be designated as a POM medicine if

(a) it needs medical supervision in use to prevent a direct or indirect danger to human health *or*
(b) it is widely and frequently misused, and so presents a danger to health *or*
(c) it is a new active substance *or*
(d) it is for parenteral administration.

The POM Order

The list of POM medicines for human use is contained in the POM Order, properly called the Prescription Only Medicines (Human Use) Order 1997, SI No. 1830.

This Order has been amended a number of times, by Prescription Only Medicines (Human Use) Amendment Orders in the following years:

1997, SI No. 2044
1998, SI No. 108
1998, SI No. 1178
1998, SI No. 2081
1999, SI No. 1044
1999, SI No. 3463
2000, SI No. 1917
2000, SI No. 2899
2000, SI No. 3231
2001, SI No. 2777
2001, SI No. 3942
2002, SI No. 549
2003, SI No. 696

and by

2001, SI No. 2889
2002, SI No. 2469
2004, SI No. 1771
2005, SI No. 765
2005, SI No. 1507

Medicinal products on prescription only

Generally the following medicinal products are POM:

(a) medicinal products consisting of or containing a substance listed in column 1 of Schedule 1
(b) controlled drugs
(c) medicinal products that are for parenteral administration
(d) cyanogenetic substances other than preparations for external use
(e) radiopharmaceuticals and generators
(f) medicinal products for human use which are licensed by the European community and classed as prescription only.

There are a number of exceptions.

Schedule 1 sets out a list of medicines together with the conditions which make a product exempt from POM.

Four categories are set out in Schedule 1. They are based on:

(1)   maximum strength
(2)   route of administration, use of pharmaceutical form
(3)   treatment limitations
(4)   maximum quantity.

Schedule 2 excludes some controlled drugs from POM when the preparation complies with the conditions.

Schedule 3 sets out the POM medicines which may be prescribed by nurses.

Schedule 4 lists a number of substances which may not be contained in a POM sold or supplied by a pharmacist under the emergency supply provisions.

Schedule 5 sets out exemptions for certain persons from the POM provisions on sale, supply or administration.

Injections
All parenteral products are POM.

Water for Injection
Sterile Water for Injection is POM. Water for Injection may be supplied without prescription by a lawful drug treatment service in 2 ml vials.

[Paragraph 7, The Medicines for Human Use (Prescribing) (Miscellaneous Amendments) Order 2005, SI No. 1507]

Administration of POMs
Section 58(2)(b) of the Act states that no one can administer a POM, except to himself, unless he is either:

● a prescriber, or
● a person acting in accordance with the directions of a prescriber.

The POM Order makes two exceptions to this blanket prohibition. The first one exempts all medicines which are not for parenteral administration (Article 9). Thus, effectively, anyone can administer to anyone else any medicines which are not injections.

Secondly, some injections are specifically exempted from the blanket prohibition (Article 7). They are ones which might be needed in an emergency:

Adrenaline injection 1 mg/1 ml
Atropine sulphate injection
Chlorpheniramine injection

Cobalt edetate injection
Dextrose injection strong BPC
Diphenhydramine injection
Glucagon injection
Hydrocortisone injection
Mepyramine injection
Promethazine hydrochloride injection
Sodium nitrite injection
Snake venom antiserum
Sodium thiosulphate injection
Sterile pralidoxime.

Thirdly, ambulance paramedics may administer a range of injections (Article 11(2) and Schedule 5 Part III).

A number of exceptions are made to allow the supply and use of POMs for research, business and in various unusual circumstances.

Prescription requirements

POM Medicines may only be supplied on prescription. The conditions which a prescription for POMs must meet are laid out in the POM Order (Article 15 as substituted by The Human Use (Prescribing) Order 2005, SI No. 765).

(1) All prescriptions must be signed in ink, with his own name, by the practitioner.
(2) Private prescriptions must be written in ink, or otherwise be indelible.
(3) NHS prescriptions, other than for Schedule 1, 2 or 3 of the MDA Regulations, may be written by means of carbon paper or similar material.
(4) No prescription may be dispensed more than 6 months after the date on which it was signed, except:

    (a) NHS prescriptions may bear a date before which they may not be dispensed. The 6 months runs from that date if it is later than the date of signing.
    (b) where a prescription contains a direction that it may be dispensed more than once, then the first dispensing must be within the 6-month period.

(5) Where a script contains directions that it may be dispensed more than once, those directions must be followed. If the number of repeats is not specified, only one repeat is allowed, except oral contraceptives may be dispensed six times in total before the end of the 6-month period.
(6) All prescriptions shall contain the following particulars:

    (a) address of the practitioner giving it
    (b) the date of signing (or start date)
    (c) an indication of whether the prescriber is a doctor, dentist, veterinary surgeon or veterinary practitioner, nurse or supplementary prescriber

(d) for prescriptions from doctors, dentists, nurses or supplementary
prescribers:

name of patient
address of patient
age of patient (if under 12 years)

(e) for vet prescriptions:

name and address of person in charge of the animal
declaration by vet that the medicine is for an animal or herd under
his care.

Electronic signatures

Electronic prescriptions may be signed with an "advanced electronic signature",
provided the prescription is transferred as an electronic communication to the person who dispenses it. Electronic prescriptions are not valid for drugs in Schedules 1,
2 and 3 of the MDR 2001.

Due diligence clause

The Order states that if the person making the sale or supply has exercised due
diligence and accordingly believes on reasonable grounds that the conditions are
fulfilled, he will not commit an offence if it turns out that the practitioner did not in
fact fulfil the conditions (Article 14).

Records of transactions

Records must be kept of the retail sale or supply of POMs. Entries must be made
in a register kept for that purpose. The entry must be made on the day of the
transaction, or on the next day. The Medicines (Sale or Supply) (Miscellaneous
Provisions) Amendment Regulations 1997, SI No. 1831, amended the original legislation in the Medicines (Sale or Supply) (Miscellaneous Provisions) Regulations
1980, SI No. 1923, so as to allow records to be kept in a computerised form.

Records are not required for:

(1) the sale or supply on a NHS prescription
(2) the sale or supply of oral contraceptives
(3) where records are made in the CD Register
(4) sale or supply to persons in respect of a drug testing scheme
(5) sale or supply in Scotland, to a doctor under the Stock Order scheme
(6) sale or supply in Northen Ireland to a doctor for NHS use by way of immediate
administration.

What details of prescriptions must be recorded?

For sale or supply of POMs on a prescription, the following details are required:

(1) date of transaction
(2) name and quantity of medicine

(3) form and strength of medicine (unless obvious)
(4) date of prescription
(5) name and address of prescriber
(6) name and address of patient (or of owner of animal).

Repeat prescriptions

When second or third supplies are made on repeat prescriptions, a shortened record may be made. The date of supply must be recorded together with a reference to the original entry.

How long must the records be kept?

The POM Register must be kept for 2 years from the date of the last entry. Prescriptions must be retained for 2 years from the date of last dispensing. The owner of the RPB is responsible for preserving the records.

Facsimile transmission of prescriptions

The requirements for a valid prescription are set out above. A fax does not comply because it is not itself "signed" by the practitioner. The RPSGB view at the time of writing is that a fax can confirm the existence of a valid prescription. The POM order does not require that the prescription itself be in the possession of the pharmacist at the time of dispensing the medicine. The Misuse of Drugs Regulations 2001 contain more stringent requirements for prescriptions for Schedule 2 and 3 medicines, in particular that the prescription must be in the handwriting of the prescriber. Accordingly, the RPSGB advise that such medicines cannot be dispensed against a fax.

Supervision of sales

The terms "supervision", direct supervision" and "personal control" are used in the legislation. They have similar but not identical meanings.

The term "supervision" is used in the MA 1968. The sale or supply of P and POM medicines must take place by or under the supervision of a pharmacist (*Section 52*).

The case of *Roberts v. Littlewoods Mail Order Stores* (1943) is usually quoted as the source of the legal meaning of "supervision". The case concerned the sale of a Part 1 poison, under the provisions of the Pharmacy and Poisons Act 1933. *Section 18* stated,

> it shall not be lawful for a person to sell any poison in Part 1 of the Poisons List unless . . . the sale is effected by, or under the supervision of, a registered pharmacist.

The sale of the poison occurred while the pharmacist was upstairs and unaware that the sale was taking place.

The court held that the statute required that the qualified person must be aware of each individual sale. The court rejected the contention that the words were sufficiently complied with by having a pharmacist in general control of the department.

In the judgment, Lord Caldicott said:

> the man who was upstairs might have been a person who was exercising personal control of a business, but I do not think that, while he was upstairs and therefore absent, he could be a person who was supervising a particular sale. It has been suggested that a man can supervise a sale without being bodily present. I do not accept that contention . . . each individual sale must be, not necessarily effected by the qualified person, but something which is shown by the evidence to be under his supervision in the sense that he must be aware of what is going on at the counter, and in a position to supervise or superintend the activities of the young woman by whom each individual sale is effected.

The judge also quoted from an earlier case, *Pharmaceutical Society* v. *Wheeldon* (1890) which concerned the Pharmacy Act 1868:

> nothing to our understanding can be clearer than that the object of the Act was beyond all other considerations to provide for the safety of the public, and to guard as far as possible, all members of the community from the disastrous consequences, so frequent in occurrence, arising from the sale of poisons by person inadequately acquainted with their baneful properties.

Although the words of the MA 1968 are slightly different, and the legislation is concerned with medicinal products rather than poisons, the meaning given above is accepted today as the law.

The NHS (PS) Regulations 2005 also use the term "direct supervision".

The Regulations 8(2) state,

> Drugs or appliances [so ordered] shall be provided by or under the direct supervision of a pharmacist.

Given the meaning of supervision outlined above it is difficult to see how the word "direct" adds anything to the meaning.

Personal control

The meaning attributed to this phrase is usually based on the judgment in the case of *Hygenic Stores Ltd* v. *Coombs* (1937). In this case the company sold drugs at 13 of its 16 shops, although there were no pharmacists employed at these shops. The company did employ three pharmacists, who worked long hours at the other three shops. The court found that there were no pharmacists in personal control at the 13 shops, and consequently the conditions for sale of drugs were not met. The Pharmacy and Poisons Act 1933 required that

> in each set of premises the business must, so far as concerns the retail sale of drugs, if not under the personal control of the superintendent, be carried on subject to the direction of the superintendent, under the personal control of a manager or assistant who is a registered pharmacist.

The court did not define what constitutes personal control. It only decided that the circumstances outlined above did not constitute personal control.

The Statutory Committee has considered the question on a number of occassions. Its views are summarized in the following sentences. It is a matter of degree. A pharmacist does not cease to be in personal control because he leaves the pharmacy for a few minutes. At the other end of the scale a pharmacist is not in personal control if he puts in only an occasional appearance. A pharmacist was held not to be in personal control when he was absent for one and a half hours a day on weekdays, and 6 hours at the weekend.

Following a decision by the chairman of the Statutory Committee in July 2003 (reported in *Pharmaceutical Journal* of, 7 August, p. 203), the Royal Pharmaceutical Society's Fitness to Practise and Legal Affairs Directorate has issued advice. In his decision the Chairman said that pharmacy premises may remain open without a pharmacist being present provided that nothing takes place that requires the presence or approval of a pharmacist.

The RPSGB advice is,

All supplies of prescription-only medicines (POMs) and pharmacy (P) medicines from registered retail pharmacy premises must be made under the supervision of a pharmacist.

Sales of general sale list (GSL) medicines do not require supervision, but do require a pharmacist to be in personal control of the premises.

Thus, if a pharmacist is not in personal control, for instance because he is late attending or he has left for the afternoon, no sales of medicines can be made, and this includes general sale list medicines.

The use of restricted titles such as "chemist" and "pharmacy" can only be used in connection with retail sales of any goods where they are being sold from registered retail pharmacy premises under the personal control of a pharmacist.

Therefore, if restricted titles are used and a pharmacist has to leave the premises, the safest option may be to close the pharmacy premises.

Where the pharmacy is in contract with a PCT to provide NHS services, the PCT should be contacted for advice

Protocols and Medicines Counter Assistants
From 1 January 1995, it has been a requirement of the RPSGB that all pharmacies have a written protocol which specifies the procedure to be followed when a medicine is supplied, and when advice on treatment is requested.

From 1 January 1996, the RPSGB has required that all staff whose work regularly involves the sale of medicines must have either completed, or be undertaking, an approved course of training. A number of such courses have been approved covering the knowledge syllabus of the National Vocational Qualification Level 2 in retail training.

Dispensing staff
From 1 January 2005 pharmacists have had a professional obligation to ensure that staff involved in dispensing are competent in the areas in which they are working

to a minimum standard equivalent to the Pharmacy Services Scottish/National Vocational Qualification level 2, or are undertaking training towards this.

Wholesaling of medicines

A Wholesale Dealers Licence is required by any person who distributes a "relevant medicinal product" by way of wholesale dealing. The person may be a real person, a body of persons or a limited company. There are certain exceptions, including a registered pharmacy business where the wholesale sales are under 5% of the total sales.

What is wholesaling?

The MA 1968 Amendment Regulations 1993, SI No. 834, altered *Section 8(7)* of the MA to define "distribution by way of wholesale dealing" as meaning: Selling or supplying it *or* Procuring, holding or exporting it for the purposes of sale or supply to a person who receives it for the purposes of selling or supplying it, or administering it, or causing it to be administered to one or more human beings in the course of business

The term "business" includes a professional practice, such as that of a medical practitioner. Thus sales to a medical or dental practitioner "for use in his practice" will be wholesale sales. Moreover, the provision of services under the NHS is considered to be the carrying on of a business by the appropriate Minister (*Section 131* Medicines Act 1968).

Certain medicinal products are outside the definition of "relevant medicinal product". Distribution of these products, for example, exempt herbal remedies, certain homoeopathic medicines, investigational medicinal products and unlicensed medicinal products for export to third countries, remains subject to the wholesale dealing controls of the Medicines Act.

Veterinary medicinal products are subject to specific legislation.

The legislation

Wholesale dealing is controlled by a combination of the Act, *Sections 8, 9, 10* and *61* (which allows for Regulations to be made limiting the persons to whom products may be sold by wholesale) and Regulations, mainly SI 1980/1923. SI 1971/1445 amended *Section 10* of the MA 1968 by adding a number of subsections. SI 1993/834 amended *Section 8*. SI 1993/833 sets out conditions for wholesalers.

The result of the interplay of this legislation is as follows.

Who may wholesale medicinal products?

Wholesaling of medicinal products may be carried out by:

(a)   the holder of a WDL *or*
(b)   the holder of a marketing authorisation *or*

(c) a retail pharmacy business or hospital pharmacy, provided the wholesale sales constitute "no more than an inconsiderable part" of the business (*Section 10(7)* MA 1968). This last phrase has been interpreted by MHRA as meaning the sales by wholesale of no more than 5% of the purchases of medicinal products

(d) a wholesale dealer handling only GSL medicated confectionery.

No licence is required where a person merely acts as a carrier.

No licence is required where an import agent imports a product to the order of another person who intends to distribute it.

No licence is required for export from the United Kingdom direct to companies outside the EC.

Who may buy?

Pharmacy only medicines

P medicines may be sold by way of wholesale dealing to:

(1) doctors, dentists, vets
(2) any person conducting a RPB
(3) persons carrying on the business of a hospital or health centre
(4) licensed wholesale dealers
(5) persons who are exempt from holding a WDL
(6) Ministers of the Crown, government departments and their officers
(7) NHS Trusts
(8) any person who requires P medicines to administer them to human beings in the course of a business where the medicines are for the purpose of being so administered
(9) any person who may sell or supply in circumstances corresponding to retail sale:

- P medicines as specified in SI 1980/1924
- certain herbal remedies
- veterinary drugs

(10) persons supplying under a Patient Group Direction (PGD).

Category (7) was added by the Medicines (Sale and Supply) (Miscellaneous Provisions) Amendment Regulations 1992, SI No. 2938 to enable P and POM medicines to be sold to ambulance trusts for use by the paramedic staff.

Prescription only medicines

POM medicines may be sold by way of wholesale dealing to:

(1) categories "1" to "7" above
(2) for the specified products, persons exempted by Schedule 5 of the POM Order
(3) registered ophthalmic opticians, for certain POMs
(4) suppliers of homoeopathic preparations
(5) those practising homoeopathy
(6) persons supplying under a PGD.

Licence types

(a) Manufacture and assembly – allows the holder to manufacture and assemble (package) medicinal products.

(b) Assembly only – allows the holder to assemble (package) medicinal products.

(c) Manufacturer "specials" (MS) – allows the holder to manufacture unlicensed medicinal products (commonly referred to as 'Specials').

(d) Full wholesale dealer – allows the holder to wholesale deal pharmacy (P), prescription only (POM) and General Sale List (GSL) medicines.

(e) Wholesale dealer (GSL) – allows the holder to wholesale deal General Sale List (GSL) medicines only.

(f) Wholesale dealer's import – allows the holder to wholesale deal medicines imported from countries outside the EEA.

Requirements for wholesalers

The Medicines (Applications for Manufacturers and Wholesale Dealers Licences) Regulations 1971, SI No. 974, sets out the information to be given on the applications for a licence.

Applicants must specify the classes of products; give the address of each site of business; a description of the facilities available; details of record keeping; details of plans for recalling defective products; and the name of a "Responsible Person".

Schedule 3 of the Medicines (Standard Provisions for Licences and Certificates) Regulations 1971, SI No. 972 (as amended), sets out the Standard Provisions for wholesalers.

The wholesaler must maintain suitable staff, premises and facilities; provide information as required; record transactions; have an emergency recall plan; only buy from licensed manufacturers and wholesalers or exempt persons and only sell to those who may lawfully handle the products.

When supplied for retail sale or supply the wholesaler must provide an invoice detailing the date of transaction, the name and pharmaceutical form of the product, the quantity supplied and the name and address of the supplier.

The Responsible Person

The RP is responsible for ensuring good distribution practice. The RP must ensure that the licence conditions the Guidelines on Good Distribution Practice are complied with.

The RP does not have to be an employee of the wholesaler, and need not be a pharmacist. If not a pharmacist then he must have relevant knowledge and experience.

Records

WDL and PL holders must keep sufficient records to enable the recall of defective medicines. Pharmacies which wholesale POMs must retain for 2 years the order or invoice relating to the transaction.

"Pseudo"-wholesale transactions

Some transactions appear on the surface to be wholesale, but on closer examination are seen not to be.

(a)   The supply of vaccines by PCTs to GPs.

PCTs may make various vaccines available to general medical practitioners in their area. Where no charge is made by the PCT to the GP for these supplies the transaction is not a wholesale transaction. There is no charge, and hence no sale – an essential element in the definition of "wholesale". Equally the transaction is not a retail sale, because it is not a sale. Neither is it a supply "in circumstances corresponding to retail sale", since *Section 132* requires that such a supply be made to persons who "receive the product for purposes other than than that of administering it or causing it to be administered. . . . "

Such a transaction may fall within the ambit of *Section 55*, which exempts from certain controls ". . . supply . . . in the course of the business of a hospital or health centre, where the product is . . . supplied for the purpose of being administered (whether in the hospital or health centre or elsewhere) in accordance with the directions of a doctor or dentist."

For *Section 55* to apply the actual supply must be made by a hospital, not just by the trust itself.

(b)   The supply by one hospital to another hospital unit owned by the same trust.

Again there is no sale, because although a nominal book charge may be made for accounting purposes, the units belong to the same body. One cannot sell to oneself.

(c)   Supply by a hospital pharmacy to wards, for administration to patients in that ward by nursing staff or doctor.

There is no sale, even though the condition of supply for the purpose of administration is fulfilled.

(d)   Co-operatives.

Sometimes groups of pharmacists are formed for the purpose of buying goods for subsequent retail sale by the individual members. Where the orders are simply bulked together the group will not normally require a WDL. However, if the group has a separate legal identity, e.g. as a limited company then a licence may be required. If the group sells its purchases to persons who buy in order to sell on (whether those persons are members of the group or not) then a licence will be required.

Importers

A person who distributes, other than by way of sale, a proprietary medicinal product for human use which is imported from a non-EC source, must be the holder of a

WDL (SI 1977/1050). There is no need for a WDL where the only activity in relation to the product is

(a)   the provision of transport facilities
(b)   the business of an import agent who imports for another person who intends to deal with it by wholesale or to otherwise distribute it.

Parallel Imports

Parallel imports (PIs) are medicines imported from another member state of the European Community. They may have been manufactured in this country, or elsewhere. They are sold "in parallel" to the brands marketed in this country by the manufacturers. The PIs may bear the same English brand name, a foreign language version or a completely different name.

Market prices for pharmaceuticals differ considerably between the countries in the EU. The price differences are due mainly to the following factors:

● The degree of price control exerted in some form by the government
● The pricing policies adopted by manufacturers to meet the competition from similar products
● Different margins at wholesale and retail level.

Legal basis for the trade

The Treaty of Rome promotes free trade between EC countries. Articles 30–34 generally prohibit restrictions on imports. The Treaty does not allow either direct restrictions such as a complete ban, or indirect restrictions such as laws which favour the sale of home-produced products rather than imported ones.

Article 36 allows import restrictions if they are justified on grounds of protection of health and life of humans, animals and plants.

In 1976 the European Court of Justice (ECJ) ruled that "national restrictions on parallel imports within the Community would be against community rules on freedom of trade" (case 104/75, *De Peijper/Centrapharm*).

The ECJ has considered parallel imports on a number of occasions since then. Parallel imports must be allowed if:

● the imported product is therapeutically equivalent to the domestic product
● it is manufactured in accordance with correct quality control standards
● it is manufactured within the same company or group of companies *or*
● subject to some conditions, it is manufactured under licence from the original manufacturer.

The medicines regulatory agency in the importing country is responsible for verifying that the imports satisfy the criteria. This is done in the United Kingdom by the MCA.

Product Licence (parallel import) PL(PI)

As only products for which a PL has been issued may be marketed in the UK, the MCA issues a version for parallel imports known as the Product Licence (parallel import) or PL(PI). This is issued subject to the following conditions:

(1) The product must be imported from an EU member state.
(2) It must be a product which is already the subject of a standard marketing authorisation issued by an EU member state.
(3) The imported product must be a "proprietary medicinal product" which is not a vaccine, toxin, serum, human blood product, radio-active isotope or homeo-pathic product.
(4) It must have the same therapeutic effect as the UK product.
(5) It must be made by, or under licence from, the manufacturer of the UK product
(6) The importer must prove that the import conforms with the specifications for the product.

Other requirements for the importer
   If the product is repacked the importer will need a ML for assembly.
   A WDL is required to distribute the product.
   Sufficient records to enable batch recalls must be kept.

Labelling

The Labelling Regulations require all medicinal products to be labelled in English.

Products with different name

In 1986 both the DOH and the RPSGB stated that pharmacists must not dispense a parallel import bearing a different brand name from that which the doctor had prescribed. The rule was challenged and the ECJ decided in 1989 that the rule was justified on public health grounds (Cases 266 and 267/87 Association of Parallel Importers).

The rule applies even where the difference in name is small and due to language problems. The rule applies to the written names. Names which are spelt differently but which sound the same are treated as different names. It makes no difference that the therapeutic effect and quality of the products are identical.

Advertising and sales promotion

The advertising of medicines is controlled by the MA 1968, and by regulations made under the Act. There are specific prohibitions on the advertising of treatments for various diseases. The Code of Ethics of the RPSGB deals with advertising by pharmacists. The use of certain titles, e.g. pharmacist, is also restricted by law. Some consumer law carries restrictions which are applicable to pharmacy.

The main Regulations dealing with the advertising of medicines are the Medicines (Advertising) Regulations 1994, SI No. 1932 – referred to as the Advertising Regulations, and the Medicines (Monitoring of Advertising) Regulations 1994, SI No.

1933 – referred to as the Monitoring Regulations. The Regulations implement the European Community Directive 92/28/EC, which concerned the advertising of medicinal products.

Both the above Regulations have been amended, mainly by the Medicines (Advertising and Monitoring of Advertising) Regulations 1999, SI No. 267.

Medicines (Advertising) Regulations 1994

These Regulations limit the advertising and sales promotion methods which may be used. They have been amended by the MAR Regulations 1994; by the Medicines (Advertising) Amendment Regulations 1996, SI No. 1552; and by the Medicines (Advertising and Monitoring of Advertising) Amendment Regulations 1999, SI No. 267. They are wide-ranging:

(1) It is an offence to advertise a medicinal product for which there is no marketing authorisation.

(2) Holders of marketing authorisations have certain duties:

- to monitor information received about their product
- to provide information about adverts to regulatory authorities on request
- to comply with directions given by regulatory authorities about advertisements
- to provide adequate training for sales representatives.

(3) The regulations make it an offence to offer or receive an inducement to prescribe or supply particular medicinal products.

(4) Regulation 3A (which was inserted by the Medicines (Advertising and Monitoring of Advertising) Regulations 1999) prohibits adverts:

- which do not comply with the SPC for the products
- which do not encourage rational use of the product by presenting it objectively and without exaggerating its properties and
- which are misleading.

What is an "advertisement"?

For the purposes of the MA 1968, an advertisement includes every form of advertising:

- in a publication
- by display of a notice
- by means of a catalogue or price list
- circular letters
- letters addressed to particular people
- in any other document
- words inscribed on an article
- photographs
- cinema film
- sound recording
- radio and television
- or in any other way.

It does not include spoken words which are not part of a recording or broadcast on radio or television, or the supply of a medicine in a labelled container.

Under the Regulations, price lists, trade catalogues, reference materials and factual informative statements or announcements are not advertisements unless they make a product claim.

Consent of marketing authorisation holder

Advertisements may only be issued by marketing authorisation holders, or with their consent.

Adverts to the public

The Regulations differentiate between advertising directed to the public and advertising aimed at health professionals.

POM medicines may not be advertised directly to the public. Where the retail sale of products has been restricted by a "safety order" under *Section 62*, then those products may not be advertised either. Products subject to the Narcotics Drugs Convention cannot be advertised.

All advertisements must clearly be such and the product must clearly be identified as a medicine. The advertisement must include

- the name of the product
- the common name of the ingredient of a single active ingredient product
- how to use it
- an invitation to read the instructions.

Prohibitions

Some claims and statements in adverts are prohibited by Regulation 9:

(a) any advert which offers a diagnosis
(b) comparative advertising
(c) suggestions that health care is improved by not taking a product
(d) adverts directed at children
(e) scientific or celebrity endorsements
(f) suggestions that a medicine is a foodstuff or cosmetic
(g) suggestions that the efficacy or safety is due to the fact that the product is natural
(h) any advert which might lead to erroneous self-diagnosis
(i) any advert which refers in improper, alarming or misleading terms to claims of recovery
(j) any advert which uses pictures in an improper, alarming or misleading manner
(k) any advert which mentions that the product has been granted a marketing authorization.

Advertising of specific diseases

The Medicines (Advertising) Amendment Regulations 2004, SI No. 1480, remove restrictions on advertising OTC medicines for some serious conditions.

The advertising to the public of products for these diseases and conditions is still banned (Regulation 6 and Schedule 1):

- Chronic insomnia
- Diabetes and other metabolic diseases
- Malignant diseases
- Serious infectious diseases including HIV-related diseases and tuberculosis
- Sexually transmitted diseases.

The advertising to the public of medicines containing psychotropic or narcotic substances controlled under the Narcotics Drugs Convention 1961 or the Psychotropic Substances Convention 1971 is prohibited (except for those products containing very small amounts) (Regulation 8).

Contraceptive products
Oral contraceptive products are POM and hence cannot be advertised to the public (Regulation 7).

Abortion
Products for abortion cannot be advertised to the public (Regulation 6).

Promotional sales to the public
Manufacturers, wholesalers and marketing authorisation holders are prohibited from selling or supplying medicinal products for promotional purposes to the public (Regulation 12).

Small-sized packs may be sold on normal business terms through normal trade outlets.

Advertisements to health professionals
The Regulations lay down certain specified particulars to be included in adverts which are intended to induce practitioners to prescribe or supply the products. The advertisements must comply with Schedule 2 of the Advertising Regulations.

The Regulations cover advertising to "persons qualified to prescribe or supply". This phrase is defined so as to include the employees of those who "in the course of their profession or in the course of a business may lawfully prescribe, sell by retail or supply in circumstances corresponding to retail sale, relevant medicinal products".

The adverts must include the PL number and details of the marketing authorisation holder, the legal classification of the product, lists of active ingredients, one or more of the licenced indications for use, the side-effects, cautions and contra-indications from the summary of product characteristics, warnings and cost.

Small, abbreviated adverts in professional publications are allowed which need only contain name of product, legal classification, name of PL holder, ingredients and an indication of where further information may be found.

Free samples   Regulation 19 limits supply of free samples to people qualified to prescribe. It does not allow supply to persons qualified only to supply. There are a number of conditions laid down. Failure to comply may be punished by a fine.

- Samples may only be supplied in limited numbers.
- There must be a signed dated written request.
- There must be a system of control and accountability.
- Only small size packs are allowed.
- Each pack must be marked "free medical sample – not for resale".
- Each sample must be accompanied by a copy of the SPC.

Samples of medicines containing psychotropic or narcotic substances controlled under the Narcotics Drugs Convention 1961 or the Psychotropic Substances Convention 1971 are prohibited (except for those products containing very small amounts).

Promotional aids

The Regulations allow for "promotional aids" such as pens and mugs to carry the name of the product and the company without any other information. "Promotional aid" means a non-monetary gift made for a promotional purpose by a commercially interested party. It should be relevant to the practice of medicine or pharmacy. The value should be less than £5.

Inducements

Regulation 21 states that it is an offence to solicit or accept any prohibited "gift, pecuniary advantage, benefit in kind, hospitality or sponsorship".

All gifts, pecuniary advantages and benefits in kind are prohibited in relation to the promotion of medicine unless they are "inexpensive and relevant to the practice of medicine or pharmacy".

Any hospitality payments must be reasonable in level, subordinate to the main purpose of the meeting and offered only to health professionals. Hospitality may include the payment of travelling or accommodation expenses at events "for purely professional or scientific purposes or "held for the promotion of relevant medicinal products".

Regulation 21(4) allows "measures or trade practices relating to prices, margins or discounts which were in existence on 1 January 1993, thus allowing most business purchase discount schemes to continue".

It is an offence both to offer prohibited inducements, and to accept them. Offering or supplying inducements is punishable with a fine and/or imprisonment and soliciting or accepting them may be punished with a fine.

Medical representatives

Medical representatives must receive adequate training. They must provide information which is as precise and complete as possible about the products. On each visit, medical representatives must give a copy of the SPC for the product they are promoting.

Summary of Product Characteristics

The SPC is a document prepared by the holder of the marketing authorisation. It must contain the information laid down in regulations (MAR Regulations 1994 as amended). Details of type size and layout are also specified.

The SPC may be distributed in the form of a compendium. The Association of the British Pharmaceutical Industry (ABPI) produces an annual compendium of SPC for products on the UK market.

Advertisements for registered homoeopathic medicinal products

Advertisements relating to a registered homoeopathic medicinal product must contain only the details in Schedule 5 and must not mention any specific therapeutic indications.

Monitoring and complaints

The Medicines (Monitoring of Advertising) Regulations 1994 give powers to monitor the form and content of advertisements, and deal with the handling of complaints. Control is based on a system of self-regulation.

Complaints about the content of advertisements may be referred by the MHRA to a suitable self-regulatory body for investigation and action. The three most important self-regulatory bodies are the Advertising Standards Authority, the Prescription Medicines Code of Practice Authority and the Proprietary Association of Great Britain. The Monitoring Regulations also set out formal procedures which allow the MHRA to take enforcement action in both civil and criminal courts.

Advertising of NHS Pharmaceutical Services

Prior to 1992 the TOS contained a restrictive clause prohibiting the advertising of NHS services. This no longer exists. Any advertising which is done is subject to the RPSGB Code of Ethics.

RPSGB Code of Ethics

The Code states in the Service Specifications:

It is in the public interest for pharmacies to provide information about their opening hours and services available. Any information or publicity material regarding pharmacy services must be accurate and honest. The public and the profession would not expect any products or services advertised or otherwise promoted to be injurious to health when properly and responsibly used.

- All information and publicity for goods and services must be legal, decent and truthful; be presented and distributed in a manner so as not to bring the profession into disrepute; and not abuse the trust or lack of knowledge of the public.
- Information and promotional material relating to professional services must be compatible with the role of pharmacists as skilled and informed advisers about medicines, common ailments, general healthcare and well-being. It should be presented so as to allow the recipient to decide independently whether or not

to use a service and should not disparage the professional services of other pharmacies or pharmacists.

- Pharmacists should not make any unsolicited approach for promotional purposes directly to the public.
- Promotions for medicines aimed at the public must emphasise the special nature of medicines; must not promote inappropriate use, must not make any medicinal claim which cannot be substantiated; be consistent with the SPC; not promote a product by way of a pharmacist endorsement.
- Pharmacists may advertise prices and discounts. Promotions which seek to persuade customers to buy in excess of need are considered to be professionally unacceptable.

Chapter 13

Supplies and Deliveries

Supply of medicines in an emergency

In an emergency a pharmacist can lawfully sell or supply most POMs, provided certain conditions are satisfied.

Section 58(2)(a) of the Medicines Act 1968 generally requires a prescription for the sale or supply of POMs. Paragraph 8 of the POM Order 1997 allows exemptions from this requirement in certain circumstances. The supply must be made by a person lawfully conducting an RPB.

Two situations are envisaged:

(1)   a request made by a prescriber
(2)   a request made by a patient.

Supply made at the request of a prescriber

The conditions that apply are

(a)   the pharmacist must be satisfied that the sale or supply has been requested by a prescriber who by reason of an emergency is unable to furnish a prescription immediately;
(b)   the prescriber has undertaken to furnish the pharmacy with a prescription within 72 hours;
(c)   the POM is sold or supplied in accordance with the directions of the prescriber requesting it;
(d)   the POM is not a CD in Schedules 1, 2 or 3 of the Misuse of Drugs Regulations 1985;
(e)   an entry must be made in the Prescription Book stating

    (i)   the name and address of the patient
    (ii)   the date on the prescription and
    (iii)   the date on which the prescription is received.

Prescriber in this case does not include a dentist. The original POM Order specified "doctor" and this has been amended to include the new classes of prescriber.

Controlled drugs

In an emergency a practitioner can personally obtain a Schedule 2 or 3 drug if he cannot immediately supply a signed requisition. This does not authorise supply direct to the patient. The practitioner must undertake to deliver a signed requisition within 24 hours of receiving the drug.

Supply made at the request of the patient

The conditions that apply are

(a) the sale or supply must be made by or under the supervision of a pharmacist.
(b) that pharmacist must have interviewed the patient and satisfied himself:

    (i) that there is an immediate need for the POM, and that it is impracticable in the circumstances to obtain a prescription without undue delay;

    (ii) that treatment with the POM requested has been previously prescribed by a doctor for the patient; and

    (iii) that the dose is appropriate.

(c) up to 5-days treatment may be sold or supplied except:

    (i) the smallest pack that the pharmacist has available may be supplied where the medicine is an original pack of an ointment or cream, an asthma aerosol, or an insulin preparation;

    (ii) a full cycle of an oral contraceptive may be supplied; and

    (iii) the smallest quantity which provides a full course of treatment may be supplied of a liquid oral antibiotic.

(d) the pharmacist makes an entry in the Prescription Book stating:

    (i) the date of the transaction

    (ii) the name, quantity, pharmaceutical form and strength of the medicine supplied

    (iii) the name and address of the patient

    (iv) the nature of the emergency.

(e) the container or package must be labelled to show:

    (i) the date of supply

    (ii) the name, quantity, form and strength of the medicine

    (iii) the name of the patient

    (iv) the words "Emergency Supply".

(f) Schedule 4 to the POM Order 1997 contains a list of drugs which may not be supplied at the request of a patient.

Despite inclusion in Schedule 3 of the Misuse of Drugs Regulations 2001, and in the above Schedule, a supply of Phenobarbital or Phenobarbital sodium may be made where it is supplied for the treatment of epilepsy. (Paragraph 8(5) of the POM Order 1997)

RPSGB has issued guidance in the Code of Ethics:

Emergencies: Increasingly the public looks to pharmacists in community practice for help and assistance, sometimes in emergencies.

(a)   Pharmacists must consider using their rights to make emergency supplies of medicines whenever a patient has an urgent need for a medicine. They must consider the medical consequences, if any, of not supplying.
(b)   Where pharmacists are not able to make an emergency supply of a medicine they should do everything possible to advise the patient how to obtain essential medical care.
(c)   Pharmacists must assist persons in need of emergency first aid or medical treatment whether by administering first aid within their competence or by summoning assistance and/or the emergency services.

The Society's booklet, "Emergency first aid: guidance for pharmacists", provides guidance on action in life-threatening situations.

Supplies under the NHS

The NHS (PS) 2005 Regulations allow a doctor to request a supply to be made to a patient in an emergency. The doctor must be known to the pharmacist. He must promise to give a prescription in 72 hours. The request must not be for a CD, except one in Schedules 4 or 5 (see Chapter 24).

There is no procedure for a patient to request an emergency NHS supply.

Supply of emergency hormonal contraception

The Prescription Only Medicines (Human Use) Amendment (No. 3) Order 2000, SI No. 3231, came into force on 1 January 2001.

This enables emergency hormonal contraception (EHC) consisting of or containing Levonorgestrel to be sold by pharmacists without a prescription. The maximum strength allowed is 0.75 mg. The tablets may only be sold or supplied exclusively for use as an emergency contraceptive in women aged 16 and over.

The RPSGB Code contains specific advice:

Pharmacists in personal control of a pharmacy must ensure that the following standards are observed in the supply of EHC as a pharmacy medicine. As with all medicines, pharmacists must have sufficient knowledge of the product to enable them to make an informed decision when requests are made.

(a)   Pharmacists must deal with the request personally and decide whether to supply the product or make a referral to an appropriate health care professional.
(b)   Pharmacists must ensure that all necessary advice and information is provided to enable the patient to assess whether to use the product.
(c)   Requests for EHC must be handled sensitively with due regard being given to the patient's right to privacy.
(d)   Only in exceptional circumstances should pharmacists supply the product to a person other than the patient.
(e)   Pharmacists should whenever possible take reasonable measures to inform patients of regular methods of contraception, disease prevention and sources of help.

Supply to women aged under 16 could be made via a PGD.

Pharmacists who choose not to supply EHC

The RPSGB advises that pharmacists who choose not to supply EHC on religious or moral grounds should advise patients of another local source of supply within the time for EHC to be effective.

Collection and delivery schemes

Certain types of collection and delivery schemes are given special exemption from the general Medicines Act requirement that the supply of medicines must be from a pharmacy.

The Medicines (Collection and Delivery Arrangements – Exemption) Order 1978, SI No. 1421, states that the restrictions of *Sections 52* and *53* of the Medicines Act 1968 do not apply where the medicine:

- is for human use
- is supplied in accordance with a prescription from a doctor or dentist
- and where the supply is as part of a collection and delivery arrangement used by a pharmacy.

Section 52 restricts supply of POM and P medicines to pharmacy premises. *Section 53* restricts the supply of GSL medicines to premises which can "be closed so as to exclude the public".

A "collection and delivery arrangement" means any arrangement whereby a person takes or sends a prescription to premises other than a pharmacy, and later collects the dispensed medicine from those premises. A common example is where a grocery shop in an isolated village acts as a collecting point for scripts written by visiting GPs. After dispensing they are held in the shop until the patient collects them.

The script must have been dispensed at a registered pharmacy, by or under the supervision of a pharmacist. The premises used must be capable of being closed so as to exclude the public.

The arrangements are not limited to the NHS. There are no other formal legal requirements.

Delivery direct from the pharmacy

Many pharmacists have a service where they collect prescriptions from a doctor, dispense them and deliver the medicines to the patient's home. These arrangements are not covered by the restrictions outlined above. They are subject to normal legal requirements in that the dispensing must be under the supervision of a pharmacist, etc. In addition the RPSGB Code of Ethics makes specific mention of such schemes in the Service Specifications:

Prescription collection
- Prescriptions must be collected by individuals acting on the instructions of the pharmacist.
- Pharmacists must ensure confidentiality and security.

- The request for the service must come from the patient or carer.
- The initial request should be recorded.
- Requests to the doctor for repeat prescriptions should be made by the patient or carer unless the pharmacy offers a repeat medication scheme complying with Service Specification 6.
- Wrongly directed prescriptions should be returned to the surgery or authorised pharmacy.

Delivery services

- On each occasion the pharmacist must use his professional judgement to decide whether a direct "face-to-face" consultation is appropriate.
- Pharmacists must ensure safe delivery of medicine.
- Pharmacists must ensure appropriate storage conditions.
- There must be a verifiable audit trail identifying the initial request for the service, and each delivery or attempted delivery.

Chapter 14

Unlicensed Products

Under the Medicines Act 1968 a company may only market, i.e advertise and sell, their products in the United Kingdom if they hold a marketing authorisation for that product. Furthermore, the therapeutic or diagnostic purposes for which the product can be marketed are limited by the terms of the authorisation. Thus a product licensed only for the treatment of gastric ulcers may not be marketed for the treatment of indigestion.

However, this legislation does not affect the clinical freedom of doctors to prescribe what they believe is best for their patient. They may use or recommend medicines which do not have a licence (unlicensed), or use medicines in ways different to those specified in the marketing authorisation (off-label).

Unlicensed products

Doctors may prescribe several categories of unlicensed products. Some substances, e.g. raw chemicals may on occasions be prescribed as medicines, although they are not normally thought of as medicines, and are not marketed as such.

Unlicensed medicines may be obtained in three ways:

(1) Prepared extemporaneously in the pharmacy
(2) Obtained from a "Specials" manufacturer
(3) Imported from another country via a wholesaler

Reasons for using unlicensed products

They may be used because:

- The medicine is prepared by the original manufacturer, but is not for sale in United Kingdom.
- It is the prescriber's own formula for a specific patient.
- It is an unusual form, e.g. liquid preparation of a medicine normally available only as capsules.
- It is an unusual strength.
- It is an unusual combination of active ingredients.
- It is an unusual formulation, e.g. no preservative eye drops, lactose free tablets.

- It is a discontinued product.
- The normal product is temporarily unavailable.

Exemptions for unlicensed medicines

Most of the relevant legislation is to be found in the Medicines for Human Use (Marketing Authorisations, etc.) Regulations 1994, SI No. 3144. These provide exemptions from the normal licensing requirements, so as to allow pharmacists to order specials and to hold stock ready for dispensing. However, much of the older legislation is still in place, and applies in certain circumstances.

Specials

The terms "named-patient medicine" and "specials" are used interchangeably to refer to an unlicensed medicine specially ordered from a manufacturer. It is usually a medicine available readymade from the manufacturer, not made up to a recipe supplied by the pharmacy or the doctor.

According to the MAR Regulations, medicinal products which have no marketing authorisation may be "placed on the market" in the following circumstances:

- The company must hold a special manufacturers licence.
- Orders must be unsolicited – no advertisements are allowed.
- The manufacture must be under adequate conditions and supervision.
- Records must be kept.
- The product must be formulated in accordance with the specification of a doctor or dentist.
- The product is supplied for use by a doctor or dentist, by his individual patients, on his direct responsibility.
- The supply must be to a doctor or dentist, or for use under the supervision of as pharmacist in a pharmacy, hospital or health centre.
- The product must be distributed by a licensed wholesaler.

Record keeping

The "Specials" manufacturer, the pharmacist and any practitioner who sells or supplies a "special" must keep records for at least 5 years, which show:

- the source of the product
- the name of the person who obtained the product
- the date of the transaction
- the quantity of each sale or supply
- the batch number
- details of any adverse reaction to the product which he knows about.

He must notify the licensing authority of any serious adverse reactions (Schedule 1, Paragraph 6, MAR Regulations 1994).

Exemption for doctors

Doctors may prepare products themselves for use on patients. They may order the products from a registered pharmacy, which may make them without any further licensing. Doctors may order products themselves from licensed specials manufacturers.

Section 9 of the Medicines Act 1968 states that the restrictions imposed by *Sections 7* and *8* of the Act (which generally require licenses) do not apply to anything which is done by a doctor or dentist which:

> relates to a medicinal product specially prepared or specially imported by him, or to his order for administration to a particular patient of his . . .

This allows a doctor to order an unlicensed product.

There are restrictions on the amount of stock held by a doctor – 5 litres of fluid and 2.5 kg of solids.

Records must be kept for 5 years of the supplier, the recipient, the date of supply, batch details and details of any suspected reaction of which the supplier is aware.

Exemption for pharmacists

The MHRA Guidance Note No. 14 states that "The supply of unlicensed medicinal products for individual patients", indicates how, in practice, MHRA will determine whether an activity is "preparation" or "manufacture".

Criteria include location of the process, nature of the activity and scale of the activity.

Dispensing to a script or formula

A pharmacist may prepare or dispense a medicinal product in a registered pharmacy: by or under the supervision of a pharmacist *and* in accordance with a specification furnished by the person to whom the product is or is to be sold or supplied, *and* the person is going to administer the product to himself or to someone under his care (*Section 10*).

Counter-prescribing

A pharmacist may prepare or dispense a medicinal product in a registered pharmacy, if the following conditions are satisfied:

- the product is for administration to a person;
- the pharmacist was requested by or on behalf of that person to exercise his judgement as to the treatment required;
- the person was present in the pharmacy at the time of the request (*Section 10*).

The exemptions allow a pharmacist to:

- Prepare or dispense a product against a prescription
- Prepare a stock in anticipation of dispensing
- Prepare or dispense a medicinal product against a specification given by the intended purchaser, where the product is to be administered to that purchaser or to someone under his care
- Prepare a product for counter-prescribing.

Conditions for counter-prescribing

The pharmacist is requested by or on behalf of the patient to use his own judgement as to the treatment required the patient is present in the pharmacy at the time of the request.

Preparation of stock

A pharmacist can prepare a stock of medicinal products in a registered pharmacy:

- with a view to dispensing them in accordance with a prescription given by a practitioner; *or*
- with a view to dispensing them in accordance with a specification from a person who is going to administer them to himself or to someone under his care.

A pharmacist may prepare a stock of medicinal products in a hospital or health centre ready for dispensing them in accordance with a prescription given by a practitioner (*Section 10*).

Regulation 3 of the MAR 1994 Regulations prohibits the placing on the market or the wholesale distribution of a relevant medicinal product unless it has a marketing authorisation. Products specially made for a particular patient will not have a marketing authorisation.

Schedule 1, Paragraph 3 allows a pharmacist to prepare or obtain a stock of an unlicensed product so that it may be supplied on prescription. The product must be prepared under the supervision of a pharmacist, and in a pharmacy, hospital or a health centre.

Imports

A further exemption allows importation of unlicensed products. The rules are contained in the Medicines (Standard Provisions for Licences and Certificates) Regulations 1971, SI No. 972, which were amended in 1999 by the Medicines (Standard Provisions for Licences and Certificates) Amendment Regulations 1999, SI No. 4.

These allow a licensed wholesaler to import an unlicensed product in response to a bona fide unsolicited order to fulfil special needs, formulated in accordance with the specification of a doctor or dentist, and for use by his individual patients on his direct personal responsibility.

There are conditions laid down in the Regulations:

(1)   The importer must give written notice to the MHRA before importing, and allow MHRA 28 days to object.
(2)   The quantity imported must not exceed 25 single doses or 25 therapeutic courses (each not to exceed 3 months).
(3)   The product must not be promoted.
(4)   Records must be kept, and the MHRA notified of any adverse reactions.

Doctors' or dentists' Personal Exemption Certificate

The Medicines (Exemption from Licences) (Special Cases and Miscellaneous Provisions) Order 1972, SI No. 1200, provides a procedure for a doctor or dentist to order medicine for use by them in their practice. A form is sent to the MHRA, which has 21 days to object to the import.

Chemist's Nostrums

The pharmacist may prepare a medicinal product (or a stock of such products) with a view to retail sale rather than to supply against an order. The sale must be from the registered pharmacy where the product was prepared. The product may not be advertised (Advertising Regulations 1994). The label must contain the standard labelling particulars (see Chapter 17).

Packing from bulk

The requirements of the Leaflet Regulations prevent a pharmacist packing small sizes of product from bulk containers.

Extemporaneous preparation in the pharmacy

Pharmacists may carry out the preparation of an unlicensed medicine to a formula specified in a prescription in the pharmacy. Following a case where a mixture was wrongly dispensed, resulting in the death of a child, the pharmacist and post-graduate trainee involved were both found guilty of a breach of *Section 64* of the MA 1968.

The RPSGB issued guidance at the time:

> Pharmacists are advised to check carefully all calculations, paying particular attention to the decimal points, and to either carry out the preparation themselves or delegate to suitably trained staff. In all cases the pharmacist should verify the formula used, the weightings or other measurements and the calculations. Where possible an independent check is advisable. The pharmacist should always undertake a final review before the product is supplied to the patient.

There is a section on extemporaneous preparation in the Code of Ethics – service specifications.

Off-label use

"Off-label" medicine describes the use of licensed medicines in a dose, age group or by a route not in the product licence specification. The product cannot be marketed for any use outside the licence conditions, but doctors are free to prescribe outside those conditions. Such use is now generally referred to by the US term "off-label use". Many medicines used for children are prescribed and used off-label. Clinical trials are rarely carried out on children, especially very young children, so the licensed use is restricted to those groups of patients where clinical trials have been carried out.

Liability issues

Special consideration should be given to issues of liability when unlicensed products are used, or when products are used off-licence. The summary of product characteristics gives some information about the use of any particular medicine, and prescribing within its limitations is unlikely to give rise to claims of negligence on the part of either doctor or pharmacist. Other information may be obtainable from specialist units.

The prescriber assumes legal liability when he prescribes unlicensed or off-label products. If a patient is harmed by the prescribing of an unlicensed or off-label product, then it may be alleged that the prescriber and/or the pharmacist has been negligent. The test of whether a doctor or pharmacist is negligent is referred to as the "Bolam test". This broadly states that a professional person will not be negligent if what he does would be approved of by a responsible body of opinion in his profession.

The liability of the manufacturer for any harm caused by off-label use remains untested in court, although theoretically there could be liability under the Consumer Safety Act 1987.

Similarly there may be a possibility that the pharmacist might be liable in circumstances where he was aware of the use, where he knew about the possibility of harm, and where he could have taken action.

Advice given to doctors

The Medical Defence Union has advised doctors in using off-label products for child patients that they must explain to those with parental responsibility that the drug is not appropriately licensed for paediatric use. Several studies recently have indicated that many doctors are unaware of the limitations for use set out in the data sheets for a product, and they may be grateful for a reminder.

The Code of Ethics

The Code of Ethics covers the use of unlicensed products, or use off-licence, in Part 3, *Section 4(d)*

> Where a product is ordered on a prescription a pharmacist must supply a product with a marketing authorisation, where such a product exists and is available, in preference to an unlicensed medicine or food supplement.

In addition a Factsheet, entitled "The use of unlicensed medicines in pharmacy" is available from the RPSGB Fitness to Practise and Legal Affairs Directorate.

Chapter 15

Traditional and Alternative Medicines

The Medicines Act makes special provision for two difficult areas: homeopathy and herbal medicines. Both present problems for the licensing system. Both represent traditional forms of treatment which have numbers of practitioners who are unable to use the exemptions from control provided for doctors and pharmacists.

The arrangements enable specified groups of medicines to be sold or supplied only by practitioners who do so after using their own judgement as to the treatment required for persons who are physically present in the premises where the supply takes place.

Additionally, certain groups of medicines may be sold in non-pharmacy outlets. Herbal products which make no medicinal claims (even if they may have a medicinal use) can be sold as foods, e.g. parsley, or as food supplements. Where an ingredient has no use other than a medicinal use the product will fall within the medicines controls.

Herbal remedies

A herbal remedy is a medicinal product consisting of:

- a substance produced by subjecting a plant or plants to drying, crushing or any other process, *or*
- a mixture whose sole ingredients are two or more substances so produced, *or*
- a mixture of one or more such substances and water or some other inert substance (*Section 132* of the Medicines Act 1968).

Special arrangements have been made to enable herbal practitioners to continue to practice and to enable the sale of simple herbs to continue. It would be impracticable to list all herbs.

Licensing of herbal remedies

Herbal medicines which meet the safety, quality and efficacy criteria in a similar manner to any other licensed medicines may have a marketing authorisation (product licence) in the same way as conventional products.

Where herbal remedies meet the conditions set out in *Section 12* of the Medicines Act 1968 they are exempt from licensing requirements.

Section 12(1) allows a person to make, sell and supply a herbal remedy during the course of their business provided the remedy is manufactured or assembled on the premises and that it is supplied as a consequence of a consultation between the herbal practitioner and the patient.

Section 12(2) allows the manufacture, sale or supply of herbal remedies where:
(a) the process to which the plant or plants are subjected consists only of drying, crushing or comminuting;
(b) the remedy is sold without any written recommendation as to its use; and
(c) the remedy is sold under a designation which only specifies the plant(s) and the process, and does not apply any other name to the remedy.

New arrangements

The Traditional Herbal Medicinal Products Directive (2004/24/EC) came into force on Friday 30 April 2004 (Article 3 of the Directive).

The purpose of the Directive is to establish within the Community a harmonised legislative framework for authorising the marketing of traditional herbal medicinal products, involving a simplified registration procedure. At present there are no specific safeguards on quality and safety for unlicensed herbal remedies. The MHRA considers that there is not enough information for the public about the safe use of unlicensed products. At the same time many companies have difficulty meeting conventional requirements to prove the product efficacy and safety needed for a marketing authorisation.

Article 2.2 provides that there is a transitional protection for existing products which legally were already on the market when the Directive came into force. This is to allow companies time to adapt to the new arrangements. This period lasts until 30 April 2011.

The Directive does not affect the provisions of *Section 12(1)* of the Medicines Act 1968.

The Directive was implemented in the UK by the Medicines (Traditional Herbal Medicinal Products for Human Use) Regulations 2005, SI No. 2750. This came into effect on 30 October 2005. There is a transition period lasting until 30 April 2011.

Herbal Medicines Advisory Committee

A new advisory committee on herbal medicines is established as a *Section 4* committee under the Medicines Act 1968. It advises Ministers directly on the registration scheme introduced under the Directive.

During the transitional period, products sold under *Section 12(2)* must continue to comply with the prevailing requirements of the Medicines Act.

Industrially produced herbal medicinal products placed on the market after 30 April 2004 require either a traditional use registration or a marketing authorisation from 30 October 2005.

Stocks products that have already been legally placed on the market before 30 October 2005 can remain legally on the market after 30 October 2005. They do not need to be recalled, but no new stock may be put on the market.

EMA Committee for Herbal Medicinal Products

The Directive set up a Committee for Herbal Medicinal Products which is part of the EMA.

The Committee will consist of one member, and an alternate member, nominated by each member state. The appointments will last for a period of 3 years, which may then be renewed. Members and alternates shall be chosen for their role and experience in the evaluation of herbal medicinal products and will represent the competent national authorities.

The Committee may also co-opt a maximum of five additional members chosen on the basis of their specific scientific competence. These members shall be appointed for a term of 3 years, which may be renewed, and shall not have alternates.

The Committee will develop Community herbal monographs and a positive list of herbal substances. Applicants will not need to demonstrate compliance with the criteria for traditional use and safety where herbal substances met the criteria set out in the positive list. The positive list of herbal substances will be accompanied by the therapeutic indication, specified strength, route of administration and any relevant safety information. The applicant would still need to demonstrate quality.

The committee will also have a role in considering the evidence of traditional use in cases where a remedy had less than 15 years' usage in the EU.

The new scheme

The simplified registration scheme will apply to herbal medicines that are taken orally, or are for external use or inhalation. The products must have been in medicinal use in the EU for 30 years at the time of the application. Evidence for up to 15 of the 30 years can relate to use outside the EU.

There is no requirement to present data on tests and trials relating to efficacy. The evidence of the medicine's use for at least 30 years will indicate the efficacy of the medicine.

Labelling

The labelling, leaflets and advertising must carry the wording:

> traditional herbal medicinal product for use in specified indication(s) exclusively based upon long-standing use.

Labelling and the user package leaflet must be in English. They must fully meet the requirements of Articles 54–65 of Directive 2001/83/EC (as amended by Directive 2004/27/EC).

Labelling and leaflets must include information and instructions about the safe use of the product, as with any licensed medicine.

It must be made clear to the consumer that the indications are based on information obtained from its long-standing use and experience. There must be advice that the user should consult a doctor or a qualified health care practitioner if the symptoms persist during the use of the medicinal product or if adverse effects not mentioned in the package leaflet occur.

Manufacturing

Manufacturers will need to meet approved standards of Good Manufacturing Practice (GMP) and have a ML.

Good Manufacturing Practice

The principles and guidelines of GMP are specified in Directive 2003/94/EC. This requires suitable premises, technical equipment and quality control facilities.

Manufacturers will in future require a Qualified Person.

Requirements for wholesale dealers

All UK wholesale dealers of traditional herbal medicinal products will require an appropriate authorisation, known as a WDL, from the MHRA.

They will need a Responsible Person.

Herbal practitioners

The MA 1968 generally requires the manufacture of, and dealing in medicinal products to be licensed. *Section 12* of the Act exempts herbal remedies from some of these requirements. The restrictions do not apply to the sale, supply, manufacture or assembly of any herbal remedy:

- in the course of business of a herbal practitioner *and*
- where the remedy is manufactured or assembled on premises of which the person carrying on the business is the occupier *and* which is able to be closed to the public.

The herbal practitioner (the person carrying on the business) may only sell or supply the herbal remedy in this way for administration to a particular person after being requested by that person to use his own judgement as to the treatment required. The person being treated must be present on the premises, but another person may make the request on his behalf.

Remedies sold under Section 12 *exemption*

The licensing restrictions also do not apply where the herbal remedy is sold or supplied in a simple way without any written recommendation as to use. In this case only the processes of drying, crushing or comminuting the plant or plants may be used to produce the herbal remedy.

Remedies sold under this section:

- must not contain non-herbal ingredients, other than inert substances such as water.
- must not be accompanied by any written recommendations in the absence of a personal consultation.
- must not be given names other than designations specifying the plants used and the processes they have undergone.

Section 52 of the MA 1968 restricts the sale of non-GSL products to pharmacies. *Section 53* lists the general conditions for the sale of GSL medicines. *Section 56* lists the situations when the restrictions in *Sections 52* and *53* do not apply to herbal remedies.

Section 53(3) allows Ministers to make an Order which narrows the effect of the exemptions in *Section 56*. The relevant order is the Medicines (Retail Sale or Supply of Herbal Remedies) Order 1977, SI No. 2130. The Order contains a three-part schedule of substances.

The effect of this interplay of the MA and the Order is

(1) Those herbal remedies which contain any of the substances listed in Parts I and II of the Schedule are restricted to pharmacies.
(2) Herbal practitioners may sell remedies containing the substances in Part III of the Schedule.
(3) Herbal practitioners may also sell GSL herbal remedies.
(4) Any shopkeeper can sell dried, crushed or comminuted herbs which are not in the Schedule, provided:

    (a) he has a manufacturing licence *or*
    (b) he has notified the RPSGB.

(5) Herbs may be sold as in (4) even if they have been tabletted, compressed, diluted with water, or made into pills.
(6) Any shopkeeper may sell GSL herbal remedies.
(7) Any shopkeeper may sell dried, crushed or comminuted herbs without a written recommendation provided the herbs are not listed in the Schedule.

Certain potent plants, e.g. Digitalis are restricted to use by medical practitioners and are classified as POM.

Nature and quality

Section 64 of the MA 1968 provides that no person shall, to the prejudice of the purchaser, sell any medicinal product which is not of the nature or quality demanded by the purchaser. Thus although there are often no applicable official standards for herbal medicines, poor quality or unsafe medicines are illegal.

Marketing Authorisation Regulations (MAR 1994 Regulations)

Regulation 1(3) of the MAR 1994 Regulations excludes herbal remedies which are manufactured or sold or supplied in accordance with *Section 12* of the MA 1968 from the definition of "relevant medicinal product". Hence the 1994 Regulations do not apply.

Homeopathic medicines

Homeopathy is a system of treatment elaborated by Samuel Hahnemann (1755–1843), a German physician. Its basis is treatment with minute quantities of the drugs capable of producing the symptoms of the disease treated. Conventional medicine is referred to as "allopathy".

Homeopathic medicines are the preparations used in homeopathy. The high dilutions are prepared from "unit preparations" which are defined as:

> a preparation, including a mother tincture, prepared by a process of solution, extraction or trituration with a view to being further diluted tenfold, or serially in multiple powers of ten, in an inert diluent, and then used either in this diluted form or where applicable, by impregnating tablets, granules, powders, or other inert substances for the purpose of being administered to human beings.

Homeopathic medicines are generally included in the GSL, although parenteral homeopathic medicines and certain strengths of some substances are restricted to POM.

Licensing

When the MA 1968 came into force, existing homoeopathic products were issued with product licences of right. These were given without any evidence of quality, safety or efficacy.

A new scheme was set up when Directive 92/73/EEC (the Homoeopathic Directive) was implemented. A codified text, including homoeopathic provisions, is now in Directive 2001/83/EEC.

Under this scheme a homoeopathic product may be given a "certificate of registration" if it meets quality and safety standards. It is not necessary to show efficacy. Because there are no demonstrations of efficacy, medical claims may not be made for the products. Certificates of registration last for 5 years. Registration under the scheme is compulsory only in respect of homoeopathic products new to the UK market.

The Directive defines a homoeopathic medicine as:

> Any medicinal product prepared from products, substances or composition called homoeopathic stocks in accordance with a homoeopathic manufacturing procedure described by the European Pharmacopoeia or, in the absence thereof, by the pharmacopoeias currently used officially in the Member States.

The Medicines (Advisory Board on the Registration of Homoeopathic Products) Order 1995, SI No. 309, established the Board in 1995. The function of the Advisory Board is to give advice to the licensing authority on the safety and quality of homoeopathic products.

The Medicines (Homoeopathic Medicinal Products for Human Use) Regulations 1994, SI No. 105, sets out the law. The safety criteria were classified in SI 1994 No. 899.

It applies to all homoeopathic products except those which are made to a "magistral or officinal" formula as defined in the Directive 2001/83/EEC.

Products which fall into this system are

- for oral or external use
- contain not more than 1 part in 10,000 of the mother tincture *or*

- if the active ingredient is POM, contain not more than 1 part in 100 of the smallest allopathic dose
- are prepared in accordance with a homoeopathic manufacturing procedure described in the European Pharmacopoeia or an official pharmacopoeia of a member state.

Products may not use a brand name or be labelled with a specific therapeutic indication.

The MA 1968 (Amendment No. 2) Regulations 1994, SI No. 276, contain a definition of a "homeopathic medicinal product":

> any medicinal product (which may contain a number of principles) prepared from products, substances or compositions called homoeopathic stocks in accordance with a homoeopathic manufacturing procedure described by the European Pharmacopoeia or in the absence thereof, by any pharmacopoeia used officially in a member state.

These Regulations mainly amend *Sections 7* and *8* of the MA 1968 so that the Medicines (HMPHU) Regulations apply to products with a certificate of registration and the existing MA 1968 provisions apply to other homoeopathic products.

Sale, supply or administration of homeopathic medicines

Many of the drugs used in homeopathy are restricted to POM when used at conventional strengths. Sale and supply is controlled by the inclusion of such drugs in the POM Order, with exceptions for diluted products.

Section 58(2)a of the MA 1968 generally restricts the sale, supply or administration of medicines containing substances specified in the POM Order to prescription.

The POM Order makes specific exemptions for medicine which contains, or consists of one or more unit preparations of highly diluted substances in the POM Order lists.

Conditions for sale (1)

Each unit preparation has been diluted to at least one part in one million (6x). The person who sells, supplies or administers the product was requested to do so. The person who requested the product was present when the seller, etc. made a judgement to supply, etc.

Conditions for sale (2)

Each unit preparation has been diluted to at least one part in one million (6c).

It should be remembered that although homeopathic practitioners claim that the more highly diluted products have greater potency, these are subject to restrictions based on conventional thinking, i.e. the lower restriction applies to the more dilute.

Standard labelling requirements for homoeopathic products

Containers and packages of homoeopathic must be labelled in clear and legible form to show a reference to their homoeopathic nature, in particular by clear mention of the words "homoeopathic medicinal product". This is in addition to any other particulars required by regulations.

Where products are placed on the market in accordance with a certificate of registration the labels of such products shall only contain the particulars set out below, which are found in the Medicines (Labelling and Leaflets) Amendment Regulations 1994, SI No. 104.

Standard labelling requirements for containers and packages of homoeopathic products marketed under a certificate of registration

(1) The scientific name of the stock or stocks followed by the degree of dilution, making use of the symbols of the pharmacopoeia used in relation to the homoeopathic manufacturing procedure described therein for that stock or stocks.
(2) The name and address of the holder of the certificate of registration and, where different, the name and address of the manufacturer.
(3) The method of administration and, if necessary, route.
(4) The expiry date of the product in clear terms, stating the month and year.
(5) The pharmaceutical form.
(6) The contents of the sales presentation.
(7) Any special storage precautions.
(8) Any special warning necessary for the product concerned.
(9) The manufacturer's batch number.
(10) The registration number allocated by the licensing authority preceded by the letters "HR" in capital letters.
(11) The words "homoeopathic medicinal product without approved therapeutic indications".
(12) A warning advising the user to consult a doctor if the symptoms persist during the use of the product.

Leaflets for homoeopathic products

The Medicines (Labelling and Leaflets) Amendment Regulations 1994, SI No. 104, also set out the requirements for Patient Information Leaflets to be supplied with homoeopathic medicines. These apply to any product placed on the market with a certificate of registration. A new Regulation 3B is inserted into the Leaflet Regulations.

Standard requirements relating to leaflets with 3B for homoeopathic products

Subject to the following provisions of these regulations, any leaflet which is enclosed in or supplied with the packaging of a proprietary medicinal product which is a homoeopathic product to which Council Directive 92/73/EEC applies and which is placed on the market in the United Kingdom in accordance with a certificate of registration, shall, in addition to clear mention of the words "homoeopathic medicinal product", contain the particulars set out in Schedule 3 to these regulations and no other particulars.

The detailed requirements are set out in Schedule 3.

Restrictions on sale for safety reasons

The MA 1968 provides various mechanisms for restricting the sale of substances considered to be harmful. The more important products and the relevant legislation are listed below.

Substances

Laetrile
A substance known variously as laetrile, amygdalin or Vitamin B17 has been used as a possible treatment for cancer. It is claimed to work by releasing cyanide in the tissues. Laetrile is a naturally occurring substance found especially in the kernels of apricots, peaches, plums and almonds. After several deaths were attributed to use of the compound it was decided that it should no longer be available freely over the counter.

The prohibition was achieved by the Medicines (Cyanogenetic Substances) Order 1984, SI 1984 No. 187, which was made pursuant to *Section 104* of the MA 1968. This section allows Ministers to extend the provisions of the Act to substances which do not ordinarily fit the definition of medicinal product. In the case of laetrile products the parts of the Act which are applied by the Order are mainly concerned with sale, supply, importing and promotion. In conjunction with the amended POM Order the effect is to restrict the sale to prescription.

The POM Order 1997:

(1) defines "cyanogenetic substances" as preparations which:

  (a) are presented for sale or supply under the name of amygdalin, laetrile or vitamin B17
  (b) are presented for sale or supply as containing amygdalin, laetrile or vitamin B17
  (c) contain more than 0.1% by weight of any substance having the fomula either: alpha-cyanobenzyl-6-ortho-beta-D-glucopyranosyl-beta-D-glucopyranoside *or* alpha-cyanobenzyl-beta-D-glucopyranosiduronic acid.

(2) includes "cyanogenetic substances" in the categories of products which are on prescription.

  The 0.1% figure corresponds with the maximum level of cyanide regarded by the Department of Health as acceptable in food, such as marzipan.

  The title of the Order refers to "cyanogenetic" substances. This is interesting example of the wrong word used in legislation. "Cyanogenetic" means "from cyanide" and not "cyanide-creating" (cyanogenic) as was presumably intended.

Chloroform

The Medicines (Chloroform Prohibition) Order 1979, SI No. 382, generally prohibits the sale or supply of medicinal products for human use which contain chloroform. There are a number of exemptions:

(1) Sales and supplies by doctors, dentists, pharmacies and hospitals. The sale or supply must be to a patient. The product must have been made by a doctor or dentist *or* to his prescription.
(2) Sale or supply as an anaesthetic. The supply must be to a doctor, dentist or hospital *or* to a wholesaler for supply as above.
(3) Sale for use solely in dental surgery.
(4) Where the medicinal product contains not more than 0.5%.
(5) Where the product is for external use, but not for use on mucous membranes, the mouth or teeth.
(6) Where the product is to be used as an ingredient in the preparation of a substance in a pharmacy or hospital, or by a doctor or dentist.
(7) For export.

This Order interacts with the POM and GSL Orders so that only items in categories (4) and (5) may be sold by retail to the public.

Bal Jivan Chamcho

Bal Jivan Chamcho is an Asian baby tonic containing high levels of lead. The product has been banned from sale, supply or importation by the Medicines (Bal Jivan Chamcho Prohibition) (No. 2) Order 1977, SI No. 670.

Aristolochia

Following concerns about the quality of various herbals products sold as aristolochia, a series of temporary orders severely restricted its sale and supply.

Following a consultation exercise the ban is to be made permanent with effect from 1 July 2001, by The Medicines (Aristolochia and Mu Tong, etc.) (Prohibition) Order 2001.

This Order prohibits the sale, supply, and importation, of any medicinal product for human use which:

(a) consists of or contains a plant belonging to a species of the genus *Aristolochia* or belonging to any of the species *Akebia quinata, Akebia trifoliata, Clematis armandii, Clematis montana, Cocculus laurifolius, Cocculus orbiculatus, Cocculus trilobus, Stephania tetrandra,* or an extract from such a plant; or
(b) is presented as consisting of or containing Mu Tong or Fangji, a plant belonging to any of the species *Akebia quinata, Akebia trifoliata, Clematis armandii, Clematis montana, Cocculus laurifolius, Cocculus orbiculatus, Cocculus trilobus, Stephania tetrandra,* or an extract from such a plant.

These prohibitions are subject to the following exceptions:

(i)   where the sale or supply is to, or the importation is made by or on behalf of, a person exercising functions in relation to the enforcement of food or medicines legislation;
(ii)   in the case of the prohibitions on importation, where the product is imported from a member State of the European Community, or, where the product originates in the European Economic Area, from a State Party to the European Economic Area Agreement which is not also a member State;
(iii) where the product is the subject of a marketing authorisation or homoeopathic certificate of registration.

Kava Kava

Kava Kava is a traditional South Sea sedative drink is made by fermentation from Kava Kava root. It was sold in Western countries as Kava root powder or as an extract put into capsules for convenience. Following evidence of liver tocicity a banning order was issued: The Medicines for Human Use (Kava Kava) (Prohibition) Order 2002, SI No. 3170.

This Order prohibits the sale, supply or importation of any medicinal product for human use which consists of or contains a plant (or part of a plant) belonging to the species *Piper methysticum* (known as Kava Kava) or an extract from such a plant.

Exceptions are products for external use, or licensed medicines.

A similar order – The Kava Kava in Food (England) Regulations 2002, SI No. 3169, prohibits the sale, possession for sale, offer, exposure or advertisement for sale, and the importation into England from a country outside the United Kingdom, of any food consisting of, or containing, Kava Kava.

A case brought by the the UK National Association of Health Stores and actress Jenny Seagrove to force the government to re-consider the ban on Kava Kava was rejected by the High Court in 2004. Mr Justice Crane agreed that the consultation process in deciding to ban kava had been "procedurally flawed" but this did not justify ordering fresh consultations.

(National Association of Health Stores, *Jennifer Ann Seagrove* v. *Secretary of State for Health*, National Assembly for Wales 2004).

Following the case the MHRA introduced The Kava Kava in Food (England) (Amendment) Regulations 2004, SI No. 455, which allow some trading activities.

Alkyl nitrites or "poppers"

Alkyl nitrites such as butyl nitrite and amyl nitrite have long been used as recreational drugs, collectively known as "poppers". The RPSGB won a test case in 1996 which established that their retail sale was illegal. The court took the view that the products were medicines and hence they could not be sold without being licensed and could not be sold from ordinary outlets.

Amyl nitrite became a POM in the Medicines (Products other than Veterinary Drugs) (Prescription Only) Amendment Order 1996. A pharmacist may still sell amyl nitrite to a person to whom cyanide salts may legally be sold, if the sale is to provide an antidote to cyanide poisoning.

Vitamins and food supplements

The Food Supplements Directive 2002/46/EC came into force in July 2002 and was implemented in England by the Food Supplements (England) Regulations 2003, SI No. 1387.

Separate, equivalent legislation has been made in Scotland, Wales and Northern Ireland. The directive and these regulations apply from 1 August 2005.

The Regulations apply to food supplements sold as food and presented as such. They do not apply to medicinal products as defined by Directive 2001/83/EC.

The regulations define a "food supplement" as: any food the purpose of which is to supplement the normal diet and which:

(a) is a concentrated source of a vitamin or mineral or other substance with a nutritional or physiological effect, alone or in combination; and
(b) is sold in dose form.

Under Regulation 4, "no person shall sell any food supplement to the ultimate consumer unless it is prepacked".

A food supplement shall be regarded as prepacked for the purposes of these Regulations if:

(a) it is ready for sale to the ultimate consumer or to a catering establishment, and
(b) it is put into packaging before being offered for sale in such a way that the food supplement cannot be altered without opening or changing the packaging.

Prohibitions on sale relating to composition of food supplements

Under Regulation 5(1) Subject to Paragraph (3), no person shall sell a food supplement in the manufacture of which a vitamin or mineral has been used unless that vitamin or mineral:

(a) is listed in column 1 of Schedule 1; and
(b) is in a form which:

    (i)   is listed in Schedule 2, and
    (ii) meets the relevant purity criteria.

If the vitamin or mineral is not listed then it can only be used if:

3 (a) the substance in question was used in the manufacture of a food supplement which was on sale in the European Community on 12 July 2002;
  (b) a dossier supporting use of the substance in question was submitted to the Commission by the Food Standards Agency or a member State other than the United Kingdom by 12 July 2005; and
  (c) the European Food Safety Authority has not given an unfavourable opinion in respect of the use of that substance, or its use in that form in the manufacture of food supplements.

The Regulations also provide a framework which can be used, if needed, to restrict the maximum and minimum levels of vitamins in food supplements.

Article 6(2) of the Directive (labelling, presentation and advertising must not attribute to food supplements the property of preventing, treating or curing a human disease, or refer to such properties) is already implemented in the Food Labelling Regulations 1996 (Regulation 40(1) and Schedule 6, Part I, Paragraph 2).

In October 2003 the National Association of Health Stores and the Health Food Manufacturers Association brought proceedings in the High Court challenging the validity of the Food Supplements Regulations.

The claimants argued that the legislation was restrictive to trade in goods, and was made on the wrong legal basis.

The judge referred the case to the ECJ requesting it to give a preliminary ruling on the validity of the underlying Directive.

On 12 July 2005 the ECJ confirmed the validity of the EC Food Supplements Directive. The case now returns to the High Court of Justice England and Wales for determination of the judicial review applications in the light of that judgment.

The court judgement can be accessed via http://curia.eu.int.

Chapter 16

Controlled Drugs

The Misuse of Drugs Act 1971 controls activities concerned with certain dangerous and harmful drugs. It covers the import, export, production, supply and possession of "Controlled drugs" (CDs).

The Act achieves control by means of extensive and detailed Regulations. It prohibits all activities with "CDs" except where the Regulations provide exceptions.

The Misuse of Drugs Act 1971 extends to Northern Ireland, although there are separate Regulations for Northern Ireland.

Basic Provisions of the Misuse of Drugs Act 1971

The Act prohibits the possession, supply, manufacture, import or export of Controlled drugs except as allowed in the Regulations, or by a licence from the S of S.

(1) *Sections 7, 10* and *22* enable and require the Home Secretary to make Regulations affecting the way health professionals and others deal with CDs.
(2) *Section 12* enables the Home Secretary to give directions to a doctor, dentist or pharmacist who has been convicted of an offence under the Act (or a related offence under the Customs and Excise Management Act). The directions can prohibit the person concerned from dealing in CDs or in authorising their administration.
(3) *Section 13* enables similar directions to be given where a doctor contravenes the Misuse of Drugs (Supply to Addicts) Regulations 1997, SI No. 1001.
(4) *Section 13* also allows for directions to be given after a tribunal has found a doctor or dentist to have prescribed CDs in an irresponsible manner.
(5) *Section 23* empowers the police or other authorised persons to enter business premises to inspect stock of CDs and related documents.

"Controlled drugs"

The drugs subject to control are listed in Schedule 2 of the Act. The Schedule is divided into three classes depending on the degree of danger the drugs present. The three classes: Class A, Class B, and Class C are used when determining penalties for offences under the Act (*Section 25*). Class A are the most harmful drugs and attract the severest penalties.

● Class A includes cocaine, diamorphine, LSD, methylenedioxymethamfetamine, morphine, opium, pethidine and Class B substances when prepared for injection.

- Class B includes oral amphetamines, barbiturates, codeine, pentazocine and pholcodine.
- Class C includes benzfetamine, buprenorphine, mebrobamate, most benzodioazepines, androgenic and anabolic steroids, cannabis and somatropin.

The list of CDs may be altered by an Order in Council approved by an affirmative resolution of both Houses of Parliament. The Advisory Council on the Misuse of Drugs must be consulted before any change.

The original list contained in the Act has been changed by the following Modification Orders: SI Sections 1973/771, 1975/421, 1977/1243, 1979/299, 1985/1995, 1986/2230, 1989/1340, 1990/2589, 1995/1966, 1996/1300, 1998/750, 2001/3932, 2003/1243 and 2003/3201.

Reclassification of Cannabis

With effect from 29 January 2004, the Misuse of Drugs Act 1971 (Modification) (No. 2) (Order 2003, SI No. 3201) reclassified cannabinol and cannabinol derivatives (previously Class A drugs) and cannabis and cannabis resin (previously Class B drugs) as Class C drugs in Schedule 2 to the Misuse of Drugs Act 1971. In addition, any substance which is an ester or ether (that is, a product) either of a cannabinol or of a cannabinol derivative (previously a Class A drug) is reclassified as a Class C drug.

International Convention

Many of the changes to both the Act and the Regulations are made because of the UK's obligations under the United Nations Single Convention on Narcotic Drugs 1961 and the United Nations Convention on Pschotropic Substances 1971. These conventions seek to regulate the world wide traffic in drugs of abuse. The Government is advised on any communication relating to the conventions by the Advisory Council.

The Advisory Council on Misuse of Drugs (ACMD)

The Advisory Council was established by the Act in 1972. Its purpose is to advise the relevant Ministers on various matters concerned with drug misuse.

The relevant Ministers are

(1) In England: the Home Secretary, Secretary of State for Health and Secretary of State for Education.
(2) In Scotland, Wales and Northern Ireland: Ministers responsible for Health and Ministers responsible for Education.

Composition of the Advisory Council

There are at least 20 members, who are appointed by the S of S after consultation with appropriate organisations. Members are required to have wide and recent experience of each of the following:

- practice of medicine
- practice of dentistry

- practice of veterinary medicine
- practice of pharmacy
- the pharmaceutical industry
- chemistry
- the social problems connected with the misuse of drugs (Schedule 1 of the Act).

Duties of the Advisory Council

The ACMD is required to keep under review the situation in the United Kingdom with respect to drugs which are being, or appear likely to be, misused. (*Section 1*) If it considers that misuse could cause harmful effects which might then constitute a social problem it must advise on the action to be taken. It must advise on measures:

- to restrict the availability of such drugs or to supervise the arrangements for their supply;
- to enable persons affected by the misuse of such drugs to obtain proper advice;
- to secure the provision of proper facilities and services for the treatment, rehabilitation and aftercare of such persons;
- to promote co-operation between the various professional and community services which it believes have a part to play in dealing with the social problems of drug misuse;
- to educate the public (particularly the young) in the dangers of drug misuse, and to publicise those dangers; and
- to promote research into, or obtain information about, any matter relevant to drug misuse prevention or the social problems of drug misuse.

The S of S is empowered to conduct such research, or to assist it (*Section 32*).

Additionally the ACMD must advise on any matter relating to drug dependence or drug misuse if asked to do so by a relevant Minister.

The ACMD must be consulted before any Regulations are made under the Misuse of Drugs Act.

The ACMD discharges these duties by holding meetings either of the full Council or of committees established by it, and by issuing reports.

Regulations concerned with misuse of drugs

Three sets of Regulations have been made under the Act, and heavily amended.

(1) The Misuse of Drugs Regulations 2001, SI No. 3998, amended by SIs 2003/1432, 2003/1653, 2003/2429, 2004/1031, 2004/1771, 2005/271, 2005/1653, 2005/2864 and 2005/3372.
(2) The Misuse of Drugs (Notification of and Supply to Addicts) Regulations 1997, SI No. 1001 as amended by SI 2005/2864.
(3) The Misuse of Drugs (Safe Custody) Regulations 1973 as amended by SIs 1984/1146, 1985/2067, 1986/2332 and 1999/1403.

The Misuse of Drugs Regulations 2001

The Misuse of Drugs Regulations 2001 provide exceptions to the blanket restrictions of the Act so that certain classes of people can produce, supply, prescribe or administer CDs in the practice of their profession.

The Regulations contain Schedules of drugs. It is these Schedules which are of most importance to practice, as they affect the degree of control to be applied to various drugs and medicines when they are used for lawful purposes.

Controlled drugs are listed in five schedules, according to the degree of control required.

Schedule 1

This Schedule contains drugs subject to the strictest controls. The drugs have little or no medical value, but cause social problems through misuse. A licence from the Home Secretary is necessary to possess, produce, supply, offer to supply, administer these drugs or cause these drugs to be administered. They include: cannabis LSD, mescaline, raw opium and coca leaf.

Schedule 2

This Schedule contains most of the drugs with medical use, including the opiates (such as heroin, morphine and methadone) and the stimulants such as amphetamines. The drugs in this schedule are subject to the full controls relating to prescriptions, safe custody and record keeping. Licences are needed for import or export. They may be manufactured or compounded by a pharmacist, doctor, dentist or vet, or by a person who holds a licence.

Schedule 3

This Schedule includes the barbiturates, diethylpropion, meprobamate, pentazocine and phentermine. Transactions do not need to be entered in the CD Register, although invoices must be retained. The requirements concerning destruction do not apply. Safe custody rules apply to temazepam, diethylpropion, buprenorphine and flunitrazepam. Other drugs in Schedule 3 are exempt from safe custody requirements.

Schedule 4

This Schedule is split into two parts. Part I contains most of the benzodiazepines plus nine other drugs. Ketamine was added by SI 2005/3372. They are subject to full import and export control. Unauthorised possession is an offence. Part II contains anabolic steroids. Drugs in Part II require a Home Office licence for import or export unless the substance is in the form of a medicinal product for personal use. Possession of listed steroids is an offence unless they are formulated as medicines.

Records need not be kept by retailers. There are no safe custody requirements.

Schedule 5

This Schedule contains dilute preparations of drugs in Schedule 2, which are not likely to produce dependence or to cause harm if they are misused. Examples are tablets and oral mixtures containing small amounts of codeine or morphine. Controls are minimal, consisting mainly of a requirement to keep invoices for 2 years. For this reason this schedule is sometimes referred to as "CD Inv".

Exempt products

Certain products, used for scientific or diagnostic purposes, and which contain an extremely small amount and proportion of controlled drugs are exempted from the prohibitions on production, supply and possession.

The Misuse of Drugs Regulations 2001 sets out the definition. An exempt product is a preparation or other product consisting of one or more components parts, any of which contains a controlled drug, where:

(a) the preparation or other product is not designed for administration of the controlled drug to a human being or animal;
(b) the controlled drug in any component part is packaged in such a form, or in combination with other active or inert substances in such a manner that it cannot be recovered by readily applicable means or in a yield which constitutes a risk to health; and
(c) no one component part of the product or preparation contains more than one milligram of the controlled drug or one microgram in the case of lysergide or any other N-alkyl derivative of lysergamide.

Import

The import of a CD is prohibited except in accordance with a licence granted by the Home Office or where the drug is exempted by Regulations. The Regulations exempt Schedule 4 Part II and Schedule 5 drugs from import controls. In addition, patients arriving in the United Kingdom with no more than a 15-day supply of a prescribed drug may do so without a licence.

Production

Production is generally prohibited by *Section 4* of the Act. "Production" means producing the drug by manufacture, cultivation or by any other method.

The Regulations provide that the following persons may lawfully produce, manufacture or compound a CD:

(a) a practitioner acting in his capacity as such;
(b) a pharmacist acting in his capacity as such;
(c) a person lawfully conducting an RPB at his registered pharmacy (Regulation 8);
(d) a person authorised in writing by the S of S may produce drugs in Schedules 3 and 4. The authority specifies the premises, and may specify other conditions;
(e) persons holding a licence issued by the S of S.

Cannabis plant

The cultivation of any plant of the genus *Cannabis* is illegal without a Home Office licence. Tha maximum penalty for conviction in the Crown Court is 14 years plus a possible fine. Merely positioning a plant in the window to secure the best light, with the objective of growing the plant, is sufficient (*Tudhope* v. *Robertson 1980*). It is a defence for the accused to show that he neither knew nor suspected nor had reason to suspect that the plant was a controlled drug.

Supply

Section 4 of the Act prohibits the supply of (or an offer to supply) Controlled Drugs except where Regulations permit. "Supply" includes distribution.

A person who is authorised by the Regulations to supply a CD may only do so:

- to another person authorised to possess *and*
- subject to any provisions of the Medicines Act 1968 (e.g. the requirements of the POM Regulations).

Various categories of persons are allowed by the Regulations to supply or distribute CDs in Schedules 2, 3, 4 and 5.

Health professionals
- a practitioner
- a pharmacist
- a person lawfully conducting a retail pharmacy business
- the person or acting person in charge of a hospital or care home providing nursing care
- the sister or acting sister of a ward, theatre or other department of a hospital or care home.

Analysts, laboratories, etc.
- a person in charge of a laboratory
- a public analyst appointed under *Section 27* of the Food Safety Act 1990
- a sampling officer within the meaning of Schedule 3 to the MA 1968
- a person employed or engaged in connection with an NHS Drug Testing Scheme.

Person in charge of a hospital or care home providing nursing care
The Regulations allow the person in charge of a publicly maintained hospital or care home to possess and supply CDs in Schedules 2–5, if no pharmacist is responsible for dispensing. The person in charge of a private hospital, care home or hospice without a pharmacist needs a Home Office licence to supply Schedule 2 CDs.

"Publicly maintained" means wholly or mainly maintained:

- by a public authority out of public funds or
- by a charity or
- by voluntary subscriptions.

Thus "publicly maintained" includes NHS Trusts, but excludes private care homes and hospitals which are operated for profit.

Sister in charge of ward or department

The sister or acting sister in charge of ward or department may only supply drugs for administration to a patient in that ward or department in accordance with the directions of a doctor. The authority only applies to drugs supplied by the person responsible for dispensing at the hospital or nursing home.

A person in charge of a laboratory

The laboratory must be recognised as one whose activities include the conduct of scientific education or research, and which is attached to a university, university college or hospital which is publicly maintained. The SoS may approve any other institution for the purpose.

Ships and oil rigs

Special arrangements are made for the unusual situations encountered on ships and oil rigs. The following persons are authorised to supply any drugs in Schedules 2–5 to anyone on the ship or rig as set out below:

- the owner or master of a ship which does not carry a doctor among the seamen employed in it
- the installation manager of an offshore installation.

The CDs may be supplied as follows:

- in order to comply with certain statutory requirements
- to return drugs to the person who lawfully supplied them
- to supply drugs to a constable for destruction.

The statutory obligations are found in:

(a) the Merchant Shipping Acts
(b) the Mineral Workings (Offshore Installations) Act 1971
(c) the Health and Safety at Work, etc. Act 1974.

Any person holding a licence under *Section 16(1)* of the Wildlife and Countryside Act 1981 may supply or offer for sale any drug in Schedule 3 for the purposes for which the licence was granted.

Possession

Various categories of persons are allowed by the Regulations to possess CDs.

Health professionals
- a practitioner
- a pharmacist
- a person lawfully conducting a retail pharmacy business
- the person or acting person in charge of a hospital or care home
- the sister or acting sister of a ward, theatre or other department of a hospital or care home providing nursing care
- paramedics when working.

Analysts, laboratories, etc.
- a person engaged in a forensic laboratory
- a person in charge of a laboratory
- a public analyst appointed under *Section 27* of the Food Safety Act 1990
- a sampling officer under Schedule 3 to the Medicines Act 1968
- a person in connection with the NHS Drug Testing Scheme.

Carriers
- a carrier
- a person engaged in the business of the Post Office
- a person engaged in conveying the drug to a person who may lawfully have it in his possession.

Various officials
- a constable in the course of his duty
- a Revenue & Excise officer in the course of his duty
- an RPSGB Inspector, under *Sections 108* and *109* of the Medicines Act.

Persons authorised by the Home Office
- a person authorised under a Home Office group authority [Schedules 2 and 3]
- a person holding a Home Office written authorisation [3–5 only].

Ships and oil rigs
The master of a foreign ship in a port in Great Britain may possess any Schedule 2 or 3 drug so far as necessary for the equipment of the ship.

Any person may possess Schedule 2 or 3 in order to comply with statutory requirements.

Possession as a patient

A person may possess a CD for his own use or for administration to another, in accordance with the directions of a doctor. This authority is negated where a patient lied in order to obtain the prescribed drug, or failed to notify the doctor that he was already being supplied with that drug by another doctor. These provisions are intended to prevent drug misusers and dealers from obtaining several prescriptions from different practitioners.

Doctors treating themselves

Doctors and dentists are allowed to possess and supply CDs when they are "acting in their capacity as practitioners". It has been held by the courts (*R v. Dunbar [1982] 1 AER 188*) that a doctor bona fide treating himself is "acting in his capacity as a doctor" for these purposes.

Confiscated illicit CDs

Illicitly obtained drugs are sometimes handed over to teachers, social workers, etc. by those who no longer require them. The Act states that in certain circumstances the person who receives them will not himself be committing an offence. The circumstances are that

(1) He knew or suspected the substance to be a Controlled Drug.
(2) He took possession for the purpose of preventing another person from committing an offence or continuing to commit an offence in connection with that drug *or* delivering it into the custody of a person lawfully entitled to take custody of it.
(3) as soon as possible after taking possession he took all steps reasonably open to him to either destroy the drug *or* deliver it into the custody of a person lawfully entitled to take custody.

Midwives

Special arrangements are made for midwives, who routinely use CDs in their professional practice.

A midwife may possess and administer any controlled drug which she may lawfully administer under the provisions of the Medicines Act. The POM Order 1997 as amended contains a list of drugs which a midwife may give by parenteral administration. This list includes pethidine, pentazocine, morphine and diamorphine. The MDA Regulations impose further conditions:

- She is a registered midwife.
- The local supervising authority has been notified of her intention to practise.
- The authority is given only so far as is necessary to her professional practice.
- Excess stocks must be surrendered to the appropriate medical officer.
- The drugs must have been obtained on a midwife's supply order signed by the appropriate medical officer.

A "midwife's supply order" means an order in writing specifying the name and occupation of the midwife obtaining the drug, the purpose for which it is required and the total quantity to be obtained. It must be signed by a doctor who is for the time being authorised in writing for the purpose of the Regulations by the local supervising authority for the region or area in which the drug is or was to be obtained.

Requirements for writing prescriptions

Regulation 15 lays out the requirements for prescriptions for CDs other than those in Schedule 4 or 5.

Prescriptions for Schedule 2 and 3 CDs must meet the following requirements:

(a) be written so as to be indelible
(b) must be signed by the prescriber with his usual signature
(c) must be dated by the prescriber
(d) specify the address of the prescriber (except for FP10 and variants)
(e) state "for dental treatment only" if issued by a dentist
(f) if issued by a vet, state that the CD is prescribed for an animal or herd under his care.
(g) where instalment dispensing is intended the script must contain a direction specifying the interval between instalments, and the amount to be given on each occasion.
(h) must specify:

- name and address of the patient
- the dose to be taken
- the pharmaceutical form and (where appropriate) the strength of the preparation of the CD
- the total quantity (in both words and figures) *or*
- the number (in words and figures) of dosage units of the preparation where the prescription is not for a preparation, then the total quantity (in words and figures) of the CD.

The changes made to s15 by the Misuse of Drugs (Amendment) Regulations 2005, SI No. 2864, allow for computer generated or type-written prescriptions.

The requirement to specify the "form" is interpreted by the Home Office as requiring the pharmaceutical form, e.g. tablets to be specified even if only one form of the product is available. It should also be specified where the brand name gives an indication of the form, e.g. MST.

There are no specific requirements for Schedule 4 and 5 CDs other than the POM regulations.

"Signed" means signed by the prescriber with his usual signature. This may be only a set of initials, or presumably a symbol such as a cross.

What the pharmacist must do

A pharmacist may only dispense a script for a Schedule 2 and 3 CDs if:

(a) the script complies with the requirements set out above;
(b) the prescriber's address is in the UK;

(c)   the pharmacist knows the prescriber's signature, and he has no reason to sup-
      pose it is a forgery, *or*
(d)   the pharmacist has taken "reasonably sufficient" steps to satisfy himself that it
      is genuine;
(e)   it is not before the date specified on the script;
(f)   it is not later than 28 days after the date on the script (legislation pending)
(g)   the script is marked, at the time of supply, with the date on which the drug is
      supplied.

With instalment prescriptions the first supply must be made not later than 28 days
after the date in the script.

The script must be marked with the date of each dispensing.

Following the 4th Report of the Shipman Inquiry the Home Office has proposed
the introduction of dedicated forms for the prescribing of Controlled Drugs in
Schedules 2 and 3, both within the NHS and in private practice. Both types of forms
will be submitted to the NHS Business Services Agency after dispensing, allowing
the creation of a central database. The forms will bear a number identifying the prescriber. No other types of form will be valid.

A maximum quantity of 30 days supply will be introduced.

There will be a new requirement for patients or people collecting medicines on
their behalf to sign for them. Patients or others collecting CDs should be asked by
the pharmacist for proof of identity.

Emergency supply

Supplies may be made to a practitioner in an emergency. He must represent that he
urgently requires a CD for professional purposes. The supplier must:

- be satisfied that the statement is true
- be satisfied that because of some emergency the practitioner is unable to furnish
  a requisition before the supply is made
- obtain an undertaking from the practitioner to furnish a requisition in 24 hours.

It is an offence for the practitioner not to produce the requisition as promised.

Emergency supplies to the patient of Schedule 2 or 3 CDs are not allowed, except
for phenobarbital for the treatment of epilepsy.

Supplies within the hospital or nursing home

The assumption is that the normal supply is by pharmacists or doctors, who are
authorised to supply drugs in Schedules 2, 3, 4 and 5. The Regulations recognise
that some institutions do not have a pharmacist available and provision is made for
other persons to possess and supply.

Supplies within the hospital or care home are governed by Regulation 14(6) of the
Misuse of Drugs Regulations 1985:

Where a person responsible for the dispensing and supply of medicines at
any hospital or care home providing nursing care supplies a CD to the sister or

acting sister for the time being in charge of any ward, theatre or other department, he shall:

(1) obtain a requisition in writing, signed by the recipient, which specifies the total quantity off the drug to be supplied;
(2) mark the requisition in such manner as to show that it has been complied with; *and*
(3) Retain the requisition in the dispensary for 2 years.

A copy of the requisition or a note of it shall be retained by the recipient for 2 years.

Hospital prescriptions

The general requirements for writing CD prescriptions apply to all hospital and care home situations, with an exception. The requirement to put on the name and address of the patient is relaxed where the prescription is written in the patient's bed card or case sheet.

Prescription requirements do not apply when medicines are administered to patients from ward stocks. This procedure is considered to be "administration in accordance with the directions of a doctor".

Storage

Schedule 2 drugs (except quinalbarbitone) and the Schedule 3 drugs buprenorphine, diethylpropion and temazepam must be kept in a CD cupboard in nursing care homes and private hospitals.

How are supplies made commercially?

Supplies may be made by pharmacies, practitioners or wholesalers. Wholesalers handling CDs require Home Office authority. A separate licence is required for each Schedule 2 CD. The Misuse of Drugs Act defines a "wholesale dealer" as someone who "carries on the business of selling drugs to persons who buy to sell again". Retail pharmacies who undertake a small amount of wholesaling to other health professionals and hospitals, etc. are not usually required by the Home Office to be separately licenced. Where the amount of wholesaling is substantial, as is the case with some NHS hospital pharmacies which are registered with RPSGB then the Home Office will require a licence to be held.

Requisitions

A wholesaler does not need a requisition in order to supply a pharmacy. The list of persons from whom a requisition is required is in Regulation 14(4).

A requisition is required where a supply is made to:

- a practitioner
- the person in charge of a hospital or care home providing nursing care
- the person in charge of a laboratory

- the owner of a ship, or the master of a ship which has no doctor on the crew
- the installation manager of an offshore installation
- the master of a foreign ship in a port in Great Britain.

Hospital requisitions

A requisition is required before a supplier can make a supply to a hospital or care home providing nursing care. In this case "supplier" means any person other than a doctor, dentist or vet.

The requisition must:

- be signed by the recipient
- state the name and address of the recipient
- state the occupation of the recipient
- state the purpose for which the drug is required
- specify the total quantity of drug to be supplied.

The supplier must be reasonably satisfied that the signature is authentic and that the person is engaged in the profession or occupation specified.

Residential homes

Residential homes cannot themselves possess or supply CDs. CDs may be prescribed for individual patients resident in the homes. Residential homes are not subject to the Safe Custody requirements.

Messengers

When a person supplies a CD on requisition, he may not give that CD to a person who claims to be a messenger unless:

- he has a written statement, which the supplier reasonably believes is genuine, from the person giving the requisition, stating that he is empowered to collect the drug;
- the messenger is otherwise authorised by Regulations.

Supplementary prescribers

The Misuse of Drugs (Amendment) Regulations 2005, SI No. 271 enable nurse and pharmacist supplementary prescribers to prescribe CDs in Schedules 2, 3 and 4.

The NHS (Primary Medical Services) (Miscellaneous Amendments) Regulations 2005, SI No. 893, enable supplementary prescribers to prescribe CDs in NHS primary care situations.

AHP supplementary prescribers may not prescribe CDs.

Patient Group Directions

The Home Office allows the supply and administration of substances on Schedule 4 (with the exclusion of anabolic steroids) and all substances on Schedule 5 on PGDs.

The Misuse of Drugs (Amendment) (No. 3) Regulations 2003, SI No. 2429/2003), came into force on 15 October 2003.

These regulations allow PGDs for the supply and administration of Schedules 4 and 5 Controlled Drugs (with the exception of anabolic steroids) plus diamorphine for the treatment of cardiac pain by nurses in accident and emergency departments and coronary care units in hospitals.

See Home Office Circular 49/2003 www.homeoffice.gov.uk/docs2/hoc4903.html.

Export

The export of a CD is prohibited except in accordance with a licence granted by the Home Office or where the drug is exempted by Regulations. The regulations exempt CDs in Schedules 4 and 5.

Doctors who wish to take emergency supplies of CDs out of the country require a licence from the Home Office, which is usually granted only when there is a real need, such as a hazardous expedition. Special arrangements are made where doctors wish to accompany pilgrims to Lourdes. Form MD50A is available from the Home Office and should be used to make the application.

Import licences may be required for the country being visited.

Patients requiring CDs when abroad

An "Open General Licence" (OGL) was introduced by the Home Office in 1987. It provides a general authority for the export of small quantities of CDs which are in medicinal products, for medical reasons. It applies to:

- a traveller carrying CDs for administration to himself
- a member of his household who is unable to administer the medicine himself
- a doctor accompanying a patient who requires treatment during a journey to or from the United Kingdom.

The CDs, and the maximum quantities which may be exported are set out in a Schedule. An explanatory leaflet is available. The CD must be under the direct personal supervision of the person importing or exporting it. Maximum quantities are based on an average 15 days' supply. Personal export of more than this amount requires a Home Office licence. No records are required to be kept of CDs imported or exported under this licence. The licence is made under *Section 3(2)(b)* of the Misuse of Drugs Act.

Records

Particulars of Schedule 1 and 2 drugs purchased or supplied must be entered in a register. The amended Regulations now state:

> "register" means either a bound book, which does not include any form of loose leaf register or card index, or a computerised system which is in accordance with best practice guidance endorsed by the Secretary of State under section 2 of the National Health Service Act 1977

The regulations specifically prohibit a loose leaf or record card system. Either a different register, or a separate part of the same register must be used for each class of drugs. Basically a class consists of a different drug together with its stereoisomers, its salts and any preparations containing them. Regulation 19(1)b states:

> he shall use a separate register or separate part of the register for entries made in respect of each class of drugs, and each of the drugs specified in paragraphs 1 and 3 of Schedule 1 and paragraphs 1, 3 and 6 of Schedule 2 together with its salts and any preparation or other product containing it or any of its salts shall be treated as a separate class, so however that any stereo-isomeric form of a drug or its salts shall be classed with that drug.

It is permissible to use separate parts of a register for different drugs or strengths within the class.

A register must not be used for any other purpose. It must be kept at the premises to which it relates, or if a computer system, be accessible from those premises. Only one register for each class must be in use at one time. Where the premises consist of several departments the Home Office may approve the keeping of separate registers in each department. Registers must be preserved for two years from the date of the last entry.

Entries in the register

All entries must be made in chronological order.

On paper, entries must be made on the day of the transaction or on the next day. Entries must not be cancelled, obliterated or altered. Corrections should be made by dated notes on the page. All entries and corrections must be in ink, or otherwise indelible. Computer systems must have an audit trail.

> Regulation 20(d) requires:
>
> (d) every such entry and every correction of such an entry shall be made in ink or otherwise so as to be indelible or shall be in a computerised form in which every such entry is attributable and capable of being audited and which is in accordance with best practice guidance endorsed by the Secretary of State under section 2 of the National Health Service Act 1977.

Who must keep a register

Any person authorised to supply Schedule 1 or 2 drugs must keep a register except that a sister or acting sister in charge of a ward, theatre or register is not required to keep a register. The person who dispenses the drugs to the ward, whether a pharmacist or a person in charge of the hospital must keep a register.

Preservation of prescriptions, etc.

Requisitions and orders for CDs in Schedules 1, 2 and 3 must be retained in the pharmacy for 2 years.

The Regulations state:

24A. For the purposes of regulations 23 and 24(6), "preserved" means kept in its original form, or copied and kept in a computerised form which is in accordance with best practice guidance endorsed by the Secretary of State under section 2 of the National Health Service Act 1977.

Invoices

Pharmacists must keep the invoices or copies when they receive and supply drugs and medicines in Schedules 3 and 5. There are similar rules for producers, wholesalers, hospitals and laboratories for the drugs they may handle. The invoices must bear the date of the transaction and the identity of the parties involved. The invoices must be kept for 2 years.

Requests for information

Certain people are authorised by the S of S to request details about stocks, supplies and receipts of Controlled Drugs. They may also inspect the stock, registers, requisitions and invoices. Confidential personal records, e.g. patient medication records need not be produced.

The authorised persons are

- Inspectors of the RPSGB
- Home Office Drugs Branch Inspectors
- Authorised Medical and Dental Officers of the Health Departments of England, Scotland and Wales.

The people required to produce the information are

- producers
- persons authorised to import and export CDs
- wholesalers
- pharmacists
- practitioners
- persons in charge of hospitals or nursing homes
- persons in charge of laboratories
- persons authorised to supply Schedule 3 and 4 drugs.

The Secretary of State or any person authorised in writing by the Secretary of State in that behalf may request that a register which is kept in computerised form be produced by sending a copy of it, in computerised or other form, to the appropriate person.

Destruction of CDs

(1) By patients – Patients may destroy any CDs in their possession, which are left over from their treatment. No records are required.
(2) By pharmacists – Pharmacists may destroy CDs which are returned by a patient or patient's representative. There is no need to make any records or have the

destruction witnessed. Medicines used for animal treatment may be similarly dealt with by vets as well as pharmacists. Other than above, pharmacists may only destroy CDs in the presence of a witness authorised by the S of S.

The persons authorised include

- Police officers
- Inspectors of the Home Office Drugs Branch
- RPSGB Inspectors (for pharmacies only)
- Chief Dental Officer of DOH, or a Senior Dental Officer to whom the authority has been delegated
- Supervisors of midwives
- Regional Medical Officers of SHHD
- Chief Administrative Pharmaceutical Officers (for their Health Board's area only)
- Deputy Chief Dental Officer of SHHD
- Regional Dental Officers of SHHD
- Regional Medical Officers of the Welsh Office
- The Pharmaceutical Advisor for Wales
- NHS Trust Chief Executives
- A PCT chief pharmacist or pharmaceutical/prescribing adviser who reports directly to the chief executive or to a director of the PCT
- A registered medical practitioner who has been appointed to the PCT Professional Executive Committee or the PCT Board with responsibility for clinical governance or risk management
- Medical director of a PCT
- Senior Trust officers reporting directly to CEO, with responsibility for health, safety and security
- Any other person who has been granted this authority by the S of S. Some members of the management of larger bodies' corporate have been authorised by the Home Office.

Authorised persons do not have the authority to delegate the task of witnessing the destruction of CDs. Where drugs are destroyed in this way a record must be made of the date of destruction and the quantity destroyed. The record must be signed by the authorised witness.

(3) Ships and Offshore oil rigs

Excess Schedule 2 drugs in the possession of a master or owner of a ship, or the installation manager of an offshore installation may not be destroyed. They should be handed to a constable or to a pharmacist or licensed dealer.

Schedules 3, 4 and 5

Schedules 3, 4 and 5 CDs may be destroyed without an authorised witness. It is not necessary to keep records of the destruction.

Re-use of Controlled Drugs

The legal position of re-use or "recycling" of CDs is the subject of some debate. The question usually relates to the use by Patient B of medicine originally prescribed for, and supplied to Patient A and which is no longer required by Patient A. This may happen in a hospice for instance.

The advice of the Home Office is that such re-use is legal, even where the pharmacist has been given the medicine in question "for destruction". The Home Office argues that the regulations do not *require* the pharmacist to destroy the medicines, they merely empower him to do so. Provided the correct records are kept the medicines may be used by him in the same way as if he had obtained them from his wholesaler. The RPSGB advise that controlled drugs returned to the pharmacy by a patient should not be returned to stock. The RPSGB Code of Ethics states that

> Medicines returned to a pharmacy from a patient's home or a nursing or residential home must not be supplied to any other patient.

Safe custody

The Misuse of Drugs (Safe Custody) Regulations 1973 (as amended) require Schedule 1, 2 and 3 CDs (with some exceptions) to be kept in a locked receptacle. Where CDs are kept in a "retail pharmacy" or in a nursing home or private hospital the receptacle must be a safe, cabinet or room which meets certain standards. These Regulations have not been amended to reflect the collective term "care home" which now includes both nursing and residential homes. Thus at present residential care homes are not legally required to use locked receptacles, though this would be good practice.

The general requirement

A person in possession of CDs must store them in a locked receptacle to which only he (and persons authorised by him) has the key. The courts have held that a car does not constitute a locked receptacle for this regulation.

Exceptions to the general requirement

This requirement does not apply to:

- a carrier in the course of his business
- a person engaged in the business of the Post Office
- a person who has been supplied with the CD on prescription, for his own use or for the treatment of another person or an animal.

In addition, a CD can remain out of the cabinet as long as it is under the pharmacist's direct personal supervision. The safe custody requirements apply to all CDs in Schedules 1 and 2 (except quinalbarbitone), and to diethylpropion, temazepam and buprenorphine.

Locked safe, cabinet or room

The Regulations specify that when CDs are kept on any premises occupied by a person lawfully conducting an RPB they must be stored in a locked safe, cabinet or room which complies with the structural standards laid down in the regulations. It is with these standards that the "CD cabinet" complies.

The requirement also applies when CDs are kept in:

(a) any premises occupied by a pharmacist engaged in supplying drugs to the public at a NHS health centre
(b) any nursing home within Part II of the Registered Homes Act 1984.

Hospitals

Regulation 3 does not apply to hospitals unless the pharmacy department is registered as an RPB with the RPSGB. Hospital wards are required to keep CDs in a locked receptacle.

Standards

The standards specify that cabinets must be made of steel sheet or welded mesh. It must be designed with a close-fitting door fitted with a dead-bolt, and a five-lever lock or equivalent. The cabinet must be rigidly attached to a wall or floor with at least two rag-bolts which pass through an internal anchor plate. Nothing shall be displayed outside a safe or cabinet to indicate that drugs are kept inside it.

There are detailed standards for secure rooms which contain CDs. The room is an alternative to the use of a cabinet or safe. Where the CDs are kept in a "retail pharmacy" the local police can issue a certificate stating that a room, safe or cabinet provides an adequate degree of security even though it does not comply with the specific standards laid down. This procedure enables the use of "money" safes which may be constructed in a different way. The certificate lasts for a year after the inspection visit, and may be renewed.

Addicts

The Misuse of Drugs (Notification of and Supply to Addicts) Regulations 1973, SI No. 1973/799, deals with the treatment of addicts by doctors.

What is an "addict"?

A person is to be regarded as an addict

> if, and only if, he has as a result of repeated administration become so dependent upon the drug that he has an overpowering desire for the administration of it to be continued.

Which drugs are affected

The Regulations apply to the following drugs: cocaine, dextromoramide, diamorphine, dipipanone, hydrocodone, hydromorphone, levorphanol, methadone, morphine, opium, oxycodone, pethidine, phenazocine and piritramide. Also included is any salt, ester or ether or stereo-isomer (except dextrorphan) of the above drugs.

Supply to addicts

If a doctor considers, or has reasonable grounds to suspect that a person is addicted to any drug listed in the Supply to Addicts Regulations then he may not prescribe cocaine, diamorphine or dipipanone (or their salts or preparations) to that person unless:

(a)   he is treating an organic disease or injury *or*
(b)   he holds a Home Office licence.

Notification

Until May 1997, doctors were required to pass on details of addicts to the Home Office. The 1997 Regulations set up a Regional Drug Misuse Database to which doctors are expected to report treatment demands.

NHS Prescriptions for addicts

Two types of NHS prescription forms are provided in E & W for doctors to use when prescribing for addicts. The forms enable addicts to receive supplies of drugs in daily instalments.

FP10 (HP)Ad

This form is used by doctors in drug addiction clinics. There are no regulations specifically covering this form, but the form itself bears the information that it may only be used for prescribing the following drugs: cocaine, diamorphine hydrochloride, dextromoramide, dipipanone, methadone hydrochloride, morphine and pethidine hydrochloride.

The prescription must state the amount to be dispensed on each instalment and the interval between instalments. Other drugs and appliances may be ordered on the same form, but the supply may be made on one occasion only.

FP10 (MDA)

Use of this form is governed by the NHS (General Medical Services Contracts) Regulations 2004. The form is issued by PCTs to any GP on request. The form may be used for the instalment prescribing of any Schedule 2 CD being used in the treatment of addiction in the patient. Only Home Office licensed doctors may prescribe diamorphine, cocaine or dipipanone (or their salts) to addicts for their addiction.

Some preparations of Schedule 2 drugs appear in Schedule 5 (e.g. tablets of dihydrocodeine) and the Home Office interpretation is that those preparations are consequently not in Schedule 2. It appears that Schedule 2 consists of a list of drugs, and Schedule 5 a list of preparations of some of the drugs in Schedule 2. An alternative interpretation would be that the word "drug" in the Instalment Prescribing Regulations refers to entries in Schedule 2, and that an additional entry in Schedule 5 is irrelevant. There has been no case law on the issue to date.

The prescription must state the amount per instalment and the interval between instalments. The Regulations restrict the supply to a maximum of 14 days per form. The number of instalments must be stated. The form may not be used for any purpose except instalment prescribing for addicts. It may, however, be used to order a single supply of a quantity of Water for Injection.

Failure to comply with the conditions for use of the form would make a doctor liable to disciplinary committee action. A pharmacist would seem to be in a slightly different position. The question remains open whether a form which does not meet the conditions of use may still be dispensed by the pharmacist without breach of his Terms of Service.

NHS repeatable prescriptions

The legislation does not allow Schedule 2 or 3 CDs to be prescribed on NHS repeat prescriptions.

Helping addicts to inject

It is not a supply to inject a person with that persons own CD. Thus where Charlie injects Snow with heroin at Snow's request, Charlie has not unlawfully supplied it – at least not by injectiong it (*R* v. *Harris 1968*).

Controls on specific drugs

In recent years the Misuse of Drugs Act and its regulations have been used to impose new controls on certain products which are subject to abuse and illicit use.

Temazepam

The Misuse of Drugs (Amendment) Regulations 1996, SI No. 1597, deal with Temazepam products. Although most benzodiazepines remain in Schedule 4, Temazepam has been moved to Schedule 3. However it is not subject to the normal prescription writing and records keeping rules which apply to Schedule 2 and 3 drugs:

- Prescriptions do not need to be in the prescriber's own handwriting.
- The date does not need to be written by the prescriber.
- No CD register entry is required.

All temazepam products, including liquids are subject to safe custody requirements.

"Magic mushrooms"

The Misuse of Drugs (Designation) (Amendment) Order 2005, SI No. 1652 and The Misuse of Drugs (Amendment) (No. 2) Regulations 2005, SI No. 1653 now make it an offence to have any dealings with (containing psilocin or an ester of psilocin) except where they are growing wild or being picked for destruction.

Steroids

The Misuse of Drugs Act 1971 (Modification) Order 1996, SI No. 1300, adds anabolic and androgenic steroids, polypeptide growth hormones and the adrenoceptor stimulant Clenbuterol to the compounds in Class C of the MDA.

The Misuse of Drugs (Amendment) Regulations 1996, SI No.1597, splits Schedule 4 into two parts. Part I contains the steroids, etc. and Part II contains mainly benzodiazepines.

Steroids are subject to the usual Schedule 4 requirements. In addition they require a Home Office licence for import or export unless the substance is in the form of a medicinal product for personal use. Possession of listed steroids is an offence unless they are formulated as a medicine.

Supply of paraphernalia to drug misusers

Section 34 of the Drug Trafficking Offences Act 1986 added a new *Section 9A* to the MDA 1971, making it an offence for anyone to knowingly sell items to drug addicts which could help them prepare or administer illicit controlled drugs.

The section states that

> It is an offence for a person to supply or offer to supply any article which may be used or adapted for use in the administration of a controlled drug to himself or another, believing that the article is to be so used, or to supply or offer to supply any article which may be used to prepare a controlled drug for administration to himself or another, believing that the article is to be so used in circumstances where the administration is unlawful.

Any administration of a controlled drug which is not in accordance with the instructions of a practitioner will be unlawful. Syringes and needles are exempt from this, by virtue of *Section 9A(2)*.

The Misuse of Drugs (Amendment) (No. 2) Regulations 2003, SI No. 1653, provides that practitioners, pharmacists and persons lawfully providing drug treatment services may supply:

(a) a swab
(b) utensils for the preparation of a controlled drug
(c) citric acid
(d) a filter
(e) ampoules of Water for Injection
(f) ascorbic acid (added by SI 2005/2864)

where the articles are believed to be used for the purposes of administering or preparing controlled drugs.

Water for Injection

The Medicines (Sale or Supply) (Miscellaneous Amendments) Regulations 2005, SI No. 1507, change the previous position and allows Water for Injection to be supplied in the course of a lawful drug treatment service. Only 2 ml ampoules may be supplied.

Drugs Act 2005

The Drugs Act 2005 amends the Misuse of Drugs Act 1971, principally to strengthen police powers in relations to drug misuse.

Chapter 17

Labelling, Leaflets and Packaging

Various Regulations and Orders have been issued under the MA 1968 to deal with the labelling of medicinal products. *Section 85* of the Medicines Act enables Ministers to regulate labelling in order to ensure descriptions are correct, to ensure that suitable instructions are given and to promote safety. The section provides that it is an offence not to comply.

Section 86 deals with leaflets relating to medicinal products.

The main regulations

The main Regulations are the Medicines (Labelling) Regulations 1976, SI No. 1726, which have been amended a number of times, and which were substantially altered by:

(a) Medicines (Labelling) Amendment Regulations 1992, SI No. 3273,
(b) Medicines (Leaflets) Amendment Regulations 1992, SI No. 3274, and
(c) Medicines for Human Use (Marketing Authorisations, etc.) Regulations 1994, SI No. 3144 [the MAR Regulations].

These 1992 Amendment Regulations implemented Directive 92/27/EEC, whose provisions are now contained in Directive 2001/83/EEC.

They apply to "relevant medicinal products" which constitute the vast majority of products. Relevant medicinal products constitute all products for human use except those prepared on the basis of a magistral or officinal formula, products intended for research or development trials, and intermediate products intended for further processing.

General provisions for labelling

All labelling of containers and packages of relevant medicinal products shall be –

(a) legible and indelible
(b) comprehensible and
(c) either in the English language only or in English and in one or more other languages provided that the same particulars appear in all the languages used.

Symbols or pictograms may be used to clarify the standard labelling requirements.

Strength of product

In any case where there is more than one pharmaceutical form or more than one strength of a product, a statement of the pharmaceutical form or strength of that product must appear on the label. This can be as part of the name of that product, but otherwise must be added immediately after the name, in the same style and size of letters as the name. "Strength" means the suitability of the product for a baby, child or adult.

The requirement for a container or package of a relevant medicinal product to be labelled to show its name is not met by the container or package being labelled to show an invented name which is liable to be confused with the common name.

Additional information useful for health education may appear on the label so long as it is not of a promotional nature. Labelling details must be approved by the licensing authority, and any changes notifies to them. The licensing authority has a 90-day period during which it may object to any changes.

Standard Labelling Requirements for medicinal products for human use

(1)   the name of the product followed, where the product contains one active ingredient and its name is an invented name, by the common name;

(2)   a statement of the active ingredients of the product expressed qualitatively and quantitatively per dosage unit or according to the form of administration for a given volume or weight, using the common names of the ingredients;

(3)   the pharmaceutical form of the product;

(4)   the contents of the product by weight, by volume or by number of doses of the product;

(5)   a list of excipients known to have a recognised action or effect. In relation to products which are injectable or are topical or eye preparations, all excipients;

(6)   the method and, if necessary, the route of administration of the product;

(7)   a special warning that the product must be stored out of reach of children;

(8)   any special warning required by the marketing authorisation for the product concerned;

(9)   the expiry date of the product (stating the month and year) in clear terms;

(10) any special storage precautions for the product;

(11) any special precautions for the disposal of any unused products or waste materials derived from such products;

(12) the name of the holder of the marketing authorisation of the product;

(13) the address of the holder of the marketing authorisation;

(14) any marketing authorisation number as allocated by the licensing authority which relates to the product, preceded by the letters "PL" in capital letters or an abbreviation of the expression "marketing authorisation";

(15) the manufacturer's batch reference;

(16) where a product is intended for self-medication, any instruction on the use of the product.

"Appropriate non-proprietary name"

Appropriate non-proprietary name means

(1) any name, or abbreviation of such a name, at the head of a monograph in one of the publications listed in *Section 103* of the MA 1968. The publications listed there are:

  (a) the European Pharmacopoeia (EP)
  (b) the British Pharmacopoeia (BP)
  (c) the British Pharmaceutical Codex (BPC)
  (d) the British Veterinary Codex
  (e) the British National Formulary (BNF)
  (f) the Dental Practitioners' Formulary (DPF)
  (g) any other compendium published under the MA 1968
  (h) the list of recommended International Non-Proprietary Names.

(2) where the product is not described in a monograph, the recommended international non-proprietary name (RINN)
(3) if none of the above apply, then the accepted scientific name or other name accurately describing the product.

This hierarchy of definitions means that wherever possible the product is labelled with a name which is clear to all users. These names are usually referred to as "generic" names.

"Appropriate Quantitative Particulars"

This means the quantity of each active ingredients, expressed in terms of weight, volume, capacity or as a percentage.

"Proprietary medicinal product"

This means a ready-prepared medicinal product marketed in the United Kingdom with a particular name and in a special pack – in other words a branded or proprietary medicine.

"Expiry date"

Since January 1990, all licensed medicinal products have been required to carry an expiry date in clear language (The Medicines (Labeling) Amendment Regulations 1985, SI No. 1558). The product "expires" at the end of the month stated, or after the date stated, e.g. "June 1992" means the product is not to be used *after* June 1992.

Braille labels

Medicines authorised after 30 October 2005 must have the name, and if appropriate, the strength of the product on the package in Braille. (Article 56(a) of Council Directive 2001/83/EC).

PILs must be made available by the manufacturer "in formats suitable for the blind and partially sighted patient."

Small containers

Ampoules and other containers of 10 ml capacity or less are not required to have all of the standard particulars on the ampoule itself. The package must bear the full standard particulars. The small container itself must have the following:

(1) name of product
(2) the contents of the product by weight, by volume or by number of doses
(3) administration route
(4) expiry date
(5) batch number.

Blister packs

Where the container of a medicinal product is a blister pack which is itself enclosed in a fully labelled package, the label on the blister pack need only include

(1) name of product
(2) expiry date
(3) the name of the holder of the marketing authorisation of the product
(4) the manufacturer's batch reference.

What is a container?

The container is the receptacle which actually contains the tablets, capsules, syrup, etc.

What is the package?

The package is the box, packet, etc. in which the container is enclosed.

GSL Medicines

The MAR Regulations 1994 contain extra requirements for some common GSL products:

(1) Products which contain aloxiprin, aspirin or paracetamol must be labelled with "If symptoms persist, consult your doctor" and the recommended dosage.
(2) Products containing aloxiprin must be labelled with "Contains an aspirin derivative".
(3) Products containing aspirin must be labelled with "Contains aspirin". This is not necessary for external products or where "aspirin" is included in the product name.

(4)   Products containing aspirin must be labelled with the "Reye's syndrome warning" (see below).
(5)   Products containing paracetamol must be labelled with "contains paracetamol", unless "paracetamol" is included in the product name.
(6)   Products containing paracetamol must also be labelled with warnings about overdose (see below).
(7)   The words "do not exceed the stated dose" must appear adjacent to the directions or dosage on paracetamol products.
(8)   The phrases above in 2, 3 and 4 may be combined where appropriate.
(9)   The phrases in 2–5 must be printed in a rectangle, in a prominent position.

Paracetamol warnings

(1)   Adult preparations must carry warnings:
      "Do not take with other paracetamol containing product" *and either* "Immediate medical advice should be sought in the event of an overdose, even if you feel well" (if there is an accompanying PIL) *or* "Immediate medical advice should be sought in the event of an overdose, even if you feel well, because of the risk of delayed, serious liver damage" (if there is no accompanying PIL).
(2)   Children's preparations must carry warnings.
      "Do not give with other paracetamol containing product" *and either* "Immediate medical advice should be sought in the event of an overdose, even if the child seems well" (if there is an accompanying PIL) *or* "Immediate medical advice should be sought in the event of an overdose, even if the child seems well, because of the risk of delayed, serious liver damage" (if there is no accompanying PIL).

"P" Medicines

A further set of requirements applies to "P" medicines, which must be labelled as follows:

(1)   All Pharmacy Only Medicines must be labelled with the capital letter "P" in a rectangle. This requirement applies to sales by wholesale also.
(2)   Products which contain aspirin, aloxiprin or paracetamol must be labelled as described above.
(3)   Some substances are exempted from POM control when present in a product below a specified level. The products must generally be labelled "Warning. Do not exceed the stated dose." Products for external use are dealt with in a different way, as are products where the substance is an antihistamine or similar substance.
(4)   Products for the treatment of asthma or bronchial spasm, and those which contain ephedrine or its salts, must be labelled "Warning. Asthmatics should consult their doctor before using this product."

(5) Antihistamine products, except those for external use, must be labelled "Warning. May cause drowsiness. If affected do not drive or operate machinery. Avoid alcoholic drink."

(6) Liquid or gel products for external use, including embrocations, liniments, lotions or antiseptics must carry the words "For external use only."

(7) Human medicines containing hexachlorophane must either be labelled "Not to be used for babies" or carry a warning that the product is not to be administered to a child under the age of two except on medical advice.

The warning phrases must be in a rectangle which does not contain any other matter.

Prescription Only Medicines

The containers and packages of POM medicines must be labelled with the letters "POM" in a rectangle. The label must also carry the appropriate warnings listed above for external medicines and for medicines containing hexachlorophane. These requirements apply when the products are sold by wholesale, which includes sale to doctors or dentists. They do not apply to dispensed medicines.

When sold by wholesale, POMs do not need to be labelled "Keep out of reach of children" but this is necessary for retail sale.

Radiopharmaceuticals

(1) The container and the package shall be labelled in accordance with the 1985 Edition (as amended in 1990) of the Regulations for the Safe Transport of Radioactive Materials recommended by the International Atomic Energy Agency.

(2) The labelling on the shielding shall explain in full the codings used on the vial and shall indicate, where necessary, for a given time and date, the amount of radioactivity per dose or per vial and the number of capsules, or for liquids, the number of millilitres in the container.

(3) The vial shall be labelled to show

    (a) the name or code of the medicinal product, including the name or chemical symbol of the radionuclide

    (b) the international symbol for radioactivity

    (c) the name of the manufacturer and

    (d) the amount of radioactivity as specified in Paragraph 2 above.

Labelling of dispensed medicinal products

A dispensed medicinal product is a medicinal product prepared or dispensed in accordance with a prescription given by a practitioner.

The container shall be labelled with

(1) the name of the patient

(2) the name and address of the person who sells or supplies the product

(3) the date of dispensing

(4)   the following details if requested by the practitioner:

    (a)   the name of the medicinal product or its common name
    (b)   the directions for use
    (c)   the precautions relating to its use.

(5)   the words "keep out of reach of children" or similar
(6)   the words "for external use only" if the product:

    (a)   is a P or POM medicine which is a liquid or gel,
    (b)   consists of an embrocation, liniment, lotion, antiseptic or other prepara-
        tion and
    (c)   is for external use.

Where the pharmacist believes that any of the particulars in (4) as requested by the practitioner are inappropriate, he may substitute those he believes to be appropriate. This may only be done after taking all reasonable steps, and failing, to consult with the prescriber.

Standard labelling requirements for homoeopathic products

Containers and packages of homoeopathic must be labelled in clear and legible form to show a reference to their homoeopathic nature, in particular by clear mention of the words "homoeopathic medicinal product". This is in addition to any other particulars required by regulations. See Chapter 14.

Pharmacists' Own Remedies

Products prepared in a pharmacy for retail sale from that pharmacy, and which are not advertised are sometimes known as "nostrums". They must be labelled with the following:

 (1)   name of product
 (2)   pharmaceutical form on the package
 (3)   appropriate quantitative details
 (4)   quantity
 (5)   directions for use
 (6)   special handling and storage requirements
 (7)   expiry date
 (8)   name and address of seller
 (9)   "keep out of reach of children"
(10)   where appropriate, the warnings for "P" medicines.

Child resistant containers

The retail sale of certain products must be in child resistant containers. The Medicines (Child Safety) Regulations 2003, SI No. 2317, cover aspirin, paracetamol and iron preparations for children. They were amended by the Medicines (Child

Safety) Amendment Regulations 1976, SI No. 1643, which made CRCs a requirement for aspirin and paracetamol used for adults.

A "child resistant container" is

(a) a reclosable container complying with BS EN 28317 or an equivalent or higher specification recognised for use within the European Economic Area

   or

(b) a non-reclosable container complying with BS 8404 or an equivalent or higher specification recognised for use within the European Economic Area.

The products covered by the Regulations are

(a) aspirin or paracetamol products in unit-dose form (except effervescent tablets containing less than 25% w/w) for human use;
(b) iron products for human use containing more than 24 mg of elemental iron.

These products must be supplied in containers that are both child resistant *and* opaque or dark tinted.

When packed for administration to children the solid dose aspirin and paracetamol products must be white, although flavours are allowed. Each container may not contain more than 25 unit doses.

Exemptions

The Medicines (Child Safety) Regulations 2003, SI 2003/2317, do not apply when the sale or supply is

(a) on prescription
(b) made by a doctor or dentist for a patient
(c) from a pharmacy by a pharmacist responding to a request from a patient to use his judgement as to treatment
(d) by a doctor or dentist to a colleague for a patient
(e) in the course of business of a hospital for use in accordance with the directions of a doctor
(f) for export or not for retail sale
(g) of products not for human use.

Warning about Reyes Syndrome

As of 1 April 2004 it has been illegal to sell or supply any aspirin product which does not bear the label

"Do not give to children aged under 16 years unless on the advice of a doctor."

In addition the PIL must carry the following:

> There is a possible association between aspirin and Reye's syndrome when given to children. Reye's syndrome is a very rare disease which can be fatal. For this reason aspirin should not be given to children aged under 16 years unless on the advice of a doctor.

Dispensed Medicines in CRCs

There is no law requiring the use of CRCs for dispensed medicines for adults. However, in 1981 the pharmaceutical and medical professions agreed that all solid-dose oral preparations should be dispensed in CRCs or in strip or blister packs. Exceptions are allowed for:

(a) original packs
(b) patients who experience difficulty in opening CRCs
(c) specific requests from patients.

The voluntary scheme became a professional requirement from 1 January 1989, and appears as a requirement in the RPSGB Code of Ethics. This was extended by a Council Statement in February 1994, which stated that from 1 January 1995 it would be a professional requirement for CRCs to be used for all liquid medicines dispensed from bulk.

Use of Ribbed or Fluted Bottles

According to the Medicines (Fluted Bottles) Regulations 1978, SI No. 40, certain medicinal products for external use must be supplied in ribbed or fluted bottles. The outer surface of the bottles must be fluted vertically with ribs or grooves recognisable by touch.

In these regulations "External use" means

> application to the skin, teeth, mucosa of the mouth, throat, nose, ear, eye, vagina or anal canal. It does not include throat sprays, nasal drops, nasal sprays, nasal inhalations, teething preparations or dental gels.

Exceptions

The regulations do not apply to:

- bottles over 1.14 litres
- containers for export
- products sold or supplied solely for scientific education, research or analysis
- eye or ear drops in a plastic bottle
- where the marketing authorisation specifies otherwise
- where there are exceptions in the Schedule.

Offences

It is an offence for any person in the course of business carried on by him to sell, supply or possess for sale any medicine which does not comply with the requirements. It is also an offence to have any leaflet which does not comply.

Medicinal products must be sold in containers. Containers, packages and leaflets must properly describe the product and must not mislead as to the nature or quality of the product. Contravention is punishable by a fine or up to £2000 and up to 2 years' imprisonment.

Patient Information Leaflets

Council Directive 92/27/EEC on the labelling of medicinal products for human use and on package leaflets was adopted by the European Commission on 31 March 1992. This is now part of Directive 2001/83/EEC. Directive 2001/83/EC was itself amended by Directive 2004/27/EC. The Directives are implemented into UK legislation via the following statutory instruments:

- The Medicines (Leaflet) Amendment Regulations 1992, SI No. 3274.
- The Medicines (Marketing Authorisations, etc.) Regulations 1994, SI No. 3144.
- The Medicines (Marketing Authorisations and Miscellaneous Amendments) Regulations 2004, SI No. 3224.

Requirement to have PIL

Regulation 7 of the MAR Regulations 1994 imposes an obligation on the holder of a UK marketing authorisation to comply with "all obligations which relate to him by virtue of the relevant Community provisions, including in particular . . . obligations relating to package leaflets."

Schedule 3 Paragraph 11 states that it is an offence for the holder of a marketing authorisation to sell or supply a product without a package leaflet which complies with the requirements of Directive 2001/83/EEC. Directive 2001/83/EEC was itself amended by Directive 2004/27/EEC.

Paragraph 12 states that any other person who, in the course of a business carried on by him, sells or supplies a product without a package leaflet is also guilty of an offence. The offence is punishable by a fine or imprisonment or both.

Requirement for a user test

Directive 2004/27/EC now states,

> The package leaflet shall reflect the results of consultations with target patient groups to ensure that it is legible clear and easy to use

The Medicines (Marketing Authorisations and Miscellaneous Amendments) Regulations 2004, SI No. 3224 implements this requirement by amending the 1994 Regulations. The amended Regulations affect all new applications from 1 July 2005. There is a transitional period for existing products up to 2008. They require a user test to ensure that the information provided in PILs is legible, clear and easy to use. They also alter the order in which information on the leaflet is presented, to comply with Directive 2004/27/EC.

Content of a PIL

The content of these patient information leaflets (PIL) is set out in the Medicines (Leaflets) Amendment Regulations 1992, which substantially amended the principal Regulations which are the Medicines Leaflets Regulations 1977.

Regulations 3 and 8 set out the content of such leaflets, which is detailed in Schedule 2 of the 1992 Regulations. The contents of the PIL must be approved by MHRA. Leaflets for "relevant medicinal products" are to be drawn up in accordance with the Summary of Product Characteristics (SPC). Leaflets may be printed in more than one language provided one is English and the same particulars appear in each language (Regulation 5(4)).

The licensing authority may direct in the marketing authorisation that certain therapeutic indications shall not appear on leaflets (new Regulation 4(7) as inserted by Regulation 5(8)).

Symbols, pictograms or other information may appear on such leaflets if there is no promotional element (new Regulation 4(8) as inserted by Regulation 5(8)).

The Regulations provide for certain information to be shown where the name of a relevant medicinal product is given, where that information does not form part of that name (new Regulation 4(9) as inserted by Regulation 5(9), Article 7.1(a) of the Directive).

Standard requirements for Patient Information Leaflets

The Leaflet Regulations require "relevant medicinal products" to have a "patient information leaflet" containing the following particulars "in a form that is understandable by the patient":

(1) For identification of the medicinal product:

    (a) the name of the product followed, where the product contains only one active ingredient and its name is an invented name, by the common name;

    (b) a statement of the active ingredients and excipients expressed qualitatively and a statement of the active ingredients expressed quantitatively, using their common names, in the case of each presentation of the product;

    (c) the pharmaceutical form and the contents by weight, by volume or by number of doses of the product, in the case of each presentation of the product;

    (d) the pharmaco-therapeutic group, or type of activity in terms easily comprehensible to the patient;

    (e) the name and address of the holder of the product licence and of the manufacturer.

(2)   The therapeutic indications.

(3)   A list of information which is necessary before taking the medicinal product as follows:

    (a)   contra-indications;
    (b)   appropriate precautions for use;
    (c)   forms of interaction with other medicinal products, with alcohol, tobacco and food, and any other form of interaction which may affect the action of the medicinal product;
    (d)   special warnings which:

        (i)   take into account the particular condition of certain categories of users;
        (ii)   mention, if appropriate, potential effects on the ability to drive vehicles or operate machinery; and
        (iii) give details of those excipients, knowledge of which is important for the safe and effective use of the medicinal product.

(4)   The necessary and usual instructions for proper use of the medicinal product which shall include:

    (a)   the dosage;
    (b)   the method and, if necessary, the route of administration;
    (c)   the frequency of administration, specifying if necessary the time at which the medicinal product may or must be administered;

and, where the nature of the product makes it appropriate, shall also include

    (d)   the duration of treatment where it should be limited
    (e)   the action to be taken in the case of an overdose
    (f)   the course of action to take when one or more doses have not been taken
    (g)   indication, if necessary, of the risk of withdrawal effects.

(5)   A description of the undesirable effects which can occur with normal use of the medicinal product and if necessary the action to be taken in such case, together with an express invitation to the patient to communicate any undesirable effect which is not mentioned in the leaflet to his doctor or pharmacist.

(6)   A reference to the expiry date indicated on the label with:

    (a)   a warning against using the product after this date
    (b)   where appropriate, special storage requirements
    (c)   if necessary, a warning against certain visible signs of deterioration.

(7)   The date upon which the leaflet was last revised.

As with labels, the particulars must be in English. Symbols and pictograms may be used to clarify information. Other information useful for health education may be included provided there is no material of a promotional nature.

Therapeutic indications need not be included if the marketing authorisation indicates that these details need not be included.

Guidelines

Article 12 of the original directive makes provision for the publication of guidelines to be used in conjunction with the Directive. The Guideline on Excipients in the label and package leaflet of medicinal products for human use became effective on 1 September 1997. This guideline is currently under review and the updated version is due to become effective in the near future. The Guideline on the readability of the label and package leaflet of medicinal products for human use became effective on 1 January 1999. MHRA published Guidance Note No. 25 in December 2002, on "Best practice guidance on labelling and packaging of medicine."

Hospital practice

Where medicines are given to patients in hospitals as individual doses e.g. on a ward, the leaflet need not be included in the packaging, but must be provided to the patient on request.

Radiopharmaceuticals

The Regulations also impose special requirements for the leaflets supplied with radiopharmaceuticals and with radiopharmaceutical-associated products (Regulation 4).

Chapter 18

Poisons and Dangerous Substances

There are a number of controls on the sale, storage, labelling and other dealings with those poisons which are not medicines. The Poisons Act 1972 sets up a mechanism to designate substances as poisons, and to lay down rules on how they are to be treated.

The Poisons Board

Section 1 of the Poisons Act creates an advisory committee (in reality a continuation of one established by earlier legislation, the Pharmacy and Poisons Act 1933).

The Board consists of at least 16 members. Five of them must be appointed by RPSGB, and one of these must be engaged in the manufacture of pharmaceuticals. Members hold office for 3 years. The Chairman is appointed by the S of S.

Poisons List

The main task of the Board is to recommend to the S of S which substances should be listed as poisons. *Section 2* of the Act creates a Poisons List, which is set out from time to time in a Poisons List Order. The list consists of two parts:

- Part I is a list of poisons which can only be retailed from a pharmacy.
- Part II is a list of poisons which can be sold from either a pharmacy or by a "listed seller".

Listed sellers

A "listed seller" is a person allowed by the local county or borough council to sell Part II poisons. The local authority can refuse permission if it believes the person is unfit. Names may also be removed from the list for non-payment of the retention fee. A court may remove a name from the list following a conviction which would make the person unfit to sell poisons.

The local authority list must include particulars of the premises and the names of the persons listed. The permission is specific to the person. Up to two deputies may be named. The list is open to public inspection without charge. The local authority is entitled to charge reasonable fees for inclusion and for retention. Listed sellers may not use any title, emblem or description which might suggest he is entitled to sell poisons other than those in Part II.

Enforcement

Enforcement is shared between the RPSGB and the local authorities, with the RPSGB dealing with pharmacies. Both appoint Inspectors, but the local authorities may appoint one of the RPSGB inspectors to work on their behalf. RPSGB Inspectors must be pharmacists.

Penalties

A person who fails to comply with the law relating to poisons is liable on conviction to a fine of up to £1000. Offences involving the misuse of titles or the obstruction of an inspector may incur a fine of £100.

When the offences are related to the sale or supply of a poison the employer remains liable even though an employee acted without his authority (*Section 8*).

Substances on the list

Only substances which appear on the Poisons List are legally poisons. Other substances, despite their toxicity, are not legally poisons. Some poisons may only be sold by listed sellers when the poison is in a specified form. Some poisons may only be sold to certain categories of purchaser

The Poisons Rules

The detail of the law is found in the Poisons Rules, which categorise poisons into a number of Schedules. There are different rules governing each of the Schedules. The current law is found in the Poisons Rules 1982, SI No. 218, as amended by the Poisons Rules Amendment Order 1985. The Rules also contain a number of general provisions which apply to all poisons.

General requirements

Generally, poisons in Part I must be sold:

- by a pharmacist or person lawfully conducting an RPB
- at the pharmacy
- by or under the supervision of the pharmacist.

Poisons in Part II must be sold

- from a pharmacy, *or*
- by a listed seller from his premises.

Listed sellers may not sell any Part II poisons which they have altered or processed in such a way as to expose the poison.

Schedule 1

Extra conditions are specified for the sale, storage and record keeping of poisons in Schedule 1.

Supervision

All Schedule 1 poisons, even those on Part II of the List, must be sold under the supervision of the pharmacist when sold from a pharmacy. When sold from "listed premises" the sale must be effected by the listed seller or one of his deputies.

Storage

Schedule 1 poisons must be stored separately from other items. They must be in:

(a)   a cupboard or a drawer used solely for poisons,
(b)   a part of the premises separated from the rest so as to exclude the public, or
(c)   on a shelf used only for storing poisons, and which has no food below it.

Schedule 1 poisons which are used in agriculture, horticulture or forestry must be kept separate from food products. If stored in a drawer or cupboard no other products may be kept with them. When poisons are transported in vehicles, adequate steps must be taken to avoid contamination of any food carried in the same vehicle.

Knowledge of the purchaser

Purchasers of Schedule 1 poisons must be known to the seller, or to a responsible person on his staff, as being "of good character". The person on the staff may be a pharmacist, or in the case of listed sellers, the person in charge of the premises or of the department.

Where the purchaser is not known, they must present a certificate stating that they are of good character. This must be in the prescribed form, and given by a householder. If the householder is not known to the seller then the certificate must be endorsed by a police officer in charge of a police station. The endorsement certifies that the householder is known to the police as a person of good character. It does not itself certify the purchaser.

Records

Sellers of Schedule 1 poisons are required to keep a "Poisons Book", and enter in it:

(1)   the date of sale
(2)   the name and address of purchaser
(3)   the name and address of person giving the certificate
(4)   the date of the certificate
(5)   the name and quantity of poison
(6)   the purpose for which the poison is stated to be required.

The format is laid down in Schedule 11 of the Poisons Rules.

The entry must be signed by the purchaser. Purchasers who require a poison for trade or professional purposes may present a signed order instead of signing the Poisons Book. A Poisons Book must be retained for 2 years after the last entry.

Signed order

A signed order must contain the following:

(1)   name and address of purchaser
(2)   trade, business or profession
(3)   purpose for which the poison is required
(4)   total quantity to be bought.

The seller must be reasonably satisfied that the signature is genuine, and that the person does indeed carry on the trade or profession stated. The seller must retain the certificate, giving it a reference number for identification. In an emergency a Schedule 1 poison may be supplied on an undertaking to supply a signed order in 24 hours.

Relaxations

The requirements relating to knowledge of the purchaser, and entries in the Poisons Book do not apply to the sale of poisons:

- for export *or*
- by wholesale.

There are specific relaxations for the sale of nicotine dusts (less than 4%), and rat poisons containing barium carbonate or zinc phosphide.

Schedule 1 poisons subject to extra controls

The following Schedule 1 poisons are subject to extra controls:

- Sodium and potassium arsenites
- Strychnine
- Fluoroacetic acid, its salts or fluoracetamide
- Thallium salts
- Zinc Phosphide.

They may only be sold or supplied:

- by wholesale
- for export *or*
- for education, research or analysis.

These poisons may also be sold or supplied in the circumstances outlined below.

Strychnine

Strychnine will no longer be approved for purchase or use for mole control from 1 September 2006. Its use falls under two EC Directives on Pesticides, Directives 91/414/EEC and 98/8/EC.

Fluoroacetic acid, its salts or fluoroacetamide may be sold to a person with a certificate authorising the use as a rodenticide. The certificate must state the quantity, and identify the place where it is to be used. It may only be used in ships, sewers, drains and dock warehouses. Certificates are issued by local authorities or port health authorities or by DEFRA.

Thallium salts may also be sold to:

(a)   local authorities or port health authorities
(b)   government departments
(c)   persons with a written authority issued by DEFRA authorising the use of thallium sulphate for killing rats, mice or moles for pest control
(d)   manufacturers who regularly use them in the manufacture of articles in the business (except thallium sulphate)
(e)   persons as an ingredient in any article not intended for consumption by persons or animals (except thallium sulphate).

Zinc phosphide may be sold:

(a)   to a local authority
(b)   to a government department
(c)   to a person for his trade or business.

Calcium, potassium and sodium cyanides may only be sold under the so-called *Section 4* "exemptions". Sales are not allowed for private purposes.

Section 4 *exemptions*

Exempted transactions of Part 1 Poisons may be made without pharmacist supervision, provided the sales are not made on retail premises: wholesale dealing, export to doctor, dentist, vet for professional purposes, for use in hospital or similar public institution, sale by wholesale to government department for education or research enables employers to meet any statutory obligation with respect to medical treatment of employees and sale to a person requiring the substance for trade or business.

The CHIP Regulations 2002

All poisons must be labelled and packaged in accordance with the Chemicals (Hazard Information and Packaging for Supply) Regulations 2002, SI No. 1689. The Regulations require the manufacturer or distributor of a "chemical" to decide if it is "hazardous" and then to label it appropriately and to supply a safety data sheet.

Classification

"Chemical" includes solids, liquids and gases, and includes pure chemical substances such as ethanol as well as preparations of chemicals such as cleaning fluid. They are classified as follows:

(1) Chemicals which are dangerous because of their physical or chemical properties: explosive, oxidizing, extremely flammable, highly flammable, flammable.
(2) Chemicals which are toxic, very toxic, harmful, corrosive, irritant or carcinogenic, mutagenic or toxic to reproduction.
(3) Chemicals which are dangerous for the environment.

Information

When classified chemicals are supplied in connection with work they must be accompanied by a "safety data sheet". Should any new safety information become available, the data sheet must be revised and copies given to anyone who obtained the chemical during the previous 12 months. There is thus an implicit requirement to keep records of sales for use in connection with work. The information in the data sheets must be given under standard headings.

Labelling

The Regulations set out details of labelling which include

- the name and address of supplier
- name of the chemical
- the type of danger
- warnings about use
- EU number
- warning pictograms.

Packaging

Chemicals must be packaged safely. Toxic, very toxic and corrosive chemicals which are sold to the public must be in containers with child-resistant closures. This applies regardless of the quantity. It also applies to solid products. Tactile danger warnings must be on containers sold to the public of chemicals which are harmful, highly flammable, extremely flammable, toxic, very toxic or corrosive.

Advertisements

Adverts must mention the type of hazard that is mentioned on the label.

Exemptions

Some products are exempt from the CHIP regulations because they are controlled in other ways, e.g. radioactive substances. The CHIP Regulations do not apply to preparations intended for use as cosmetics or medicinal products.

The Environmental Protection Act 1990

This Act places a duty of care on "waste producers" to dispose of "controlled waste" legally. Waste producers are persons in business, but not householders where their own waste is concerned.

The Special Waste Regulations 2005, SI No. 894, came into effect on 16 July 2005. Under these Regulations, cytotoxic and cytostatic medicines are automatically classed as "hazardous".

Every person who produces or stores hazardous waste must notify the Environment Agency, except where the premises are "shop premises" and the waste arises as a result of the activity of the shop. Thus a pharmacy which dispenses prescriptions and accepts waste from individuals and households will be exempt from notification requirements. Different types of hazardous waste may not be mixed. Hazardous waste may not be mixed with non-hazardous waste.

COSHH

The Control of Substances Hazardous to Health (COSHH) Regulations 2002, SI No. 2677, affect the use of hazardous substances in a work situation, by laying down measures which an employer must take to control hazardous substances and to protect people who are exposed to such substances.

Regulation 6 requires that an employer may not carry on any work that is liable to expose any person to any substance hazardous to health, unless a suitable and sufficient assessment of the risks has been made.

What is a substance hazardous to health?

A substance hazardous to health is defined as:

> any natural or artificial substance: solid, liquid, gas, vapour or hazardous micro-organism, and certain dust levels.

Substances hazardous to health can include

(1)   any substance classed as toxic, very toxic, harmful, corrosive or irritant
(2)   any micro-organism
(3)   any dust
(4)   any substance which has a prescribed maximum exposure limit, e.g. formaldehyde
(5)   any other substance which can adversely affect the health.

Helpfully, the Regulations state that a substance is *not* hazardous when it is at a level that nearly all the population can be exposed to it, repeatedly, without ill effect.
Certain situations are specifically excluded from COSHH:

(a)   those covered by the Control of Lead at Work Regulations 1980
(b)   those covered by the Control of Asbestos at Work Regulations 2002
(c)   when the hazard is radio-activity
(d)   when the hazard is the explosive or flammable properties of the substance

(e) underground mines

(f) medicines administered to patients.

What must the employer do?

The employer must first of all decide whether or not any substance is potentially hazardous. This must be done by a competent person.

The employer must then:

(1) assess the risk to health from the use of the substance in the workplace
(2) decide what precautions are needed
(3) introduce appropriate measures to control the risk
(4) tell employees about the risk, and about what precautions must be taken
(5) ensure that precautions are taken
(6) if appropriate, monitor the exposure and carry out health surveillance.

Assessment

The assessment must be carried out by a competent person. The results of the assessment must be made available to staff.

If the assessment indicates a risk, then the employer must take steps to prevent exposure. If prevention is impossible then the exposure must be reasonably controlled (Regulation 7).

Packaging waste

The Producer Responsibility Obligations (Packaging Waste) Regulations 1997, SI No. 648, implement the European Directive 94/62/EEC on the recycling of waste. The Regulations are made under the Environment Act 1995.

The Regulations place a "producer responsibility" on businesses involved in the packaging chain to recover and recycle certain percentages of packaging waste. The obligation applies to businesses with a turnover of more than £5 million a year and which handle more than 50 tonnes of packaging a year. Packaging which contained "special waste" is partially exempted from the regulations. Smaller businesses are subject to a requirement to keep records of the tonnage of waste handled each year and of any steps taken to promote the recovery of this packaging.

Dangerous Substances and Explosive Atmospheres Regulations 2002

These Regulations require businesses to carry out risk assessments when using potentially dangerous substances. They must provide measures to eliminate or reduce as far as possible the identified explosion or fire risks.

Food Safety Act 1990

The Food Premises (Registration) Regulations 1991 require all premises which sell food to be registered with the local authority. It is an offence to use unregistered premises for a food business. Food includes packed baby foods, confectionery, etc.

The General Food Regulations 2004 require food retailers to keep records of the source of food items. Details of the purchaser must be kept if the supply is a wholesale supply. Food includes baby foods, baby milks and dietary supplements which are not medicinal products.

The Offensive Weapons Act 1996

Section 6 of the Act prohibits the sale of knives and similar objects to people under 16-year old. The prohibited items include "any knife blade or razor blade" and "any other article which has a blade or is sharply pointed and which is made or adapted for causing injury to the person". Items in pharmacies which might fall within these wide definitions include corn knives, metal nail files, scissors and the like.

Chapter 19

Patient Group Directions

What are Patient Group Directions

Patient Group Directions (PGDs) (formerly termed "Group Protocols") are written instructions for the supply or administration of named medicines to groups of patients who are not individually identified before they present for treatment. They are documents which make it legal for medicines to be given to groups of patients – for example in a mass casualty situation – without individual prescriptions having to be written for each patient. They can also be used to authorise persons who are not "prescribers", for example paramedics, to legally supply and to administer the medicine in question.

The POM Order contains the following definition in Article 1.

"Patient Group Direction" means,

(a) in connection with the supply of a prescription only medicine as referred to in Article 12A(2), 12B, 12C, 12D or 12E, a written direction relating to the supply and administration of a description or class of prescription only medicine; or

(b) in connection with the administration of a prescription only medicine as referred to in Article 12A(2), 12B, 12C, 12D or 12E, a written direction relating to the administration of a description or class of prescription only medicine,

and which, in the case of either (a) or (b),

(i)   is signed by a doctor or dentist, and by a pharmacist; and
(ii) relates to supply and administration, or to administration, to persons generally (subject to any exclusions which may be set out in the Direction).

The legislation introducing PGDs applies mainly to the NHS. It includes activity in the private and voluntary sectors which is funded by the NHS. It covers treatment provided by NHS Trusts, PCTs, HAs, GP practices, dental practices, Walk-in Centres, NHS-funded family planning clinics, and police and prison services. Apart from those situations where services are funded by the NHS it does not apply to private hospitals or other private or voluntary services.

Differences between PGDs and Written Directions

Article 12 of the POM Order allows for "Written Directions" to authorise the supply or administration of a POM within the course of business of a hospital. Such directions are patient-specific.

PGDs allow a range of specified health care professionals to supply or administer a medicine directly to a patient with an identified clinical condition without them necessarily seeing a prescriber. The health care professional working within the PGD is responsible for assessing that the patient fits the criteria set out in the PGD.

A patient specific direction is used once a patient has been assessed by a prescriber. The prescriber (doctor, dentist or independent nurse prescriber) then instructs another health care professional in writing to supply or administer a medicine directly to that named patient or patients.

Generally speaking, patient-specific directions are a direct instruction and do not require an assessment of the patient by the health care professional instructed to supply or administer the medicine.

Types of PGD

At present there are five main types:

(1) PGD which authorises specified health professionals to supply medicines on behalf of an NHS body;
(2) PGD which authorises persons assisting in providing primary care NHS services;
(3) PGD authorising the owner of a pharmacy to supply a medicine;
(4) PGD authorising the supply and administration of prescription only medicines by independent hospitals, clinics and agencies;
(5) PGD authorising health professionals to assist the provision of health care by or on behalf of the police, the prison services or the armed forces.

Background

The legal framework for medicines control was traditionally based on the principle that doctors prescribe for individual patients. Over time the definition of prescriber has been widened. Some health professionals, e.g. paramedics are authorised to use medicines in defined circumstances.

In some cases, the legal necessity to have a prescription signed by a doctor and dispensed by a pharmacist restricted the development of new services that were both safe and effective.

To facilitate the development of patient-focused services, organisation within the NHS began to use "group protocols" under the previous Article 12. Group protocols enabled nurses, and other health care professionals to supply or administer medicines directly to certain groups of patients.

In 1998 a report on the Supply and Administration of Medicines under Group Protocols was published. The Report recommended that the legal position about protocols for supply should be clarified, and in August 2000 the relevant medicines legislation was amended in respect of the NHS and those services funded by the NHS that were provided by the private, voluntary or charitable sector.

Subsequently, the legislation was further amended to permit the sale, supply or administration of medicines under PGDs in specified healthcare establishments throughout the United Kingdom provided through the private, charitable or voluntary sector, and in certain UK Crown establishments.

PGDs do not extend to independent and public sector care homes or to those independent sector schools that provide healthcare entirely outside the NHS. They cannot produce PGDs for use within their individual institutions. However, health care professionals who visit patients in nursing and care homes in their routine practice can use PGDs authorised by their own organisations for domicillary visits.

The law

The relevant modifications to the provisions about sale or supply in and under the MA 1968 are contained in: The Prescription Only Medicines (Human Use) Order 1997, SI No. 1830, which has been amended by:

- The Prescription Only Medicines (Human Use) Amendment Order 2000, SI 2000 No. 1917
- The Prescription Only Medicines (Human Use) Amendment (No. 2) Order 2000, SI No. 2899
- The Prescription Only Medicines (Human Use) Amendment Order 2003, SI 2003 No. 696
- The Prescription Only Medicines (Human Use) Amendment (No. 2) Order 2004, SI 2004 No. 1189.

The legislation about wholesaling to persons using PGDs is contained in The Medicines (Sale or Supply) (Miscellaneous Provisions) Regulations 1980, SI No. 1923, which has been amended by:

- The Medicines (Sale or Supply) (Miscellaneous Provisions) Amendment (No. 2) Regulations 2000, SI 2000 No. 1918
- The Medicines (Sale and Supply) (Miscellaneous Provisions) Amendment Regulations 2003, SI 2003 No. 698.

Changes made to The Medicines (Pharmacy and General Sale – Exemption) Order 1980, SI No. 1924 by:

- The Medicines (Pharmacy and General Sale – Exemption) Amendment Order 2000, SI 2000 No. 1919
- The Medicines (Pharmacy and General Sale – Exemption) Amendment Order 2003, SI No. 697
- The Medicines (Pharmacy and General Sale – Exemption) Amendment (No. 2) Order 2004, SI No. 1190 deal similarly with GSL medicines.

All the Orders can be accessed on www.hmso.gov.uk.

Schedule 7 of the POM Order, as amended, sets out information which is required for a legal PGD.

Information in the PGD itself

The legislation specifies that each PGD must contain the following information:

- the name of the business to which the direction applies;
- the date the direction comes into force and the date it expires;
- a description of the medicine(s) to which the direction applies;
- class of health professional who may supply or administer the medicine;
- signature of a doctor or dentist, as appropriate, and a pharmacist;
- signature by an appropriate organisation;
- the clinical condition or situation to which the direction applies;
- a description of those patients excluded from treatment under the direction;
- a description of the circumstances in which further advice should be sought from a doctor (or dentist, as appropriate) and arrangements for referral;
- details of appropriate dosage and maximum total dosage, quantity, pharmaceutical form and strength, route and frequency of administration, and minimum or maximum period over which the medicine should be administered;
- relevant warnings, including potential adverse reactions;
- details of any necessary follow-up action and the circumstances;
- a statement of the records to be kept for audit purposes.

(Part I of Schedule 7 of the POM Order, inserted by The Prescription Only Medicines (Human Use) Amendment Order 2000, SI 2000 No. 1917.)

The groups who may supply or administer

The qualified health professionals who may sell, supply or administer medicines under a PGD are nurses, midwives, health visitors, optometrists, pharmacists, chiropodists, radiographers, orthoptists, physiotherapists, ambulance paramedics, dietitians, occupational therapists, speech and language therapists, prosthetists and orthotists. They must be named individuals, either in the PGD or in a separate document. They must be registered members of their profession and act within their own council's code of professional conduct and as described in the PGD.

The signatures required

The PGD must be signed by a senior doctor (or, if appropriate, a dentist) and a pharmacist, both of whom should have been involved in developing the direction. Additionally, the PGD must be authorised by the relevant appropriate body as set out in the legislation.

Who signs for the appropriate body

Healthcare provider – Person by whom or on whose behalf the Direction must be signed.

An independent hospital, clinic or medical agency (England, Wales and Scotland only) – The registered provider and the manager if there is a relevant manager for the hospital, clinic or agency.

A nursing home (Northern Ireland only) – The registered provider and the manager if there is a relevant manager for the home that manager.

A police force in England or Wales – The chief officer of police for that police force and a doctor who is not employed/engaged or providing services to any police force.

A police force in Scotland – The chief constable of that police force and a doctor who is not employed/engaged or providing services to any police force.

The Police Service of Northern Ireland – The Chief Constable of the Police Service of Northern Ireland and a doctor who is not employed/engaged or providing services to any police force.

The prison service in England and Wales – The governor of the prison in relation to which the health care in question is being provided.

The prison service in Scotland – The Scottish Prison Service Management Board.

The prison service in Northern Ireland – The Northern Ireland Prison Service Management Board.

Her Majesty's Forces:

(i)   the Surgeon General,
(ii)   a Medical Director General, or
(iii)   a chief executive of an executive agency of the Ministry of Defence.

These requirements are set out in Part II of Schedule 7 of the POM Order, as amended by The Prescription Only Medicines (Human Use) Amendment Order 2000, SI 2000 No. 1917.

Organisations where PGDs may be used

- a Special Health Authority
- an NHS or Primary Care Trust
- a doctor's or dentist's practice, in the provision of NHS services
- a body not run by an NHS body, but providing treatment under an arrangement made with one of the NHS bodies in 1 or 2 above (e.g. a family planning clinic, health centre or Walk-In Centre)
- healthcare services provided by the Prison Services in the United Kingdom
- healthcare services provided by police forces in the United Kingdom
- healthcare services provided by the Defence Medical Services
- healthcare services provided by independent hospitals, clinics and medical agencies as defined in the Care Standards Act 2000, the Regulation of Care Act (Scotland) 2001 and equivalent arrangements in Northern Ireland.

PGDs can be used by all NHS organisations. In addition, those services funded by the NHS but provided by the private, voluntary or charitable sector can also use PGDs.

Labelling of supplied products

The EC Labelling and Leaflet Directive 92/27 applies to all supplies of medicines, including those supplied under PGDs. A PIL should be made available to patients treated under a PGDs.

Medicines without a Marketing Authorisation

The POM Order requires that only licensed medicines may be supplied under a PGD – e.g. Article 12A "at the time at which the product is supplied, a product licence, a marketing authorisation or a homoeopatic certificate of registration has effect in respect of it".

Exceptional products

Black triangle drugs (i.e. those recently licensed and subject to special reporting arrangements for adverse reactions) and medicines used outside the terms of the SPC (e.g. as used in some areas of specialist paediatric care) may be included in PGDs provided such use is exceptional, justified by current best clinical practice and that a direction clearly describes the status of the product. Where the medicine is for children, particular attention will be needed to specify any restrictions on the age, size and maturity of the child. Each PGD should clearly state when the product is being used outside the terms of the SPC and the documentation should include the reasons why, exceptionally, such use is necessary.

Controlled drugs

The Home Office have agreed to allow the supply and administration of substances on Schedule 4 (with the exclusion of anabolic steroids) and all substances on Schedule 5 to be included in PGDs. The Misuse of Drugs (Amendment) (No. 3) Regulations 2003, SI No. 2429, came into force on 15 October 2003.

These regulations also allow nurses to use PGDs for the supply and administration of Schedule 4 and Schedule 5 Controlled Drugs (with the exception of anabolic steroids) plus diamorphine for the treatment of cardiac pain by nurses in accident and emergency departments and coronary care units in hospitals. For full details see Home Office Circular 49/2003 www.homeoffice.gov.uk/docs2/ hoc4903.html.

Radiopharmaceuticals

The administration of radiopharmaceuticals continues to be regulated by the Medicines (Administration of Radioactive Substances) Regulations 1978 and should not be included in PGDs.

Guidance

For the NHS, guidance was issued in 2000 – HSC 2000/026.

The RPSGB issued guidance and a resource pack – http://www.rpsgb.org.uk/pdfs/pgdpack.pdf.

The relevant parts of the POM Order now read as follows:

Exemptions for the supply and administration of prescription only medicines by national health service bodies

12A – (1) The restrictions imposed by *Section 58(2)(a)* (restrictions on sale and supply) shall not apply to the supply of a prescription only medicine by:

(a)   the Common Services Agency
(b)   a Health Authority or Special Health Authority
(c)   an NHS trust
(d)   a Primary Care Trust or
(e)   where sub-paragraphs (a)–(d) do not apply, a person other than an excepted person, pursuant to an arrangement made with one of the persons specified in those sub-paragraphs for the supply of prescription only medicines, where the medicine is supplied for the purpose of being administered to a particular person in accordance with the written directions of a doctor or dentist relating to that person notwithstanding that those directions do not satisfy the conditions specified in Article 15(2).

(2) The restrictions imposed by *Section 58(2)* (restrictions on sale, supply and administration) shall not apply to the supply or, as the case may be, the administration of a prescription only medicine by –

(a)   the Common Services Agency
(b)   a Health Authority or Special Health Authority
(c)   an NHS trust
(d)   a Primary Care Trust or
(e)   where sub-paragraphs (a)–(d) do not apply, a person other than an excepted person, pursuant to an arrangement made with one of the persons specified in those sub-paragraphs for the supply or, as the case may be, the administration of prescription only medicines, and where the medicine is supplied for the purpose of being administered, or, as the case may be, is administered, to a particular person in accordance with a Patient Group Direction and where the conditions specified in Paragraph (3) are satisfied.

(3) The conditions referred to are that

(a)   the PGD relates to the supply or, as the case may be, the administration, by the person who supplies or administers the medicine, of a description or class of prescription only medicine, and the Direction has effect at the time at which the medicine is supplied or, as the case may be, is administered;
(b)   the PGD contains the particulars specified in Part I of Schedule 7 to this Order (but with the omission of Paragraph (c) of that Part in the case of a Direction which relates to administration only);
(c)   the PGD is signed on behalf of the person specified in Column 2 of the Table in Part II of Schedule 7 to this Order ("the authorising person") against the entry in Column 1 of that Table for the class of person by whom the medicine is supplied or administered;
(d)   the individual who supplies or, as the case may be, administers the medicine belongs to one of the classes of individual specified in Part III of Schedule 7 to this Order, and is designated in writing, on behalf of the authorising person, for the purpose of the supply or, as the case may be, the administration of prescription only medicines under the PGD; and
(e)   at the time at which the medicine is supplied or, as the case may be, is administered, a product licence, a marketing authorization or a homoeopathic certificate of registration has effect in respect of it.

(4) In this article, "excepted person" means

(a)   a doctor or dentist; or
(b)   a person lawfully conducting an RPB within the meaning of *Section 69*.

Exemption for health professionals who supply or administer prescription only medicines under a Patient Group Direction in order to assist doctors or dentists in providing national health services

12B – (1) The restrictions imposed by *Section 58(2)* (sale, supply and administration) shall not apply to the supply or, as the case may be, the administration of a prescription only medicine by an individual belonging to one of the classes specified in Part III of Schedule 7 to this Order where:

(a)   the individual supplies or, as the case may be, administers the medicine in order to assist a doctor or dentist in the provision of, respectively, NHS primary medical services or NHS primary dental services;
(b)   the medicine is supplied for the purpose of being administered, or, as the case may be, is administered, in accordance with a Patient Group Direction; and
(c)   the conditions specified in Paragraph (2) are satisfied.

(2) The conditions referred to are that

(a)   the PGD relates to the supply or, as the case may be, the administration of a description or class of prescription only medicine in order to assist the doctor or dentist in question in providing the services referred to in Paragraph (1)(a) (whether or not it also relates to such supply or administration in order to assist any other doctor or dentist);
(b)   the PGD has effect at the time at which the medicine is supplied or, as the case may be, is administered;
(c)   the PGD contains the particulars specified in Part I of Schedule 7 to this Order (but with the omission of Paragraph (c) of that Part in the case of a Direction which relates to administration only);
(d)   the PGD is signed:

    (i)   by the doctor or dentist in question or, alternatively, where the Direction also relates to supply or administration in order to assist one or more other doctors or dentists, as referred to in sub-paragraph (a), by one of those other doctors or dentists; and
    (ii) on behalf of the health authority:

        (a)   in the case of the provision of general medical services or general dental services, with which an arrangement has been made for the provision of those services; or
        (b)   in the case of the performance of personal medical services or personal dental services, which is a party to the pilot scheme under which those services are provided;

(e)   the individual referred to in Paragraph (1) is designated in writing for the purpose of the supply or, as the case may be, the administration of prescription only medicines under the Patient Group Direction, by the doctor or dentist in question, or, alternatively, where the Direction also relates to supply or administration in order to assist one or more other doctors or dentists, as referred to in sub-paragraph (a), by one of those other doctors or dentists; and

(f)   at the time at which the medicine is supplied or, as the case may be, is administered, a product licence, a marketing authorization or a homoeopathic certificate of registration has effect in respect of it.

(3) In this article:

(a)   a reference to the provision of NHS primary dental services shall be construed as a reference to:

   (i)   in relation to England and Wales, the provision of general dental services under Part II of the National Health Service Act 1977, or the performance of personal dental services in connection with a pilot scheme under the National Health Service (Primary Care) Act 1997[16];

   (ii)   in relation to Scotland, the provision of general dental services under Part II of the National Health Service (Scotland) Act 1978, or the performance of personal dental services in connection with a pilot scheme under the National Health Service (Primary Care) Act 1997; and

   (iii) in relation to Northern Ireland, the provision of general dental services under the Health and Personal Social Services (Northern Ireland) Order 1972[17], or the performance of personal dental services in connection with a pilot scheme under the Health Services (Primary Care) (Northern Ireland) Order 1997[18];

(b)   a reference to the provision of NHS primary medical services shall be construed as a reference to:

   (i)   in relation to England and Wales, the provision of general medical services under Part II of the National Health Service Act 1977, or the performance of personal medical services in connection with a pilot scheme under the National Health Service (Primary Care) Act 1997;

   (ii)   in relation to Scotland, the provision of general medical services under Part II of the National Health Service (Scotland) Act 1978, or the performance of personal medical services in connection with a pilot scheme under the National Health Service (Primary Care) Act 1997; and

   (iii) in relation to Northern Ireland, the provision of general medical services under the Health and Personal Social Services (Northern Ireland) Order 1972, or the performance of personal medical services in connection with a pilot scheme under the Health Services (Primary Care) (Northern Ireland) Order 1997.

Exemption for persons conducting a retail pharmacy business who supply or administer prescription only medicines under a Patient Group Direction
12C – (1) The restrictions imposed by *Section 58(2)* (restrictions on sale, supply and administration) shall not apply to the supply or, as the case may be, the

administration of a prescription only medicine by a person lawfully conducting a retail pharmacy business within the meaning of *Section 69* where:

(a) the medicine is supplied or, as the case may be, is administered by such a person pursuant to an arrangement made with:

    (i)   a body referred to in Article 12A(a)–(d),

    (ii)   an authority or person carrying on the business of an establishment or agency referred to in Article 12D(1),

    (iii) a force or service referred to in Article 12E(1)(a)(i)–(iii), or

    (iv)   Her Majesty's Forces, for the supply or, as the case may be, the administration of prescription only medicines;

(b) the medicine is supplied for the purpose of being administered or, as the case may be, is administered, to a particular person in accordance with a PGD; and

(c) the conditions specified in Paragraph (2) are satisfied.

(2) The conditions referred to are that

(a) the PGD relates to the supply or, as the case may be, the administration of a description or class of prescription only medicine by the person lawfully conducting a retail pharmacy business who supplies or, as the case may be, administers the prescription only medicine, and the Direction has effect at the time at which the medicine is supplied or, as the case may be, is administered;

(b) the PGD contains the particulars specified in Part I of Schedule 7 to this Order (but with the omission of Paragraph (c) of that Part in the case of a Direction which relates to administration only);

(c) the PGD is signed:

    (i)   in the case of an arrangement with a body referred to in Article 12A(a)–(d), on behalf of that body,

    (ii)   in the case of an arrangement with an authority or person carrying on the business of an establishment or agency referred to in Article 12D(1), by or on behalf of the relevant provider and, if there is a relevant manager for the establishment or agency, that manager,

    (iii) in the case of an arrangement with a prison service, by or on behalf of the person specified in Column 2 of the Table in Part IIA of Schedule 7 to this Order against the entry in Column 1 of that Table for that service,

    (iv)   in the case of an arrangement with a police force or the Police Service of Northern Ireland –

        (a) by or on behalf of the person specified in Column 2 of the Table in Part IIA of Schedule 7 to this Order against the entry in Column 1 of that Table for that force or service, and

        (b) a doctor who is not employed or engaged by, and who does not provide services under arrangements made with, any police force or the Police Service of Northern Ireland, and

    (v)   in the case of an arrangement with Her Majesty's Forces, by or on behalf of a person specified in Column 2 of the Table in Part IIA of

Schedule 7 to this Order against the entry in Column 1 of that Table for Her Majesty's Forces; and

(c) where the prescription only medicine is administered by the person lawfully conducting a retail pharmacy business within the meaning of *Section 69*, the individual who administers the medicine belongs to one of the classes of individual specified in Part III of Schedule 7 to this Order, and is designated in writing:

    (i) in the case of an arrangement with a body referred to in Article 12A(a)–(d), on behalf of that body,

    (ii) in the case of an arrangement with an authority or person carrying on the business of an establishment or agency referred to in Article 12D(1), by or on behalf of the relevant provider or, if there is a relevant manager for the establishment or agency, that relevant manager,

    (iii) in the case of an arrangement with a force or service referred to in Article 12E(1)(a)(i)–(iii), by or on behalf of the person specified in Column 2 of the Table in Part IIA of Schedule 7 to this Order against the entry in Column 1 of that Table for that force or service, or

    (iv) in the case of an arrangement with Her Majesty's Forces, by or on behalf of a person specified in Column 2 of the Table in Part IIA of Schedule 7 to this Order against the entry in Column 1 of that Table for Her Majesty's Forces, for the purpose of the administration of prescription only medicines under the PGD; and

(d) at the time at which the medicine is supplied or, as the case may be, is administered, a product licence, a marketing authorization or a homoeopathic certificate of registration has effect in respect of it.

Exemption for the supply and administration of prescription only medicines by independent hospitals, clinics and agencies

12D – (1) The restrictions imposed by *Section 58(2)* (restrictions on sale, supply and administration) shall not apply to the supply or, as the case may be, the administration of a prescription only medicine in the course of the business of:

(a) in England, Wales or Scotland:

    (i) an independent hospital
    (ii) an independent clinic or
    (iii) an independent medical agency or

(b) in Northern Ireland, a nursing home,

where the medicine is supplied for the purpose of being administered, or, as the case may be, is administered, to a particular person in accordance with a PGD and where the conditions specified in Paragraph (2) are satisfied.

(2) The conditions referred to are that

(a)   the PGD relates to the supply or, as the case may be, the administration, by the person who supplies or administers the medicine, of a description or class of pre-scription only medicine, and the Direction has effect at the time at which the medi-cine is supplied or, as the case may be, is administered;

(b)   the PGD contains the particulars specified in Part I of Schedule 7 to this Order (but with the omission of Paragraph (c) of that Part in the case of a Direction which relates to administration only);

(c)   the Patient Group Direction is signed:

    (i)   by or on behalf of the registered provider, and

    (ii)   if there is a relevant manager for the independent hospital, clinic or agency, or nursing home, by that manager;

(d)   the individual who supplies or, as the case may be, administers the medicine belongs to one of the classes of individual specified in Part III of Schedule 7 to this Order, and is designated in writing:

    (i)   by or on behalf of the registered provider, or

    (ii)   if there is a relevant manager for the independent hospital, clinic or agency, or nursing home, by that manager,

for the purpose of the supply or, as the case may be, the administration of pre-scription only medicines under the Patient Group Direction; and

(e)   at the time at which the medicine is supplied or, as the case may be, is administered, a product licence, a marketing authorization or a homoeo-pathic certificate of registration has effect in respect of it.

Exemption for health professionals who supply or administer prescription only medicines under a Patient Group Direction in order to assist the provision of health care by or on behalf of the police, the prison services or the armed forces

12E – (1) The restrictions imposed by *Section 58(2)* (sale, supply and administration) shall not apply to the supply or, as the case may be, the administration of a prescription only medicine by an individual belonging to one of the classes specified in Part III of Schedule 7 to this Order where:

(a)   the individual supplies or, as the case may be, administers the medicine in order to assist the provision of health care by, on behalf of, or under arrange-ments made by –

    (i)   a police force in England, Wales or Scotland,

    (ii)   the Police Service of Northern Ireland,

    (iii) a prison service, or

    (iv)   Her Majesty's Forces;

(b)   the medicine is supplied for the purpose of being administered, or, as the case may be, is administered, in accordance with a Patient Group Direction; and

(c)   the conditions specified in Paragraph (2) are satisfied.

(2) The conditions referred to are that

(a) the Patient Group Direction relates to the supply or, as the case may be, the administration of a description or class of prescription only medicine in order to assist the provision of health care by, or on behalf of, or under arrangements made by the police force or service, the prison service or, as the case may be, Her Majesty's Forces;

(b) the Patient Group Direction has effect at the time at which the medicine is supplied or, as the case may be, is administered;

(c) the Patient Group Direction contains the particulars specified in Part I of Schedule 7 to this Order (but with the omission of Paragraph (c) of that Part in the case of a Direction which relates to administration only);

(d) the Patient Group Direction is signed:

  (i)   by or on behalf of a person specified in Column 2 of the Table in Part IIA of Schedule 7 to this Order ("the authorising person") against the entry in Column 1 of that Table for the police force or service, the prison service or Her Majesty's Forces by whom, or on whose behalf, the health care is provided, or with whom arrangements are made for the provision of such care; and

  (ii) in the case of a police force or the Police Service of Northern Ireland, by a doctor who is not employed or engaged by, and who does not provide services under arrangements made with, any police force or the Police Service of Northern Ireland;

(e) the individual referred to in Paragraph (1) is designated in writing, by or on behalf of the authorising person, for the purpose of the supply or, as the case may be, the administration of prescription only medicines under the Patient Group Direction; and

(f) at the time at which the medicine is supplied or, as the case may be, is administered, a product licence, a marketing authorization or a homoeopathic certificate of registration has effect in respect of it.

Chapter 20

Non-Medical Prescribing

Background

The final report of the Review of Prescribing, Supply and Administration of Medicines (1999) recommended that two types of prescriber should be recognised:

(1) an independent prescriber who would be responsible for the assessment of patients with undiagnosed conditions and for decisions about the clinical management required, including prescribing;

(2) a dependent prescriber who would be responsible for the continuing care of patients who have been clinically assessed by an independent prescriber.

Continuing care

The Report envisaged that this continuing care might include prescribing, which would be informed by clinical guidelines and be consistent with individual treatment plans, or might consist of continuing an established treatment by issuing repeat prescriptions, with the authority to adjust the dose or dosage form according to the patients' needs.

The Review recommended that there should be provision for regular clinical review by the assessing clinician.

The term "Dependent Prescriber" used in the Report has been replaced by the term "Supplementary Prescriber".

The review is available at
http://www.dh.gov.uk/assetRoot/04/07/71/53/04077153.pdf.

Supplementary prescribing

According to the DOH the supplementary prescribing program is designed "to ease the burden on doctors and improve access to medicines."

Supplementary Prescribing involves a voluntary partnership between an independent prescriber, who must be a doctor or dentist, and a supplementary prescriber to implement an agreed patient-specific clinical management plan (CMP) with the patient's agreement.

Supplementary Prescribing has two tiers:

(1) doctors or dentists ("independent prescribers") are responsible for the diagnosis of the patient, and for determining the class or description of medicines that may be prescribed by the supplementary prescriber under a clinical management plan for the patient; and

(2) other health professionals ("supplementary prescribers") who are responsible for the continuing care of the patient in accordance with a Clinical Management Plan. They have authority to prescribe specific medicines for particular medical conditions in accordance with the Plan.

The supplementary prescriber may be a:

- nurse
- midwife
- pharmacist
- physiotherapist
- chiropodist/podiatrist
- radiographer
- optometrist.

Legislation

Section 63 of the HSC Act 2001 enabled the Government to extend prescribing responsibilities to other health professions. It also enabled the introduction of new types of prescriber, including the concept of a supplementary prescriber, by allowing Ministers to make regulations which attach conditions to their prescribing.

Section 42 (for England and Wales) and *Section 44* (Scotland) of the Act relate to the dispensing by community pharmacists of prescriptions written by these new prescribers.

Amendments to the POM Order and to NHS regulations enabled the introduction of supplementary prescribing for first level registered nurses, registered midwives and registered pharmacists from April 2003.

Amendments in April 2005 enabled chiropodists/podiatrists, physiotherapists and radiographers to become supplementary prescribers. Further amendments in July 2005 enabled optometrists to become supplementary prescribers.

The definition of "supplementary prescriber" was inserted in the POM (Human Use) Order 1997 by SI 2003/696 and amended by SI 2004/1771, SI 2005/765 and SI 2005/1507. It now reads:

Supplementary prescriber means

(a) a first level nurse
(b) a pharmacist
(c) a registered midwife
(d) a person whose name is registered in the part of the register maintained by the Health Professions Council in pursuance of Article 5 of the Health Professions Order 2001 relating to

  (i) chiropodists and podiatrists
  (ii) physiotherapists or
  (iii) radiographers: diagnostic or therapeutic or

(e) a registered optometrist

against whose name is recorded in the relevant register an annotation signifying that he is qualified to order drugs, medicines and appliances as a supplementary prescriber.

Definition of supplementary prescribing

The working definition of supplementary prescribing is

> a voluntary partnership between an independent prescriber (a doctor or dentist) and a supplementary prescriber to implement an agreed patient-specific Clinical Management Plan with the patient's agreement.

The Clinical Management Plan

Before supplementary prescribing can take place, it is obligatory for an agreed CMP to be in place (written or electronic) relating to a named patient and to that patient's specific condition(s) to be managed by the supplementary prescriber. This should be included in the patient record.

The POM (Human Use) Order 1997, as amended by 2003/696, defines a CMP:

A "clinical management plan" means a written plan (which may be amended from time to time) relating to the treatment of an individual patient agreed by:

(a) the patient to whom the plan relates
(b) the doctor or dentist who is a party to the plan and
(c) any supplementary prescriber who is to prescribe, give directions for administration or administer under the plan.

The Regulations specify that the CMP must include the following:

- The name of the patient to whom the plan relates.
- The illness or conditions which may be treated by the supplementary prescriber.
- The date on which the plan is to take effect, and when it is to be reviewed by the doctor or dentist who is party to the plan.
- Reference to the class or description of medicines or types of appliances which may be prescribed or administered under the plan.
- Any restrictions or limitations of strength or dose of any medicine which may be prescribed or administered under the plan, and any period of administration or use of any medicine or appliance which may be prescribed or administered under the plan. Relevant warnings about known sensitivities of the patient to, or known, difficulties that the patient may have with particular medicines or appliances.
- The arrangements for notification of:

    (a) Suspected or known reactions of clinical significance to any medicine which may be prescribed or administered under the plan, and suspected or known clinically significant adverse reactions to any other medicine taken at the same time as any medicine prescribed or administered under the plan, and

(b) Incidents occurring with the appliance which might lead, might have led or has led to the death or serious deterioration of state of health of the patient.

- The circumstances in which the supplementary prescriber should refer to, or seek the advice of, the doctor or dentist who is party to the plan.

What may be prescribed by supplementary prescribers

Nurse and pharmacist supplementary prescribers are able to prescribe any medicines that are listed in an agreed Clinical Management Plan.

These may include any:

- General Sales List, Pharmacy or Prescription Only Medicine prescribable at NHS expense
- Antimicrobials
- "Black triangle" drugs and those products suggested by the BNF to be "less suitable" for prescribing Controlled Drugs (except those listed in Schedule 1 of "The Misuse of Drugs Regulations 2001" that are not intended for medicinal use).
- Products used outside their UK licensed indications (i.e. "off-label" use). Such use must have the joint agreement of both prescribers and the status of the drug should be recorded in the CMP.
- Unlicensed drugs (that is, a product that is not licensed in the UK).

There are no legal restrictions on the clinical conditions that may be dealt with by a supplementary prescriber.

The DOH advises that supplementary prescribing is primarily intended for use in managing specific long-term medical conditions or health needs affecting the patient. However, acute episodes occurring within long-term conditions may be included in these arrangements, provided they are included in the CMP.

Controlled drugs

The Misuse of Drugs Regulations 2001 were amended by the Misuse of Drugs (Amendment) Regulations 2005 No. 271 which came into force on 14 March 2005. This enabled nurse and pharmacist supplementary prescribers to prescribe CDs in Schedules 2, 3 and 4.

The GMS/PMS regulations which came into effect on 14 April 2005 enable supplementary prescribers to prescribe CDs in NHS primary care situations. AHPs supplementary prescribers may not prescribe CDs.

Unlicensed medicines

The Medicines for Human Use (Marketing Authorisations, etc.) Amendment Regulations 2005, SI No. 768, came into affect on 14 April 2005 and allows supplementary prescribers to prescribe unlicensed medicines.

Registration conditions for undertake supplementary prescribing

A nurse supplementary prescriber must be a 1st level Registered Nurse or Registered Midwife whose name in each case is held on the NMC professional register, with an annotation signifying that the nurse has successfully completed an approved programme of preparation and training for supplementary prescribing.

A pharmacist supplementary prescriber must be a registered pharmacist whose name is held on the membership register of the RPSGB, with an annotation signifying that the pharmacist has successfully completed an approved programme of training for supplementary prescribing.

A supplementary prescriber who is a chiropodist/podiatrist, physiotherapist or radiographer must be a registered professional whose name is held on the relevant part of the Health Professions Council membership register, with an annotation signifying that the individual registrant has successfully completed an approved programme of training for supplementary prescribing. A supplementary prescriber who is an optometrist must be a registered optometrist whose name is entered in the register of optometrists maintained under *Section 7(a)* of the Opticians Act 1989.

Independent prescribing

District nurses and health visitors are able to prescribe independently from a limited formulary, mostly dressings. This Formulary is referred to as the Nurse Prescribers Formulary for District Nurses and Health Visitors. It is set out in the BNF and in the Drug Tariff. It contains 13 POMs, some P medicines and GSL medicines.

Registration

A definition of "district nurse/health visitor prescriber" was inserted into the POM Order by The Prescription Only Medicines (Human Use) Amendment Order 2002, SI No. 549 as:

a person who –

(i)   is registered in Part 1 or 12 of the professional register, and

(ii) has a district nursing qualification additionally recorded in the professional register under rule 11 of the Nurses, Midwives and Health Visitors Rules 1983[4]; or

(b) a person who is registered in Part 11 of the professional register as a health visitor, against whose name (in each case) is recorded in the professional register an annotation signifying that he is qualified to order drugs, medicines and appliances for patients.

Independent Nurse Prescribers

Nurses who have undertaken further training are able to independently prescribe from a larger range of medicines. All 1st level nurses and registered midwives may undertake the training.

The Nurse Prescribers Extended Formulary (NPEF) was introduced in April 2002, originally for four therapeutic areas: minor injuries, minor ailments, health promotion and palliative care. It was expanded in 2003 and again in May 2005, to cover an extended range of medicines and conditions outside the original therapeutic areas, mainly for emergency care and first contact care. At the time of writing the NPEF now contains around 240 Prescription Only Medicines (POMs) – including some controlled drugs and over 6,100 Extended Formulary Nurse Prescribers can diagnose, prescribe for and manage 110 medical conditions.

There are currently about 6000 Extended Formulary Nurse Prescribers.

Registration

A definition of "extended formulary nurse prescriber" was inserted into the POM Order by The Prescription Only Medicines (Human Use) Amendment Order 2002, Sl No. 549, and altered by the POM (Human Use) Amendment Order 2003, Sl No. 696. It now reads as:

a person –

(a) who is a first level nurse; and
(b) against whose name is recorded in the professional register an annotation signifying that he is qualified to order drugs, medicines and appliances from the Extended Formulary.

In the same Order a "first level nurse" is defined as "a person registered in Parts 1, 3, 5, 8, 10, 11, 12, 13, 14 or 15 of the professional register."

Use of NHS prescriptions

The same Order altered the definition of "health prescription" to allow the use of NHS prescription forms.

Further extension of prescribing

In March 2006 the DOH announced that later in the year it would introduce legislation to allow Extended Formulary Nurse Prescribers (and pharmacist independent prescribers) to prescribe any licensed medicine for any medical condition. The Extended Formulary will then cease to exist.

The nurse prescribers will be known as Independent Nurse Prescribers.

Under the new scheme the nurses prescribing from the Nurse Prescribers Formulary for District Nurses and Health Visitors will in future be called "Community Practitioner Nurse Prescribers".

Prescribing limitations

The 2002 POM Amendment Order inserted Article 3A:

Prescribing by extended formulary nurse prescribers

3A. – (1) Subject to Paragraph (2), the description and classes of medicinal products in relation to which extended formulary nurse prescribers are appropriate practitioners are those prescription only medicines which consist of, or contain, one or more of the substances specified in column 1 of Schedule 3A, but which do not contain any other substance or combination of substances which is a prescription only medicine not included in Schedule 3A.

(2) An extended formulary nurse prescriber may –

(a) give a prescription for a medicinal product referred to in paragraph (1); or
(b) if that medicinal product is for parenteral administration –

(i) administer that medicinal product, or
(ii) give directions for the administration of that medicinal product,

only where he complies with any condition as to the cases or circumstances in which he may do so that is specified by virtue of Paragraph (3).

(3) If the entry in column 2 of Schedule 3A relating to a substance specifies one or more requirements as to use, route of administration or pharmaceutical form, it is a condition for the purposes of paragraph (2) that a medicinal product which consists of, or contains, that substance is administered, or is prescribed or directed for administration, in accordance with the specified requirements.

INPs can prescribe borderline substances but DOH guidance will restrict these to the substances on the ACBS list.

INPs can prescribe for off-label and off-licence use but should do so only where it is best practice.

INPs must talke full responsibility for such prescribing.

INPs can prescribe the CDs that are currently on the Extended Formulary.

INPs cannot prescribe unlicensed medicines except as part of a supplementary prescribing arrangement within a Clinical Management Plan.

Independent Pharmacist Prescribers

Similar legislation will apply to Independent Pharmacist Prescribers. Pharmacist prescribers will have their names in the RPSGB Register annotated to indicate their status as prescribers.

Administration

Medicines legislation does not specifically address the issue of administration of medicines except where the product is for injection. Then it may only be:

- self-administered;
- administered by a doctor or, subject to certain limitations, an independent nurse prescriber or supplementary prescriber;
- administered by anyone acting in accordance with the Patient Specific Directions of a doctor or, subject to certain limitations, an independent nurse prescriber or supplementary prescriber. See Articles 3b, 3c of the POM Order (inserted by The POM (Human Use) Amendment Order 2003 SI No. 696).

Chapter 21

Rights of Access

Access to Pharmacies

Because of the complex nature of community pharmacy, as a business, as a profesion and as retailers, many organisations have statutory rights of access to pharmacies. As well as entry to premises some persons are able to access records and information stored there.

RPSGB Inspectors

Under *Section 108* of the MA 1968. The RPSGB has a duty and is given powers to enforce provisions relating to the retail sale and supply of medicinal products. Any person authorised in writing by the RPSGB has a power to enter premises to ascertain whether there is, or has, been any contravention of the provisions of the Act. The persons authorised also have a power to inspect, take samples and to seize goods and documents. *Sections 109* and *110* deal respectively with arrangements in Scotland and Northern Ireland.

The RPSGB Inspectors are also authorised by the Medicines and Healthcare Regulatory Products Agency, in relation to wholesale and manufacturing matters, within pharmacies. Those RPSGB Inspectors who are pharmacists are also authorised under the Poisons Act 1972, which provides powers at all reasonable times, to enter any premises for the purpose of enforcement of the Poisons Act 1972 and the Poisons Rules 1982. They also enforce certain provisions, relating to membership certificates, of the Pharmacy Act 1954. The RPSGB Inspectors can apply to a Magistrate for a warrant if it is necessary to enter premises other than those where medicines are sold or supplied.

Regulation of Investigatory Powers Act 2000 (RIPA)

This Act sets out a legal framework for the interception of communications, surveillance in the course of authorised investigations and related matters. It provides exemptions from the general human rights set out in the Human Rights Act 1998, which make it unlawful for a public authority to act in a way, which is incompatible with any of the Convention rights, including the right to privacy.

The Society is listed in Part II of Schedule 1 of RIPA as a public authority, which can authorise directed covert surveillance under *Section 28*, as part of investigations to detect or prevent crime, or in the interests of public safety or public health, among other purposes. The Director of Fitness to Practise and Legal Affairs and the Director of Practice and Quality Improvement are named in secondary legislation (SI 2003/3171) as officers of the Society who can authorise covert surveillance. No other member of staff is permitted to provide authorisation.

Under the Act, directed surveillance is defined under *Section 26(2)* as covert surveillance which does not entail the presence of individuals or use of monitoring devices on residential premises or in private vehicles. The surveillance must also be proportionate and be carried out for the purposes of a specific investigation. It may only be authorised by the Society for one of these three reasons:

(1) for the purpose of preventing or detecting crime or for preventing disorder
(2) in the interests of public safety
(3) for the purpose of protecting public health.

Authorisations have to be given in writing, other than in urgent cases, and must specify the nature of the surveillance, the circumstances in which it is to be carried out and the nature of the investigation being undertaken. Oral authorisations expire after 72 hours, unless renewed; written authorisations are valid for 3 months, unless renewed. Authorisation is necessary for investigations which might lead to either criminal action or Statutory Committee proceedings.

The Act is in force in England and Wales, but by virtue of the Regulation of Investigatory Powers (Authorisations Extending to Scotland) Order SI 2000/2418 (as amended) the Society's authority extends to Scotland.

Covert Human Intelligence Sources (CHIS)

The Society is not permitted to authorise the use of a CHIS, i.e. person who establishes or maintains a personal or other relationship for the purpose of (i) covertly using the relationship to obtain information or provide access to information about another person or (ii) covertly disclosing information obtained by the use of such a relationship.

Intrusive surveillance

The Society is not permitted to authorise "intrusive surveillance". This is defined in the Act as covert surveillance carried out in relation to anything taking place on any residential premises or in any private vehicle *and* involves the presence of an individual *on* the premises or *in* the vehicle or is carried out by means of a surveillance device. This does not preclude Society inspectors carrying out directed covert surveillance on a person and noting vehicle registration plates and movements in and out of residential properties.

Test purchases

Test purchases do not require authorisation under RIPA. These are usually undertaken when the Society has received allegations that sales of restricted medicines (e.g. P medicines and POMs) are being made in the absence of a pharmacist. Test purchases involve a member of the inspectorate entering a pharmacy in an area where they are unknown in order to purchase a restricted medicine and make a request to speak to the pharmacist on duty. Test purchases may also be used as a means to test a pharmacist's competence.

Primary Care Trust

Paragraph 37 of the TOS for Chemists provides that the PCT, or any person acting on its behalf, may at any reasonable time on request, inspect the premises of pharmacies providing NHS pharmaceutical services. This is for the purpose of satisfying itself that those services are being provided.

A pharmacy undertaking NHS pharmaceutical services must also, on request, make available to the PCT any information required to audit, monitor and analyse the provision for patient care and the management of the services provided.

PPI Forums

Patient and Public Involvement Forums are set up within each PCT under the NHS Reform and Health Care Professions Act 2002. One of their functions is to monitor and review the range and operation of health services provided under arrangements made by a PCT. They are able to visit pharmacies to carry out this monitoring activity.

The TOS for Chemists require that the pharmacy complies with the obligations set out in the Patients' Forums (Functions) Regulations 2003. These Regulations provide for the entry and inspection of premises, either owned or controlled by a Chemist or where pharmaceutical services are provided.

Under those regulations persons who are authorised in writing by a PPI Forum may at any reasonable time enter and inspect the above premises except where in the Chemist's opinion this would compromise the effective provision of health services or patient's safety, privacy or dignity. Guidance is being prepared for members of PPI Forums, to ensure that they are mindful of the limits that may be placed on their entry to premises, and also the care that must be taken to avoid unnecessary interference with the rights of privacy of patients.

Although the powers of entry and inspection appear to cover the whole of the premises it is generally understood that they would restrict their interest to those areas from which pharmaceutical services are provided under the NHS Act 1977. They do not have any right of access to any part of the premises used for residential accommodation without obtaining consent of the person whose accommodation it is.

NHS Counter Fraud Service

The Counter Fraud Service was established in September 1998 and is now part of the NHS Business Services Authority which is a Special Health Authority. Its role is to reduce all losses to fraud and corruption in the NHS. The Pharmaceutical Fraud team carry out most of their investigations from their offices, and by contacting patients and other health professionals.

The counter fraud specialists can enter pharmacies, with police officers on a Magistrate's warrant, providing they have been included on the warrant. If they are not mentioned on the warrant, they can enter the premises only with the consent of the pharmacist (or any other person in charge).

Police Controlled Drugs Inspectors (CDI)

These officers are sometimes referred to as Chemist Inspection Officers. The Misuse of Drugs Act 1971 authorises a police officer (or any other person authorised by the Secretary of State) to enter pharmacy premises and to demand production of any books or documents relating to dealing in controlled drugs. He may inspect books, documents and stocks of controlled drugs. This applies to all controlled drugs, not just those in Schedule 2 to the Misuse of Drugs Regulations 2001.

In addition, the Misuse of Drugs Regulations requires the pharmacy to produce any register, book or document required to be kept under the Regulations. The position of the private prescription register is peculiar. It is not required to be kept under the Regulations and there is no automatic right to examine it under these Regulations. However the officer can demand production under the general rights of enforcement given by the Act.

The Controlled Drugs Inspectors are also charged with the task of alerting the Home Office of any trends involving misuse of other products which ought to be scheduled under the Misuse of Drugs Act 1971.

The Healthcare Commission

The Healthcare Commission is the independent inspection body for the NHS. It was established under the Health and Social Care (Community Health and Standards) Act 2003, and publishes reports on NHS organisations in England and Wales.

At present the Commission's work includes routine inspections (clinical governance reviews) and investigating serious service failures. It does not normally inspect pharmacies, although it has the power to do so.

Persons authorised in writing by the Commission may at any reasonable time enter and inspect premises owned or controlled by a service provider and used for purposes connected with the services provided. The entry and inspection must be for the purpose of conducting a clinical governance review or an investigation.

The persons authorised by the Commission are not able to demand admission to premises unless reasonable notice has been given of the intended entry. Like the Patients' Forum, persons authorised by the Commission cannot enter premises used as residential accommodation without having first obtained the consent of the persons residing in the accommodation. A person authorised by Commission may inspect and take copies of any documents which appear to him necessary for the purposes of the review, inspection or investigation.

HM Revenue and Customs

This department resulted from the 2005 merger of the Inland Revenue and Customs & Excise. Customs officers continue responsibility for VAT, but are also concerned with the legislation relating to excise duties (e.g. spirits, including IMS and ethanol use in medicines).

For the purpose of exercising any powers under the Finance Acts an authorised person may at any reasonable time enter premises used in connection with the carrying on of a business and inspect any goods found on them. An authorised person can also demand to see, and can seize, any documents relating to the goods or services provided.

An authorised person can apply to a Magistrate for a warrant, which will allow entry at any time stated within the warrant and using force if necessary. During entry under a warrant, the officer can seize and remove any documents or other things which he has reasonable cause to believe may be required as evidence. He may also search persons on the premises that he has reasonable cause to believe may be in possession of any such documents or other things.

Health and Safety Inspectors

Health and safety is enforced by inspectors both from the Health and Safety Executive (HSE) and from the local authority. Inspectors have the right to enter any workplace without giving notice. They can inspect the workplace, the work activities, the management of health and safety, and check that the owner is complying with health and safety law. They have a right to speak to employees, take photographs, and make copies of documents. They can also take away equipment for examination or as evidence. They must, on request, produce their identification, before being allowed entry to the premises.

The inspector may provide employees with information where necessary for the purpose of keeping them informed about matters affecting their health, safety and welfare. Some matters of health and safety, e.g. fire precautions in the workplace, are enforced by other enforcement bodies. In the case of fire precautions, the fire service can appoint Inspectors to enforce the Fire Precautions Act 1971 and in particular the Fire Precautions (Workplace) Regulations 1997. As well as giving advice, these Inspectors can issue enforcement notices requiring immediate attention.

Trading Standards (Weights and Measures)

Trading Standards Officers, formerly known as 'weights and measures' Inspectors, enforce legislation relating to foodstuffs, consumer protection and fair trading. This legislation includes

- Consumer Protection Act 1987
- Health and Safety at Work Act 1974
- Trade Descriptions Act 1968
- Food Safety Act 1990
- Business Names Act 1985
- Supply of Goods and Services Act 1982
- Sale and Supply of Goods Act 1994
- The Sale and Supply of Goods to Consumers Regulations 2002
- Unfair Contract Terms Act 1977
- Unfair Terms in Consumer Contracts Regulations 1999
- Sunday Trading Act 1994
- Weights and Measures Act 1985
- others not so relevant to pharmacy.

The Inspectors are appointed locally and are restricted to working within their geographical area.

Because the officers enforce a wide range of provisions, they have powers under the different legislative regimes. For example, under the Food Safety Act 1990, an authorised officer on producing, if required, an authenticated document showing his authority has a right at all reasonable hours to enter any premises within the authority's area for the purpose of ascertaining whether there is or has been any contravention of the provisions of the Food Safety Act or its regulations.

Admission to any private dwelling-house requires 24 hours' notice of the intended entry to be given to the occupier. A Magistrate's warrant will authorise entry without notice, and by force if necessary.

An authorised officer may inspect any records relating to a food business and, where kept by means of a computer, may require the records to be produced in a form in which they may be taken away. Similar provisions apply to the other Acts.

Trading standards officers enforce some parts of the MA 1968 and the Poisons Act 1972 in non-pharmacy premises.

Disclosure of confidential information

Disclosure of confidential information is usually a breach of confidence. It is authorised in certain circumstances by the following laws:

Police and Criminal Evidence Act 1984
PACE allows police to access medical records for the purpose of a criminal investigation, provided they make an application to a circuit judge.

Road Traffic Act 1988
The police are entitled on request any person to provide information, e.g. name and address, which might identify a driver alleged to have committed a traffic offence. However, clinical information should not normally be disclosed without the patient's consent or a court order.

NHS (Venereal Diseases) Regulations 1974
It allows limited disclosure of information for contact-tracing in the case of sexually transmitted diseases. Such disclosure can only be made to a doctor, or to someone working on a doctor's instruction in connection with treatment or prevention. It forbids those working in a genito-urinary clinic to inform an insurance company of a patient's sexually transmitted disease – even with the patient's consent. GPs are not routinely informed of the patient's attendance at such clinics, although the patient may request that the GP be informed.

Children Act 1989
Regulates many aspects of childcare including professionals' duties when there is suspicion of child abuse.

Prevention of Terrorism (Temporary Provisions) Act 2000
All citizens must inform the police, as soon as possible, of any information that may help to prevent an act of terrorism, or help in apprehending or prosecuting a terrorist.

Chapter 22

Confidentiality

The professional relationship between a patient and the pharmacist depends in part on trust. The confidentiality of information held by pharmacists is a matter both of law and of ethics.

The Data Protection Act 1998

The Data Protection Act (DPA) 1998 controls the use of "personal data", which is data relating to an identifiable living person. The Act came into effect in March 2000 and there is a transition period up to October 2001, by which time all systems must comply. The DPA 1998 implements an EC Directive 95/46/EEC, which requires Member States "to protect the fundamental rights and freedoms of natural persons, in particular their right to privacy with respect the processing of personal data".

Personal data covers both facts and opinions about the individual. It also includes information regarding the intentions of the data controller towards the individual, although in some limited circumstances exemptions will apply.

"Data" is information which is being processed by equipment operating automatically in response to instructions given for that purpose:

- is recorded with the above intention,
- is recorded as part of a structured filing system, or
- forms part of accessible record, e.g. a health record.

The DPA 1998 applies both to computerised data and to paper records and filing systems. All computer records come within the terms of the DPA 1998 if they can be used to identify the individual the record refers to, no matter how they are filed. Manual records will be covered if specific information relating to particular individuals is readily accessible.

Data controller

The data controller is the person responsible for determining how any personal data is processed. The data controller is responsible for ensuring that the terms of the DPA 1998 are followed.

The data processor

The data processor is any person (other than an employee of the data controller) who processes the data.

Processing

Processing includes obtaining, recording or holding information and the organisation, alteration, retrieval, accessing, disclosure or erasure of the data, whether in a manual or electronic form.

Information Commissioner

The DPA 1998 is administered by the "Information Commissioner", created by the Act to maintain a register of data users (those who hold or process the information).

Registration

All businesses that process personal data (such as prescription data) must notify the Information Commissioner of their processing activity. Notification can be undertaken online at www.dataprotection.gov.uk. It is an offence to hold or process personal data unless registered with the Commissioner. The use of computers for labelling medicines or for stock control does not require registration. However, the keeping of patient medication records on computer must be registered. The data controller must notify the Commissioner of:

- The name and address of the data controller (and a representative if one is nominated)
- The description of the data being processed
- The purposes of the processing
- Other parties who may have access to the data.

Offences

Failure to comply with the notification requirements of the Act is a criminal offence and a conviction can result in a maximum fine of £5000 in the Magistrates Courts and unlimited fines in Crown Courts.

The Principles

Section 2 of the Act requires data users to comply with a set of "Principles" which are found in Schedule 1 of the Act. These state that personal data shall be

- fairly and lawfully processed
- processed for limited purposes
- adequate, relevant and not excessive
- accurate

- not kept longer than necessary
- processed in accordance with the data subject's rights
- secure
- not transferred to countries without adequate protection.

These principles apply to the handling of all data. The general effect is that data may not be processed at all unless either the subject has given permission, or a series of other conditions are met.

Sensitive personal data

The Act imposes extra requirements for "sensitive personal data". "Sensitive personal data" means personal data consisting of information as to:

(a) the racial or ethnic origin of the data subject
(b) his political opinions
(c) his religious beliefs or other beliefs of a similar nature
(d) whether he is a member of a trade union (within the meaning of the Trade Union and Labour Relations (Consolidation) Act 1992)
(e) his physical or mental health or condition
(f) his sexual life
(g) the commission or alleged commission by him of any offence or
(h) any proceedings for any offence committed or alleged to have been committed by him, the disposal of such proceedings or the sentence of any court in such proceedings.

Health data is classified by the Act as "sensitive personal data". This includes information about the subject's racial or ethnic origin, his physical or mental health or condition, and his sexual life. Where sensitive personal data are health data, including health records, the subject must give explicit consent to the processing of his health data, unless it is necessary for medical purposes and is undertaken either by a health professional or by a person with a similar duty of confidentiality.

What is a "Health record"?

A "Health record" is a record which consists of information relating to the physical or mental health or condition of an individual which has been made by or on behalf of a health professional in connection with the care of that individual.

The individual must be identifiable from that information, or from that together with other details held by the record holder.

It is clear, therefore, that many of the records being held by pharmacies, surgeries, NHS Trusts and other health care institutions will constitute "health records" and will therefore fall within the scope of the 1998 Act's subject access provisions. The definition of a "health record" could apply to material held on an X-ray, an MRI scan or a blood pressure monitor printout, for example.

What are "Medical purposes"?

"Medical purposes" include the purposes of preventative medicine, medical diagnosis, medical research, the provision of care and treatment, and the management of healthcare services.

Generally sensitive personal data requires that the subject give explicit consent, but this is not required when the data is processed for a health professional and is for medical purposes.

The subject's rights

The DPA 1998 gives seven main rights to the data subject.

Right of access

Section 7 of the DPA 1998 gives a right of access to all information held about a person. A copy may be obtained by applying in writing to the data user. A period of 40 days is allowed for the copy to be supplied. A fee of up to £10 may be charged. Unauthorised disclosure may entitle the person to compensation. There are various exemptions to the right of access, e.g. where data is held for taxation purposes.

Right to prevent processing likely to cause damage or distress

An individual can serve written notice prohibiting a controller from processing data that can cause substantial damage or distress. The controller has 21 days to either comply or to give reasons why the request is unreasonable.

Right to prevent processing for direct marketing

Individuals can prevent their data being used for marketing purposes.

Other rights

The Act also gives individuals rights to compensation when they have suffered damage as a result of a contravention of the Act, and rights to rectification of incorrect records. Individuals can also ensure that decisions which affect them are not based solely on automated processing. They can ask the Commissioner to assess compliance with the Act.

Use of personal data for research or analysis

Personal data may be used for research without explicit permission where:

- the data is used exclusively for that purpose
- the analysis does not identify individuals
- the analysis is not in support of decisions relating to particular individuals
- no damage or distress is caused to any individual.

Non-computerised records

The DPA covers many types of manual records and files. A manual record is subject to the Act if:

- There is a "set" of information about individuals, with a common theme or element. The set need not all be kept in one place.
- There is a "structure" to the set. This may be either by reference to individual's name or a code number or other identifier, or by reference to criteria such as age, purchases, illness, etc.
- The structure allows specific information to be "readily accessible".

The Act also covers personal data which is recorded with the intention that it should be processed by means of a computer. Thus information obtained by, e.g. customer survey forms will be subject to the Act even before it has been inputted.

Two earlier Acts deal with specific circumstances where a patient may wish to access medical records held about them.

Access to Health Records Act 1990

The DPA 1998 only covers the records of living patients. If a person has a claim arising from the death of an individual, he or she has a right of access to information in the deceased's records necessary to fulfil that claim. These rights are set out in the Access to Health Records Act 1990 or Access to Health Records (Northern Ireland) Order 1993.

Access to Medical Records Act 1988

The Access to Medical Records Act 1988 gives a patient a right to view the clinical information contained in his or her own medical history when released by the GP as a medical report for insurance or employment purposes. A medical report is a "report relating to the physical or mental health of the individual prepared by a medical practitioner who is or has been responsible for the clinical care of the patient".

The GP may charge a "reasonable fee" if a copy is provided. The rights given under this Act relate solely to records prepared by a GP. There is no direct effect on pharmacists and the information is included to give a complete picture.

Use of anonymised data for research

In the case of *R* v. *Department of Health, Ex Parte Source Informatics Limited* 1999, the Court of Appeal held that the disclosure by pharmacists of anonymised prescription data does not amount to a breach of confidentiality.

Source Informatics, a division of IMS, obtained information from pharmacies on doctors' prescribing habits in order to sell the data on to pharmaceutical companies so that the companies might market their products more effectively. Source was interested in the doctors' names and the products they prescribed but not the names or identities of the patients concerned. They marketed this data from NHS patients in an aggregated and anonymised form.

A DOH policy document issued in July 1997 stated that the sale of such data breached patient confidentiality. Source Informatics challenged that view and sought a declaration that it was wrong in law. They initially lost the case and appealed. The Court of Appeal held that participation in Source's scheme by doctors and pharmacists would not expose them to any serious risk of successful breach of confidence proceedings by a patient. Therefore pharmacists could sell anonymised information if they wished. The court said if the DOH viewed such schemes as operating against the public interest then it should make laws to control the situation.

The DOH later indicated that their original position had not been fully thought through in regard to its consequences for the collection of research information. However, they promptly introduced new law for this area.

Control of patient information under the Health and Social Care Act 2001

The HSC Act 2001 enables the Secretary of State to regulate the sharing of medical information to improve patient care, or in the public interest.

Under *Section 60*, the S of S may make regulations which require or regulate the processing of patient information in prescribed circumstances. This, for instance, makes it possible for patients to receive more information about their clinical care and for confidential patient information to be lawfully processed without informed consent to support prescribed activities such as cancer registries.

Safeguards

The HSC 2001 Act built in a number of safeguards over the use of this power, to protect patients' interests.

First, regulations can only provide for the processing of patient information for medical purposes where there is a benefit to patient care or where this is in the public interest. Medical purposes means

(a) preventative medicine, medical diagnosis, medical research, the provision of care and treatment, and the management of health and social care services;

(b) informing individuals about their physical or mental health or condition, the diagnosis of their condition or their care and treatment.

Secondly, regulations can only require the processing of confidential patient information, where there is no reasonably practicable alternative. The Secretary of State can only make following consultation with those likely to be affected and with the new Patient Information Advisory Group.

Thirdly, any such regulations can only be made under the affirmative resolution procedure, requiring the consent of both Houses of Parliament.

Fourthly, all the controls of the DPA 1998 remain in place.

The Health Service (Control of Information) Regulations 2002

The Health Service (Control of Patient Information) Regulations 2002, SI No. 1438, were introduced to achieve this control. They allow the DOH to collect certain information for specified purposes, but do not otherwise alter the Source Informatics judgement.

Patient Information Advisory Group

The DOH set up the Patient Information Advisory Group to advise it on the processing of patient information. The advice must be published. There is an Annual Report.

The terms of reference of the Group are

- To advise the S of S on use of powers provided by *Section 60* of the Health and Social Care Act 2001, and in particular on:
    - applications and proposals for use of these powers;
    - draft regulations made under *Section 60(1)* of the Act;
    - proposals to vary or revoke such regulations following the S of S's required annual review of existing provisions.

- To advise the S of S on key issues, particularly those of national significance, relating to the processing of patient information.

Confidentiality and children

A child's right to confidentiality is as important as the adult's right, even in the face of parental enquiries.

The RPSGB advises that when the patient is a child, the pharmacist may have to decide whether to release information to parents or guardians without the consent of the child, but in the child's best interests. Much will depend on the maturity of the child concerned and his or her relationship with parents or guardians. Such decisions are particularly difficult when the issue concerns contraception. The courts have laid out some helpful guidance in this area, following the Gillick case in 1985 (see later).

Confidentiality is not normally breached if parents seek advice in relation to their children who are under 16 years of age. If the young person is the client, the visit and discussions are confidential, even in the face of parental enquiries.

Medical records

Young people under 16 have the right of access to personal information (including medical records) stored on computers, and to their written medical records providing that the holder of the records considers them capable of understanding the nature of the request. A parent or guardian will not be given access unless the young person consents or is incapable of understanding the nature of the request and the granting of access would be in their best interests (Data Protection Act 1998).

Human Rights Act 1998

Article 8 of the HRA sets out a "right to respect for private and family life". This reinforces the duty to preserve confidentiality.

The Caldicott Review 1997

This Review was commissioned by the Chief Medical Officer of England owing to increasing concern about the ways in which patient information is used in the NHS in England and Wales and the need to ensure that confidentiality is not undermined.

The review set out a list of principles for handling patient information.

Caldicott Principles

Principle 1 – Justify the purpose(s)
Every proposed use or transfer of patient-identifiable information within or from an organisation should be clearly defined and scrutinised, with continuing uses regularly reviewed by an appropriate guardian.

Principle 2 – Do not use patient-identifiable information unless it is absolutely necessary. Patient-identifiable information items should not be used unless there is no alternative.

Principle 3 – Use the minimum necessary patient-identifiable information
Where use of patient-identifiable information is considered to be essential, each individual item of information should be justified with the aim of reducing identifiability.

Principle 4 – Access to patient-identifiable information should be on a strict need to know basis. Only those individuals who need access to patient-identifiable information should have access to it, and they should only have access to the information items that they need to see.

Principle 5 – Everyone should be aware of their responsibilities
Action should be taken to ensure that those handling patient-identifiable information – both clinical and non-clinical staff – are aware of their responsibilities and obligations to respect patient confidentiality.

Principle 6 – Understand and comply with the law
Every use of patient-identifiable information must be lawful. Someone in each organisation should be responsible for ensuring that the organisation complies with legal requirements.

Caldicott Guardian

Recommendation 3 of the Review was that a senior person, preferably a health professional, should be nominated in each health organisation to act as a guardian, responsible for safeguarding the confidentiality of patient information. This person has become known as the "Caldicott Guardian".

The RPSGB has stated that all NHS pharmacies should appoint a Caldicott Guardian and comply with the recommendations of the report.

Department of Health Code of Practice

On 1 April 2005 the DOH issued Directions to PCTs and SHAs that require compliance with the NHS Confidentiality Code of Practice. The Code was issued in 2003 and is available on the DOH website.

Ethical obligations placed on pharmacists

Section A2 of Part II requires that effective measures are in place in pharmacies for protecting the confidentiality of person identifiable data.

Section C of Part II repeats the general requirements of the Data Protection legislation. It specifies that pharmacy computer and manual systems which include patient-specific information should incorporate access control systems to minimise the risk of unauthorised or unnecessary access to data.

The Service Specifications in Part III include a section on Patient medication records.

The RPSGB has issued a Guidance note on confidentiality.

Persons with legal rights to access confidential information

Some persons are given legal rights to access data that would otherwise be confidential. A pertinent pharmacy example is the right of inspection of CDs registers, which is given to people appointed by the Home Office, e.g. policemen. The right is specific to information recorded in the CD Register or in the private prescription register, and does not extend to other information about that patient contained, e.g. in the PMR.

Disclosure may be ordered by a coroner, a court, or by the Crown Prosecution Office or by the Procurator Fiscal in Scotland.

Sharing data within the NHS family

It is often considered that sharing information between health professionals who are each bound by professional rules of confidentiality does not require consent. The Health Service Commissioner has stated that this is too wide. In the Commissioner's view, a patient's record could not be made generally available to a patient's previous doctor, who has ceased to have care of that patient.

The BMA accepts that the exchange of identifiable information between health professionals caring for a patient is essential, unless the patient has expressly prohibited it. However, the BMA does not accept that such data can be routinely circulated to others simply because they are health professionals or are members of the NHS family. A need to know justification applies to the sharing of information necessary to provide care or treatment for an individual patient.

Patients should be made aware that health teams need to share essential relevant information in order to ensure that the safety and effectiveness of treatment are maximised.

Records

Pharmacies keep various records which include personal details of patients. Some records are kept because of a legal requirement, e.g. CD register, some by a contractual requirement, e.g. PMRs for the elderly, and some for professional reasons only, e.g. PMRs for children.

The following are likely to be encountered:

- CD Register
- NHS Patient Medication Records (written)

- NHS Patient Medication Records (on Computer)
- Private PMRs (written)
- Private PMRs (computer)
- Prescription book.

Various legal issues arise in relation to the different types of record.

CD register

The legal requirements are dealt with in Chapter 16.

NHS Patient medication records

The arrangements made by a PCT include the provision of patient medication records.

Prescription book

The following details must be recorded about the sale or supply of POMs:

(1) date of sale or supply
(2) name and quantity of medicine (where it is not apparent from the name, the strength and pharmaceutical form must also be included).
(3) date of the script
(4) name and address of prescriber
(5) name and address of patient (or owner of animal).

Repeat prescriptions
It is sufficient to record the date of supply, together with a reference to the original entry.

Keeping the prescription book

The book used to record POM supplies must be kept for 2 years after the last entry.

Keeping the prescriptions

The prescriptions must be retained for 2 years after they were dispensed.

Computer records

The Medicines (Sale or Supply) (Miscellaneous Provisions) Amendment Regulations 1997, SI No. 1831, amended the law to permit records of private prescriptions and emergency supplies to be held on computer. The same details are required as for paper records. The computer records must be kept for 2 years. The RPSGB has advised that the computer records should contain an accurate audit trail of entries.

Chapter 23

Consent

It is sometimes wrongly assumed that informed consent is necessary only for surgery or invasive procedures. Consent is necessary in any professional relationship between a patient and a healthcare provider. For major procedures or treatments involving risk to the patient, such as surgical procedures, it is usual for informed consent to be obtained in writing.

Consent is necessary for all treatment, but it is often is implied in the interaction, e.g. in the normal pharmacist–patient interaction where the patient seeks and accepts the advice of the pharmacist on treatment. Examples would be buying an OTC or having a prescription dispensed.

For some services now being provided by pharmacists, explicit consent is required. It is especially important where touching is concerned, as for instance when a blood sample is taken.

Definition of consent

The Department of Health's Mental Health Act 1983: Code of Practice (1999) gives the following definition of consent (15.13):

> 'Consent' is the voluntary and continuing permission of the patient to receive a particular treatment, based on an adequate knowledge of the purpose, nature, likely effects and risks of that treatment including the likelihood of its success and any alternatives to it. Permission given under and unfair undue pressure is not 'consent'.

Explicit consent

Explicit consent can be verbal or written. When explicit consent is obtained the patient should have the procedure adequately explained. The attendant risks should also be explained. In order to give valid consent the patient must have understood, and must have the legal capacity to consent.

Implicit consent

Implicit consent occurs when the patient agrees to the procedure simply by being a patient and by not objecting to therapeutic procedures about which they have received general information, for instance by holding out an arm for an injection.

Basis for the consent concept

The bases for the concept of informed consent lie in civil and criminal law, and in the ethical concept of autonomy.

Criminal law

Strictly, it is unlawful to touch or even threaten to touch a person without their permission. Such a touch would constitute "battery", and there are remedies in both civil and criminal courts. It is not necessary to prove that there was any damage. Therefore treatments or investigations performed without consent constitute "battery". There are exceptions, such as emergency life-saving procedures.

Civil law – negligence

Consent is part of the agreement between the patient and the professional. Without consent there can be no agreement. Indeed the first case brought by a patient claiming that he did not consent to the procedure took place in 1767.

Consent must be based on adequate information especially about the risks. If inadequate information is given a patient may win a negligence claim. A court may regard any consent as invalid if it is based on inadequate information (*Chatterton* v. *Gerson 1981*).

How much information must be given to the patient

The professional standard with regard to the provision of information was dealt with in two legal cases:

(1) *Bolam* v. *Friern Hospital Management Committee*
(2) *Sidaway* v. *Board of Governors of the Bethlem Royal and the Maudsley Hospital.*

Generally the amount of information to be given is at the discretion of the doctor, provided he follows recognised good practice.

To make an informed and valid consent a patient must be given the information relevant to the decision he is going to make. The case law indicates that this should be the information that a responsible body of professional opinion would consider necessary.

The courts have said that patients should be told of risks which are "obviously necessary to an informed choice on the part of the patient that no reasonably prudent medical man would fail to make it". Questions asked by the patient must be truthfully answered.

In Bolam a patient was given ECT without relaxant drugs. He was not given any warning of any risk by the treating physician. An unusual fracture occurred during treatment. The judgment sets out the "Bolam" test which is applied to conduct alleged to be negligent. A professional person should act in accordance with a responsible body of professional opinion.

In Sidaway a spinal operation was properly performed but the nerve root was damaged – a known risk. Unfortunately the surgeon had only informed the patient of possible damage to the spinal cord itself, and further he had not told the patient that the operation was one of choice. It was not a necessary operation. The patient's claim for negligence was upheld.

Qualifications of the person seeking the consent

Consent is often given because the patient recognises the qualifications of the person seeking the consent. For instance hairdressers are allowed to touch clients in situations where other people might not get consent.

The patient may make assumptions about the status of the other person that affects consent. Some patients may be confused about supplementary prescribing. They may assume that anyone who "prescribes" is a doctor, and therefore they consent to accepting the prescription on that basis. They may feel differently about accepting a prescription from a pharmacist. Any pharmacist undertaking prescribing in such a situation should make his profession clear to the patient at the outset.

Is the patient capable of making an informed decision?

Consent is based on the assumption that the patient is capable of making an informed and voluntary decision. There are two aspects to this:

(1) the information given about what is to happen and
(2) the patient's ability to make a decision.

Adult patients are normally presumed to be competent to make decisions about their health, and therefore to accept or refuse treatment. However this presumption can be challenged in court, especially where the patient does not have the mental capacity to make reasoned decisions.

How to determine whether a person can validly consent

The courts have suggested three tests to determine capacity:

(1) Did the patient understand what was said to him?
(2) Did he believe it?
(3) Did he consider the information, and balance needs and risks before reaching his decision?

In Regulation C 1994, an elderly paranoid schizophrenic had delusions that he was a doctor. The courts held that nevertheless he was capable of refusing consent for an amputation to treat gangrene, because he understood the information about treatment.

Generally speaking, a mentally competent patient has the right to refuse medical treatment, regardless of consequences and how beneficial or necessary treatment may be. As the judge in Sidaway put it *"a competent adult has a right to refuse treatment . . . for reasons which are rational or irrational, or for no reason"*.

Regulation C can be contrasted with Regulation T 1992 where the courts found that a woman had been influenced by her Jehovah's Witness mother into refusing a necessary blood transfusion. The court declared that she had not been fully rational when she refused, due to the influence of her mother, and partly due to the medications received.

Consent by children

The above cases concerned adults. Children may also be considered competent to take decisions about their health.

The Family Reform Act 1969 lowered the age of majority to 18 years and gave 16- and 17-year-olds the same right to consent to treatment as adults. *Section 8(1)* says

> the consent of a minor who has attained the age of sixteen . . . shall be as effective as it would be if he were of full age; and where a minor has . . . given an effective consent to any treatment it shall not be necessary to obtain any consent for it from his parent or guardian.

Children under 16

The parental right to determine whether a child below the age of 16 has medical treatment ends if, and when, the child achieves sufficient understanding and intelligence to comprehend fully what is proposed.

It is for the doctor to use his clinical judgement to decide whether the child has reached such a level of understanding and intelligence.

The Gillick case established broad principles on the capacity of children aged under 16 (*Gillick* v. *West Norfolk and Wisbech Area Health Authority [1985] 3 All ER 402*).

The Gillick case

The Department of Health and Social Security issued a circular stating that in exceptional circumstances doctors could give contraceptive advice and prescriptions to girls under 16 without the consent of the parents.

Mrs Gillick sought an assurance from her local health authority that her daughters would not be given advice on contraception without her prior consent. When this was refused, she challenged the legality of the circular. The House of Lords gave judgment in 1985 (*Gillick* v. *West Norfolk and Wisbech Area Health Authority [1985] 3 All ER 402*).

This case established the following broad principles:

- Parental rights exist for the benefit of the child, not the parent.
- The parental right to determine whether a child below the age of 16 has medical treatment ends if, and when, the child achieves sufficient understanding and intelligence to comprehend fully what is proposed.
- It is for the doctor to use his clinical judgement to decide whether the child has reached such a level of understanding and intelligence.

The Gillick decision is reinforced by the Children Act 1989, under which parental rights yield to children's rights to make their own decisions once they have enough understanding and intelligence to make up their own minds.

Consent to contraception

A girl under 16 can consent to contraceptive advice and treatment, and the doctor can proceed without her parent's knowledge or consent if satisfied that

- she understands the advice;
- she cannot be persuaded to inform her parents, or to allow the doctor to do so;
- she is likely to have sexual intercourse with or without contraceptive treatment;
- unless she has contraceptive advice or treatment her health (physical or mental) will suffer;
- her best interests require that she receive contraceptive advice and treatment without the knowledge or consent of her parents.

Application to pharmacists

The phrases used in the judgment are directed at doctors. Similar conditions will apply to the supply of OTC products by pharmacists. It may be more difficult for pharmacists to satisfy the criteria, especially number (4).

Refusal of consent by the child

The Gillick case concerns the giving of consent. It does not apply where a Gillick competent child refuses to give consent. There may be a more limited right to refuse to give consent. Under the Children Act 1989, *the "child's welfare shall be the court's paramount consideration"*. The Act itself gives young people who understand what is happening a limited right to refuse certain treatments in circumstances connected to care proceedings. The right to refuse treatment is also limited by two judgments Re R and Re W. In both cases the child's refusal to accept treatment was overruled and the parents' wishes for treatment prevailed.

Both in the United States, and in the United Kingdom, courts have ordered necessary blood transfusions for a child whose parents objected because they were practising Jehovah's Witnesses. UK courts have also overridden the wishes of the parent in order to facilitate a procedure of benefit to the child, but which was refused by the parents.

Clinical trials and children

In clinical trials the Clinical Trials Regulations supercede the Gillick judgment and require that written informed consent from a parent or guardian is always required.

The law in Scotland

Gillick is English law and does not apply in Scotland, which is covered by the Age of Legal Capacity (Scotland) Act 1991.

Chapter 24

The European Union

The law of the European Union, commonly referred to as European Community law, is automatically part of UK law, and consequently it is necessary for pharmacists to have some knowledge of the European Union and the way it works.

The EEC was established by the Treaty of Rome in 1957. The original members were Belgium, France, Germany, Italy, Luxembourg and the Netherlands. The United Kingdom joined in 1972, along with Denmark and the Republic of Ireland. They were then joined by Greece, Portugal and Spain.

In 1994 the European Free Trade Area (EFTA) countries of Austria, Finland and Sweden joined to form the European Economic Area. Ten more countries joined in 2004, making a total so far of 25.

The original treaty was modified in 1972 by the "Maastricht treaty on European union". In 1992 a new treaty gave new powers and responsibilities to the Community institutions and created the European Union.

Law-making institutions

The Treaty of Rome established several institutions to deal with the law-making process of the Community.

The Council of the European Union

This was formerly called the Council of Ministers. It is the legislative and decision-making body of the EC. It is composed of ministers from each of the member governments, normally the Foreign Ministers but it may be any appropriate minister. One minister attends from each state. Most decisions are taken on a majority basis. The Presidency rotates between the states, in alphabetical order, at 6-month intervals.

The Committee of Permanent Representatives (known by the French acronym COREPER) consists of senior civil servants from each state, and it acts as the administrative arm of the Council. The members are the heads of the permanent delegations in Brussels. Disputes are often sorted out here.

The European Council is the name given to the regular meetings of heads of governments, which discuss broad policy.

The Commission

The Commission is charged with seeing that the treaties are implemented. There are 25 Commissioners with a large supporting staff. Commissioners are appointed for a 5-year term, serve the EC as a whole, and can only be removed from office by the European Court of Justice or by the European Parliament (which can only dismiss the entire Commission on a two-third majority vote). Each Commissioner is responsible for an area of policy. The staff are organised into Directorates-General.

The Commission is

(a)   a policy-planning body
(b)   a mediator between governments
(c)   the executive arm of the Community
(d)   the prosecutor of those who breach the treaty rules.

The European Parliament

The Parliament is composed of directly elected representatives of the citizens of the member states. It has three main roles:

(1)   It has little direct power of legislation, but it examines new law.
(2)   It controls the Commission's budget.
(3)   It exercises democratic supervision over the other EU institutions.

There are 732 members, with the numbers reflecting the size of each country's population.

The European Court of Justice

The Court is based in Luxembourg. It is responsible for ensuring that Community legislation is correctly interpreted and applied. Cases may be brought by a member state, a community institution or an individual. The court reponds to requests from national courts for an interpretation of Community law. It has the power to impose fines. Member states in breach of community law are required to comply with the orders of the court. Judges are appointed from each country.

There is a Court of First Instance which has jurisdiction relating to competition policy and to cases brought by individuals, companies and some organisations. The European Civil Service Tribunal gives rulings on employment disputes of the Commission staff.

Economic and Social Committee

This influential committee known as "Ecosoc" advises the Commission and the Council on economic matters. It is made up of representatives of the employers, workers and other interest groups in the member states. The representatives are proposed by the governments, and appointments are made by the Council.

Community law

There are four categories of Community law:

"Regulations" are laws issued by the Community which have effect throughout the Community as they stand. There is no need for the EC law to be "transposed" into national law.

"Directives" are binding on the Member States. They lay down the result to be achieved but leave to the national authorities the task of enacting the necessary national legislation. This may be done by creating new primary legislation, e.g. Acts of Parliament, or secondary legislation, e.g. Regulations or Orders.

"Recommendations" are merely advisory statements.

"Decisions" are binding on the individuals or institutions to whom they are addressed.

Directives affecting pharmacy

Community law overrides national laws of the member states.

A number of Directives have been issued concerning medicines. They are based on Articles 100 and 100A of the Treaty of Rome. The majority of the medicines Directives are concerned with the licensing process, laying down the procedures to be adopted, the types of data to be required and giving definitions.

One codification exercise means that legislations about the quality, safety and efficacy of medicines is mainly in Directive 2001/83/EC and in Regulation (EEC) 726/2004.

Directive 2001/83/EC

The main Directive replaced Directive 65/65/E. It was amended by Directive 2004/27/EC. It sets out the most important aspects of the marketing of medicines. These include the common principles which should be adhered to by each Member State with regard to the conditions for granting a marketing authorisation, manufacture and quality control procedures, labelling and information leaflets, and detailed guidance on data requirements.

The Directive requires that a marketing authorisation (product licence) is granted on grounds of safety, efficacy and quality – the same grounds as are laid down in the MA 1968.

The Directive 2001/83/EC applies to "medicinal products" which are defined as

> any substance or combination of substances presented for treating or preventing disease in human beings. Any substance or combination of substances which may be administered to human beings with a view to making a medical diagnosis or to restoring, correcting or modifying physiological functions in human beings.

Directive 2001/83/EC and Directive 2004/27/EC are put into UK law by the Medicines (Marketing Authorisations and Miscellaneous Amendments) Regulations 2004.

Regulation EC 726/2004

Regulation EC 726/2004 lays down Community procedures for the authorisation and supervision of medicinal products. It also establishes the European Medicines Agency.

The "Transparency" Directive

Directive 89/105/EEC is known as the "Transparency Directive". It requires Member States which impose controls on the prices of medicinal products, or on the profits of the pharmaceutical industry to publish their criteria, and the reasons for the decisions. The intention is to ensure that all procedures are operated in accordance with the Treaty, i.e. they are fair and are not discriminatory.

Article 1 states

> Member States shall ensure that any national measure, whether laid down by law, regulation or administrative action, to control the prices of medicinal products for human use or to restrict the range of medicinal products covered by their national health insurance systems complies with the requirements of this Directive.

Later articles lay down a timetable of 90 days for the authorities to make a decision about a product.

The Directive applies to the Selected List scheme, the ACBS approval scheme, and by virtue of Article 5, to the PPRS scheme.

Free movement of pharmacists

Three Directives of the Council of the European Communities are concerned with pharmacy qualifications.

The Directives are

(1)   Directive 85/432/EEC (Known as the "Training Directive") which is concerned with ensuring a common minimum standard of training for pharmacists in the EC.
(2)   Directive 85/433/EEC (known as the "Recognition Directive") which is concerned with the mutual recognition of qualifications, and which gives certain rights to practise pharmacy.
(3)   Directive 85/584/EEC took account of the accession of Spain and Portugal to the EC.

These Directives have been implemented in Great Britain by an Order-in-Council, the Pharmaceutical Qualifications (EEC Recognition) Order 1987 (SI 1987/2202).

The Order mainly amends the Pharmacy Act 1954, but also amends the MA 1968, the NHS Act 1977 and the NHS (Scotland) Act 1978. The main amendment to the Pharmacy Act 1954 inserts a new *Section 4A* into the Act. This provides that EC nationals who hold one of the listed "Qualifying European Diplomas in Pharmacy are entitled to registration as a pharmacist in Great Britain. The diplomas are now listed in Schedule 1A to the Act.

The "Greek derogation"

During negotiations on the Directive it was agreed that for a period, Greece was allowed to derogate from the requirement to recognise the qualifications of other member states. The Directive allowed the individual state to decide whether it would in return refuse to fully recognise Greek qualifications. The UK government decided that for the period of the Greek derogation, the UK authorities would recognise qualifications obtained in Greece only for employees. Greek pharmacists are consequently prohibited from becoming the proprietor of a UK pharmacy.

Qualifying European Diploma

The new *Section 4A* designates the RPSGB and the PSNI as "competent authorities". Together the two organisations cover the whole of the United Kingdom. The Free Movement Directive lays down a procedure by which nationals of one member state are entitled to registration as pharmacists in another member state. This procedure depends upon the possesion of either a certificate or diploma (Qualifying European Diploma) where the training conforms with the Directive's requirements, or a certificate of training together with a period spent in practice. The competent authority can confirm the applicability of the relevant criteria.

Statutory Committee

Section 4A also provides that the Statutory Committee of RPSGB, when exercising its disciplinary powers, may take account of disqualifications to practise incurred in another Member state.

Personal control of "new" pharmacies

Article 3 of the Order amended *Section 70* MA 1968 so as to impose a condition that a pharmacy which has been registered for less than 3 years should not be under the personal control of a pharmacist who qualified in another member state. This is the so-called "Prag Amendment" (after the Euro-MP who proposed it) which was intended to soften the expected impact of migrating pharmacists. At the time of the debate on the Directive several countries, including the United Kingdom, had no controls on entry to practice. In the United Kingdom at the time an application to dispense NHS prescriptions was automatically granted. This is no longer the case, although of course there are no restrictions of that nature on the establishment of a non-NHS pharmacy.

Linguistic ability

Article 4 of the Order amended the NHS Act 1977 to enable PCTs to be satisfied that the linguistic competence of EC-trained applicants for NHS contracts is adequate for the provision of services in the locality. Article 5 inserted a similar provision into the NHS (Scotland) Act 1978. Linguistic ability is now covered by Regulation 11 of the NHS (PS) Regulations 2005.

The Council of the RPSGB has made the following statement about competence in the English language:

> Pharmacist must ensure that pharmacists and other staff employed by them are sufficiently competent in English.

Titles

Pharmacists from other EC states are entitled to use the titles by which they are known in their own state, provided this does not cause confusion.

RPSGB Bye-laws

Section XIX of the Society's Byelaws deals with registration of overseas pharmacists. The Byelaws list the evidence which the Council of RPSGB requires, and the fees to be paid.

The evidence required is of:

(1)   identity
(2)   good character
(3)   good physical and mental health
(4)   the holding of a relevant EC diploma

Many EC nationals hold diplomas which were granted before the states agreed the basic core knowledge of the course. They may be registered in the United Kingdom if they have lawfully practised pharmacy in another EC state for a period of at least 3 consecutive years during the last 5 years. The evidence for this is a certificate from the competent authorities of the member state. This process is referred to as the "acquired rights" route.

Other professions

Similar Directives cover doctors, dentists, nurses, midwives and vets. A Directive issued in 1989 deals with the principle that a person fit to practise a professional activity in one state should in principle be allowed to practise in any other. Generally, professional qualifications achieved after a course of training equivalent to university are to be recognised. Where differences are substantial, a short test of ability may be imposed.

Chapter 25

The Pharmacy Profession

History

Chemists and druggists

The history of pharmacy as a profession distinct from the practice of medicine begins in 1794. Until then medicines had been dispensed by physicians and apothecaries as part of an ancillary service, but the compounding of prescriptions became more complex, and expensive new avenues of supply were explored. Chemists and druggists had started to appear, with the primary purpose of dispensing the prescriptions of medical men.

An association

In response to the commercial threat posed by this new breed of merchant, the apothecaries formed a pharmaceutical association to restrain chemists and druggists from dispensing prescriptions and interfering with what was perceived as the legitimate business of apothecaries. The association was formed in 1794. When the association failed to stem the chemists and druggists, the apothecaries tried to enlist help at Westminster. In the original draft of the Apothecaries Act 1815 the apothecaries sought to prohibit the dispensing of medicines other than by apothecaries licensed under the provisions of the Act. After much intense lobbying by the chemists and druggists the proposal was abandoned. *Section 28* of the Apothecaries Act expressly preserved "the trade or business of a chemist and druggist in the buying, preparing, compounding, dispensing, and vending drugs, medicines, and medicinal compounds, wholesale and retail". This was the first recognition of the pharmacy profession in an Act of Parliament.

Training

There was nevertheless a problem. Whereas the apothecaries could practise only after passing examinations required by the Apothecaries Act 1814, there was no equivalent requirement for chemists and druggists. Yet the measuring and compounding of medicines was a skilled and exact science. Compulsory pharmaceutical training was required in other European countries such as France, Germany and Sweden, and there was genuine concern that chemists and druggists in this country were neither licensed nor trained. On a number of occasions enterprising individuals tried to introduce an improved system, but few chemists and druggists supported ideas for reform.

The Hawes Bill

The introduction of a medical Bill by Mr Hawes provided the necessary catalyst for reform in 1841. The Hawes Bill sought to give supervision of chemists and druggists to medical practitioners, who would set up a system of education and licensing along European lines. In order to oppose the Bill leading chemists in London formed a Society, the Pharmaceutical Society, the object of the Society being to improve the education of pharmaceutical chemists.

Royal Charter

The Hawes Bill failed, but the legislative attempt achieved its purpose. Following discussions with London University, the College of Physicians and the College of Surgeons, the Pharmaceutical Society established an educational programme and founded its own Board of Examiners. The Pharmaceutical Society's membership grew from 668 members (not including associates and apprentices) in 1841 to 1640 in 1843 when a Royal Charter was granted. The Royal Charter declared that existing chemists and druggists could be admitted as members, but assistants, apprentices and students would be admitted only after being examined and certified as qualified for admission. After a few years, the Pharmaceutical Society obtained the introduction of a Bill in order to place the education and certification of pharmaceutical chemists on a statutory footing. The Society of Apothecaries did not oppose the Bill.

Statutory regulation

The Pharmacy Act 1852 confirmed the Royal Charter, empowering examiners appointed by the Pharmaceutical Society to grant or refuse certificates of competent skill and knowledge to exercise the business of pharmaceutical chemist. It became a criminal offence fraudulently to exhibit a certificate purporting to be a certificate of membership.

In the 150 years which have followed, the Pharmaceutical Society has grown in strength. The Royal Charter was superseded by a second Charter in 1953 and then on 7 December 2004 a third new Royal Charter came into force.

The Pharmacy Act 1852 was repealed and replaced by the Pharmacy Act 1954, and together these provisions govern the education and organisation of the modern profession. Members of the Pharmaceutical Society were divided into pharmaceutical chemists, and chemists and druggists, but the latter class was abolished in 1953. In 1988 the Queen permitted the Society to be known as the RPSGB. At the time of writing, the RPSGB currently have approximately 44,000 persons on the Register of Pharmaceutical Chemists. Some 23,000 members work in community pharmacy, with around 6,000 employed in hospital pharmacy.

Contemporary challenges

The RPSGB is responding to a number of different challenges, in particular:

(i)   the challenges set by government in the development of pharmacy and the way in which the profession is to be regulated;
(ii) the regulatory challenges presented by Internet pharmacy, and its impact on Community pharmacy in general.

The Royal Pharmaceutical Society of Great Britain

Objects

The main objects of the RPSGB under the 2004 Charter are as follows:

- to advance knowledge of, and education in, pharmacy and its application, thereby fostering good science and practice;
- to safeguard, maintain the honour and promote the interests of pharmacists in their exercise of the profession of pharmacy;
- to promote and protect the health and well being of the public through the regulation and professional leadership and development of the pharmacy profession and regulation of other persons engaged in related activities;
- to maintain and develop the science and practice of pharmacy in its contribution to the health and well-being of the public.

These objects were defined to similar effect, albeit with less emphasis on the promotion of well-being of the public, in the 1953 Royal Charter and have been considered in detail by the courts on two occasions.

Not a trade association

In the first case, *Jenkin* v. *Pharmaceutical Society (1921)*, the court decided that the RPSGB's objects were not intended to cover activities normally associated with a trading association. It followed that the RPSGB was unable:

(1)   to regulate the terms of employment (hours, wages and conditions) between employer and employee members of the RPSGB;
(2)   to expend its funds in the formation of an industrial council committee to further these purposes;
(3)   to insure its members against insurable risks.

A distinction had to be drawn between activities which promoted the interests of those engaged in the exercise of the profession of pharmacy as a whole and the promotion of the interest of an individual or individuals. The formation of an industrial council committee was an activity which fell into the latter category and therefore could not be said to promote the exercise of the profession of pharmacy within the meaning of the Charter. Although decided under the 1843 Royal Charter, the same decision would almost certainly be reached today.

The National Pharmaceutical Association

Shortly after this decision, the National Pharmaceutical Union was formed to represent pharmacists on the trading aspects of pharmacy. Now known as the National Pharmaceutical Association, the Association offers indemnity insurance through the Chemists' Defence Association which is operated under its auspices.

No power to restrain trade

In the second case, *Pharmaceutical Society* v. *Dickson (1970)*, the RPSGB had sought to include in the Code of Ethics a rule which, amongst other things, would confine the trading activities of new pharmacies to pharmaceutical and "traditional" goods. The sale of "non-traditional" goods, such as jewellery, beachwear, handbags, Thermos flasks, etc. was, in the Society's opinion, degrading the quality and status of the profession. As in *Jenkins*, the House of Lords held that the proposed restrictions went outside the expressed objects of the Society. In the absence of evidence to show that professional standards had been eroded by reason of the trade in "non-traditional" goods, the proposed restraint could not be said to be necessary to maintain and safeguard the honour of the profession or to promote the interests of members in the exercise of the profession.

The Council of the RPSGB

The Council of the RPSGB manages the affairs of the Society. It meets six times every year to discuss key issues affecting pharmacy and to decide on policies and practice. The Council is advised on particular areas of pharmacy policy by a number of committees and subcommittees as well as by a number of membership and special interest groups.

Under the 2004 Charter the reformed Council took office on 25 May 2005. The new Council of 30 members comprises 17 elected pharmacists with 3 places reserved for the constituencies of England (with the Isle of Man and the Channel Islands), Scotland and Wales together with 14 unreserved places with one pharmacist appointed by the universities awarding pharmacy degrees accredited by the Society and two pharmacy technicians. A further 10 lay members are appointed by the Privy Council.

The Council elects its own president. Elected members serve on the Council for 3 years, although those elected in the first election (2005) will have terms of 1 year, 2 years and 3 years, allocated on the number of votes received.

Membership

Members of the RPSGB are defined as those whose names are registered as pharmaceutical chemists with the RPSGB.

Register of pharmaceutical chemists

Under *Section 1* of the Pharmacy Act 1954 the Council of the RPSGB is obliged to appoint a registrar. The registrar's principal duty under the Act is to maintain a register of pharmaceutical chemists. The register must contain the names and addresses of all persons who are entitled to have their names registered, and the registrar must publish a list known as the "annual register of pharmaceutical chemists" every year. Registration is essential to a practising pharmacist. Only a registered pharmacist is entitled to buy and sell drugs and to compound and dispense medicines. Similarly, only a registered pharmacist can run an RPB. Every registered pharmaceutical chemist must pay an annual fee to the RPSGB. A person is entitled to have his name included in the register if he satisfies the registrar that he is qualified, whether by examination or under bye-laws made by the RPSGB, to receive a certificate of competence to practise.

Section 16 of the Pharmacy Act 1954, together with bye-laws made under the Act, have the effect of prescribing a maximum number of attempts to pass the pharmacy registration examinations. Although the practice constituted a restraint of trade, it is justifiable in the interests of safeguarding the public and preserving the integrity of the profession – see *R* v. *RPSGB ex parte Mahmood (2000).*

Certificate of registration

The Council of the RPSGB is obliged under *Section 5* of the Pharmacy Act 1954 to issue to a qualified pharmacist a certificate of registration. Under the MA 1968 a pharmacist is bound to "conspicuously exhibit" his certificate of registration at each premises in respect of which he has personal control. It is a criminal offence fraudulently to exhibit a certificate purporting to be a certificate of membership of the RPSGB. It is further a criminal offence to forge a certificate or allow it to be used by any other person.

Removal of name from the register

The Council may direct the registrar to remove the name of a pharmaceutical chemist from the register if he has failed to pay the annual fee within 2 months of the date of demand. The Statutory Committee may also direct the removal of the name of a pharmaceutical chemist from the register if he has been guilty of a crime or professional misconduct.

Registration of premises

Under *Section 75* of the MA 1968 the registrar is obliged to keep a register in which he enters any premises in respect of which an application for registration is made. The registrar must be satisfied that at the time of the application the applicant is a person lawfully conducting an RPB or entitled to conduct an RPB lawfully from the premises. The meaning of these terms has been explained earlier in Chapter 9.

Infringements

During 1999 the Ethics Infringements Committee and the Law Infringements Committee combined to form a new Infringements Committee. The Infringements Committee is made up of eight council members. Five are professional pharmacist members and the remaining three are the lay members of Council nominated by the Privy Council. If cases need to be heard involving registered pharmacy technicians or technicians applying to join the voluntary register, two expert technician members will be co-opted onto the Committee for expert advice. The quorum of the Committee is four, including one Privy Council nominee and at least two pharmacist members.

In accordance with the Infringements Committee (Procedure) Rules 2005 the Committee conducts investigations into allegations of misconduct, infringements of ethical standards and/or unlawful activity.

The Committee is required to consider all allegations brought before it and on the most appropriate course of action to deal with such infringements. In doing so it acts as a mechanism for the filtering of cases and has to be mindful of a number of competing desirables:

- The need to ensure protection of the public
- The need to ensure maintenance of the reputation of, and public confidence in the profession
- The legitimate expectations of the public, and of complainants in particular, that allegations of misconduct will be fully and fairly investigated
- The need for legitimate safeguards for the practitioner, who, as a professional person, maybe considered particularly vulnerable to, and damaged by, unwarranted allegations against him (see RPSGB IC Guidance).

This filtering exercise is necessary in order to ensure that the only cases that are referred to the Statutory Committee (see below) are those in which there is a real prospect of establishing misconduct which would render the person concerned unfit to remain on the register.

With consideration of the above factors the Committee will need to decide whether to:

- inform the person concerned that it will take no further action on this occasion, but that should any fresh allegation be made against the person concerned within 5 years from the date of the Committee's decision, the Committee will consider the original alleged infringement together with the further alleged infringement;
- write a letter of advice to the person concerned, and to such other person or body the Committee considers appropriate in the circumstances of the case;
- where the alleged infringement is admitted, issue a warning to the person concerned;
- instruct the Society's Fitness to Practise Directorate to initiate criminal proceedings against the person concerned;
- refer the case to the Statutory Committee; or
- take no further action.

Since 25 September 2000 the RPSGB has been empowered to conduct covert surveillance under the Regulation of Investigatory Powers Act 2000. The RPSGB is included in a list of public authorities allowed to authorise directed surveillance as part of an investigation into the detection or prevention of crime. Directed surveillance is defined as covert surveillance which does not entail the presence of individuals or use of monitoring devices on residential premises or in private vehicles. The surveillance must be proportionate and be carried out for the purposes of a specific investigation.

Although covert surveillance has been used to a fairly limited extent to date the inclusion of the RPSGB as an authorised public authority might encourage its use in the investigation of the most serious cases.

The Statutory Committee of the RPSGB

Introduction

The professional conduct of pharmaceutical chemists is supervised by a committee of the RPSGB known as the Statutory Committee. The Statutory Committee exercises its supervisory and disciplinary jurisdiction pursuant to *Section 7* of the Pharmacy Act 1954, and its procedures are governed by statutory instrument, i.e. the Pharmaceutical Society (Statutory Committee) Order of Council 1978, SI 1978 No. 20. In accordance with *Section 8* of the latter Act, the Statutory Committee considers any convictions received by, or allegations of misconduct made against, a pharmacist or a person applying for registration with the RPSGB.

Under *Section 80* of the Medicines Act 1968, the Statutory Committee additionally considers cases against companies carrying on a retail pharmacy business where:

- the company has committed an offence under medicines legislation;
- a director, officer or employee of the company has been convicted of an offence, or is alleged to have committed misconduct.

In 2004 the Statutory Committee ordered the erasure of 16 pharmacists from the register and issued 20 reprimands. The Committee also restored five former pharmacists to the register but decided not to restore to the register three further pharmacists who had applied.

Composition

The Statutory Committee consists of six members appointed by the Council of the RPSGB and the chairman who must be legally qualified. The chairman is appointed by the Privy Council. Members of the Statutory Committee hold office for 5 years. The quorum for a meeting of the Statutory Committee is three, but the chairman must be present. The Council of the RPSGB also appoints a secretary who is usually present at all Statutory Committee meetings. The Statutory Committee sits 3 to 4 days each month.

Reference to the Statutory Committee

If information concerning the criminal conviction or professional misconduct of a registered pharmacist or one of his employees comes to the attention of the RPSGB (either as a result of the activities of the inspectors or by complaint from a member of the public), the information may be passed to the secretary of the Statutory Committee. On receipt of the information the secretary must submit to the chairman a report which summarizes the information or complaint. The chairman may direct the secretary to write to the person affected by the complaint to invite that person to submit an answer or an explanation of the conduct in question.

After considering the totality of the information available to him, the chairman must direct himself as follows:

- If he considers that the case is outside the Statutory Committee's jurisdiction, or is otherwise frivolous, or that it should be disregarded due to lapse of time or some other circumstance, the chairman must decide that the case is not to proceed further.
- If he considers that the conviction or alleged professional misconduct is not of a serious nature, or for some other reason may be disposed of without an inquiry, he may, after consulting the other members of the Statutory Committee, decide that the case is not to proceed further, but he may direct the secretary to send a reprimand to the person affected and caution him as to his future conduct.
- In any other case the chairman must direct the secretary to take the necessary steps to hold an inquiry by the Statutory Committee into the matter. In this event, the secretary must instruct a solicitor to investigate the facts of the case. If the solicitor reports that there is insufficient evidence to prove the criminal conviction or alleged misconduct, the Statutory Committee must consider his report and decide whether to hold an inquiry.

Notice of inquiry

The secretary must send notice to the person affected that the Statutory Committee is to inquire into the circumstances of a criminal conviction or his alleged misconduct. The notice must be sent not less than 28 days before the date of the inquiry.

Procedure at the hearing

An inquiry is held in public, although the Statutory Committee may direct the public to be excluded if it appears that exclusion is in the interests of justice or there is some other compelling reason. The person affected and the complainant (in effect, the RPSGB) may be represented by a solicitor or barrister at the hearing. If the person affected does not attend the inquiry, the Statutory Committee may proceed in his absence or adjourn the hearing. At the hearing the case is presented against the person affected, and witnesses are called to give evidence. The witnesses may be cross-examined. This will be followed by evidence from the person affected. The Statutory Committee has a wide discretion to receive evidence orally or in writing. However, the Statutory Committee is bound to disregard evidence from a person who is present but refuses to submit for cross-examination.

The decision

After hearing the evidence and submissions, the Statutory Committee retires to consider its decision. The Statutory Committee must decide:

- whether the conviction or misconduct is proved;
- if so, whether the conviction or misconduct is such as to render the person with regard to whom it is proved unfit to be on the register;

- if so, whether one of the statutory directions should be made;
- whether any reprimand or admonition should be addressed to the person affected.

The statutory directions are set out in *Section 8* of the Pharmacy Act 1954 and *Section 80* of the MA 1968. By *Section 8* of the Pharmacy Act 1954 the Statutory Committee may direct the removal of a registered pharmaceutical chemist, or person employed by him, from the register. *Section 80* of the MA 1968 gives the same power to direct removal from the register of a limited company which carries on an RPB and any member of the company's board or any officer employed by the company. In either case a statutory direction does not take effect until 3 months after notice of the direction has been given or, where an appeal to the High Court is brought against the direction, until the appeal is determined or withdrawn.

The chairman must announce the decision in public, and the decision must be communicated to the person affected and the registrar, who must act on any statutory direction which has been given.

Application for restoration

A person whose name has been removed from the register as a result of criminal conviction or misconduct may apply to have his name restored to the register. The application must be supported by a statutory declaration made by the applicant and accompanied by at least two certificates of his identity and good character. One must be given by a registered pharmaceutical chemist. The other certificate may be given by a registered pharmaceutical chemist, a fully registered medical practitioner, a justice of the peace or a legally qualified holder of a judicial office – Regulation 31 of the Pharmaceutical Society (Statutory Committee) Order of Council 1978.

In addition, any applicant seeking restoration to the register is advised to provide, in support of the application, detailed evidence demonstrating the applicant's fitness to return to the register. This may include evidence of activities designed to address or learn from the original offence or misconduct, and evidence of learning activities designed to keep up to date with skills and knowledge, and with developments in practice. The applicant should also provide evidence demonstrating insight into the gravity of the offence or misconduct which resulted in the removal of his name from the register.

In the past the application has been considered by the Statutory Committee in private, unless the chairman directed otherwise. However, the Statutory Committee can determine its own procedure, and in November 1990 the Statutory Committee changed its procedure. The chairman stated that the application will now always be held in public, unless there was some special reason for the application to be heard in private. Unless the Statutory Committee decides to grant the application without a hearing, the applicant is entitled to appear before the Statutory Committee and be represented by a solicitor or barrister. If the statutory direction had been given at the inquiry following a complaint, the complainant may be given an opportunity of being heard or submitting written evidence. The secretary must communicate the decision of the Statutory Committee to the applicant and to any objector, and also to the registrar who must act on any direction which has been given.

Purpose of sanction imposed by the statutory committee

When considering an application for restoration, the purpose of the original sanction of removal from the register must be borne in mind. The purpose of the sanction is threefold, namely

(1) the protection of the public
(2) the maintenance of public confidence in the profession and
(3) the maintenance of proper standards of behaviour.

Principles to be applied when considering a restoration application

Removal from the register is the most serious sanction available to the Statutory Committee. Once removed from the register, a former practitioner is considered no longer fit to be a member of the profession. In ordinary circumstances, the Statutory Committee will not entertain an application for restoration within any period shorter than 3 years from the date that the removal from the register took effect.

Guidance on the approach to be adopted is provided in the following cases. The Master of the Rolls in *Bolton* v. *Law Society, 1994* stated,

> It often happens that a former solicitor appearing before the tribunal can adduce a wealth of glowing tributes from his professional brethren. He can often show that for him and his family the consequences of striking off or suspension would be little short of tragic. Often he will say, convincingly, that he has learned his lesson and will not offend again. On applying for restoration after striking off, all these points may be made, and the former solicitor may also be able to point to real efforts made to re-establish himself and redeem his reputation. All of these matters are relevant and should be considered. But none of them touches the essential issue, which is the need to maintain among members of the public a well founded confidence that any solicitor whom they instruct will be a person of unquestionable integrity, probity and trustworthiness. [. . .] The reputation of the profession is more important than then fortunes of any individual member. Membership of a profession brings many benefits, but that is a part of the price.

In *Gosai* v. *General Medical Council, 2003*, these points were reiterated by the Privy Council:

> The Professional Conduct Committee accepted that the appellant was making real efforts to demonstrate his fitness to practise. However, the Professional Conduct Committee was entitled to conclude, in relation to . . . the refusal of restoration . . . that the efforts he had made were outweighed by other factors. These included the seriousness of the original offence when the Professional Conduct Committee stated that the appellant had "fallen lamentably below the professional standards to which patients were entitled," "demonstrated clinical importance of the most basic kind", and [had] "not been truthful."

The Statutory Committee will give careful consideration to all the circumstances of an individual case and the representations made by the applicant. However, the applicant will need to present a strong argument and will be required to demonstrate his suitability to be restored to the register.

Appeals

A person or a limited company affected by a decision of the Statutory Committee to remove them from the register or not restore them to the register may, within 3 months from the date of the decision, appeal to the High Court. The RPSGB may appear on the hearing of an appeal as the respondent. On appeal the High Court may make any order as it thinks fit, including an order as to the costs of the appeal. The registrar is bound to make such alterations in the register as are necessary to give effect to the High Court's order on appeal. An affected person who has been reprimanded may also appeal to the High Court, but by way of judicial review. Again the appeal has to be lodged promptly and within a maximum time limit of 3 months from the date of decision.

It is difficult to appeal successfully against the Statutory Committee's decision. The function of the High Court is not to impose its own view in substitution for a view taken by the Statutory Committee unless it came to the conclusion that the Committee was plainly wrong or had misdirected itself in reaching its conclusion – see *Thobani* v. *Pharmaceutical Society of Great Britain, 1990*, and *Singh* v. *General Medical Council, 2001*.

Furthermore, *Section 11(2)* of the Pharmacy Act 1954 stipulates that in a situation where an applicant has previously appealed to the High Court against the decision to remove his name from the register and the appeal was dismissed, any direction by the Statutory Committee to restore his name to register shall not take effect unless it is approved by the Privy Council.

The standards of professional conduct

Code of Ethics

The RPSGB maintains a Code of Ethics and Standards for its members with the aim of safeguarding and promoting the interests of the public and the profession. The public places great trust in the knowledge, skills and professional judgement of pharmacists. This trust requires pharmacists to ensure and maintain, throughout their career, high standards of personal and professional conduct and performance, up-to-date knowledge and continuing competence relevant to their sphere of practice whether or not they work in direct contact with the public. The Code of Ethics and Professional Standards are reproduced on the RPSGB's website (www.rpsgb.org.uk).

Key responsibilities

The Code of Ethics identifies the key responsibilities of a pharmacist in the following terms:

> Pharmacists understand the nature and effect of medicines and medicinal ingredients, and how they may be used to prevent and treat illness, relieve symptoms or assist in the diagnosis of disease. Pharmacists in professional practice use their knowledge for the well-being and safety of patients and the public.

- At all times pharmacists must act in the interests of patients and other members of the public, and seek to provide the best possible health care for the community in partnership with other health professions. Pharmacists must treat all those who seek pharmaceutical services with courtesy, respect and confidentiality. Pharmacists must respect patients' rights to participate in decisions about their care and must provide information in a way in which it can be understood.
- Pharmacists must ensure that their knowledge, skills and performance are of a high quality, up to date, evidence based and relevant to their field of practice.
- Pharmacists must ensure that they behave with integrity and probity, adhere to accepted standards of personal and professional conduct and do not engage in any behaviour or activity likely to bring the profession into disrepute or undermine public confidence in the profession.

Principles

There are a number of guiding principles which stand at the core of the Code of Ethics. Apart from minor amendments these principles do not differ from the principles set out in the Code of Ethics approved by Council in 1984. The principles are as follows.

(1) A pharmacist's prime concern must be for the welfare of both patients and public.
(2) A pharmacist must uphold the honour and dignity of the profession and not engage in any activity which may bring the profession into disrepute.
(3) A pharmacist must at all times have regard to the laws and regulations applicable to pharmaceutical practice and maintain a high standard of professional conduct. A pharmacist must avoid any act or omission which would impair confidence in the pharmaceutical profession. When a pharmaceutical service is provided, a pharmacist must ensure that it is efficient.
(4) A pharmacist must respect the confidentiality of information acquired in the course of professional practice relating to patients and their families. Such information must not be disclosed to anyone without the consent of the patient or appropriate guardian unless the interests of the public or the patient require such disclosure.
(5) A pharmacist must keep abreast of the progress of pharmaceutical knowledge in order to maintain a high standard of professional competence relative to his sphere of activity.
(6) A pharmacist must neither agree to practise under any conditions of service which compromise his professional independence nor impose such conditions on other pharmacists.
(7) Publicity for professional services is permitted provided that such publicity does not create an invidious distinction between pharmacists or pharmacies, is dignified and does not bring the profession into disrepute.
(8) A pharmacist offering services directly to the public must do so in premises which reflect the professional character of pharmacy.
(9) A pharmacist must at all times endeavour to cooperate with professional colleagues and members of other health professions so that patients and the public may benefit.

Obligations

The Council formed the view that it was necessary to elaborate on the nine principles so as to form a brief summary of the pharmacist's obligations in each area. Any complaint of misconduct would be based upon an alleged breach of these obligations and, by inference, of the principle which governs them.

Guidance

In order to assist pharmacists in the practical discharge of their professional obligations, the Council has set out some guidance which is intended to reflect the standards which pharmacists should meet in their daily lives.

A practical example

The operation of the Code of Ethics can be demonstrated by a consideration of a practical example which arises almost daily in a retail pharmacy. A customer wishes to purchase two bottles of codeine linctus cough mixture. The pharmacist recognizes the customer, and believes that she bought two bottles of the same mixture 3 days earlier. It would not be unlawful to make the sale. But what does the Code of Ethics say?

> *Principle 1.* A pharmacist's prime concern must be for the welfare of both the patients and public.
>
> *Obligation*: A pharmacist must exercise professional judgment to prevent the supply of unnecessary and/or excessive quantities of medicines and other products, particularly those which are liable to abuse or which are claimed to depress appetite, prevent absorption of food or reduce body fluid. Guidance on Obligation Many POMs and CDs have a potential for abuse or dependency. Care should be taken over their supply even when it is legally authorized by prescription or signed order. A pharmacist should be alert to the possibility of drug dependency in health care professionals and patients and should be prepared to make enquiries to ensure that such medicines are to be used responsibly.
>
> Some over-the-counter medicines and non-medicinal products are liable to be abused, which in this context usually means (a) consumption over a lengthy period and/or (b) consumption of doses substantially higher than recommended. Requests for such products should be dealt with personally by the pharmacist and sales should be refused if it is apparent that the purchase is not for a genuine medicinal purpose or if the frequency of purchase suggests over-use. A pharmacist should not attempt on his own to control an abuser's habit, but should liaise with bodies such as drug abuse clinics in any local initiative to assist abusers.

An up-to-date list of products known to be abused nationally appears in the Medicines, Ethics and Practice Guide. The products which are abused are subject to change, and pharmacists should keep abreast of local and national trends. The professional requirements for the provision of needle and syringe exchange schemes are set out in Standard 17. It is clear from this guidance that the pharmacist should not make the sale because the frequency of purchase suggests overuse. The pharmacist would err in his professional judgement if he made the sale because he would be supplying an excessive quantity of medicine which is liable to abuse. This error, particularly if it was repeated on more than one occasion, would render the pharmacist open to a finding of misconduct by the Statutory Committee.

Part 3 of the Code of Ethics and Standards: Service Specifications

The application of the key professional responsibilities described in Part 1 to the following activities indicates that the provision of these services should incorporate the following professional requirements. The following service specifications cover a wide cross-section of service specifications some of which are core services which will be provided by the majority of pharmacies whilst others are additional professional services which pharmacists may choose to be involved in.

There are 23 areas covered by the service standards, as follows.

(1) standards for premises – appearance, safety, condition and tidiness of premises, environment, size of dispensary, and hygiene;
(2) standards for dispensary design and equipment – suitability of dispensary, work surface and shelves, floor covering, water supply, waste disposal, and dispensing equipment;
(3) standards for procurement and sources for materials – responsibility for procurement, sources of supply, safe systems of work, and medical gases;
(4) standards of manufacturing and quality assurance – good manufacturing practice, quality assurance and control, batch numbers, manufacturing formulae, and documentation, equipment and sources of supply for manufacturing;
(5) standards for dispensing procedures – dispensing procedures, supervision of dispensing and sales, safety in dispensing procedures, forged prescriptions, dispensing containers, re-use of containers, re-use of medicines, labels, storage, recalls, and personal hygiene;
(6) standards for professional indemnity;
(7) standards for education, training and development – competency, self-assessment, legislative changes and new services;
(8) standards for relationships with patients and the public;
(9) standards for relationships with other health care professionals;
(10) standards for administration and management;
(11) standards for community pharmacists providing a repeat medication service.
(12) standards for the sale of non-prescribed medicines – request for medicine by name, pharmacist's involvement, special purchasers or users, medicines requiring special care.
(13) standards for pharmacists providing services to nursing and residential homes.
(14) standards for pharmacists providing instalment dispensing services.
(15) standards for the home delivery of medicines.
(16) standards for pharmacists providing domiciliary oxygen services.

(17)   standards for pharmacists providing needle and syringe exchange schemes.
(18)   standards for the collection and disposal of pharmaceutical waste by community pharmacies.
(19)   standards for the provision of on-line pharmacy services: security/confidentiality, request for supply of medicines, information and advice, record keeping.
(20)   standards for pharmacists dispensing extemporaneously prepared products.
(21)   standards for pharmacists serving drug users.
(22)   standards for pharmacists providing aseptic dispensing services from non-licensed units.
(23)   standards for pharmacists involved in writing and/or approving patient group directions.

Council statements

The Council has issued two Council statements which supplement the obligations set out in the Code. The first statement prohibits any involvement in petitions promoting self interest to the detriment of other existing pharmacy contractors. The second concerns the circumstances in which a dog may be present on pharmacy premises.

Professional Standards Fact Sheets

The RPSGB has also prepared a series of Professional Standards Fact Sheets addressing areas of practice which are frequently the subject of enquiry. At the time of writing, sheets were available on the following subjects:

(1)   controlled drugs and community pharmacy
(2)   controlled drugs and hospital pharmacy
(3)   the export of medicines
(4)   the use of unlicensed medicines in pharmacy
(5)   advertising
(6)   prescription collection, home delivery and repeat medication services
(7)   pharmacy and the Internet
(8)   labelling of MDS and compliance aids
(9)   patient group directions
(10)   dealing with dispensing errors
(11)   confidentiality, the Data Protection Act 1998 and the disclosure of information
(12)   the Medicines for Human Use (Marketing Authorisations, etc.) Regulations 1994, and the effect thereof
(13)   employing a locum/working as a locum.

The fact sheets are reproduced on the RPSGB's website (www.rpsgb.org). The RPSGB has also prepared a series of guidance documents on issues that pharmacists and registered pharmacy technicians might be required to deal with as part of their professional practice. The titles are:

● raising concerns – guidance for pharmacists and registered pharmacy technicians
● maintaining running balances of Controlled Drug stock.

Further guidance on issues such as counter-prescribing for self-limiting minor illness and common conditions and the supply of emergency hormonal contraception as a pharmacy medicine can be found in the professional pharmaceutical publication, Pharmaceutical Journal.

Breach of the Code

A breach of the Code of Ethics could form the basis of a complaint of misconduct but the Council, in considering whether or not action should follow, takes into consideration the circumstances of an individual case and does not regard itself as being limited to those matters which are mentioned in the Code. In law, the arbiter of what constitutes misconduct is the Statutory Committee. Misconduct does not necessarily involve some sort of moral censure; rather, misconduct may be defined as "incorrect or erroneous conduct of any kind provided that it is of a serious nature", i.e. judged according to the rules written or unwritten of the pharmaceutical profession (see *R* v. *Statutory Committee of the Pharmaceutical Society of Great Britain, ex parte Sokoh, 1986*). Moreover, in that case the High Court held that it was possible that just one error may constitute misconduct, if the error was sufficiently serious.

The incorrect or erroneous conduct must, however, be regarded as so serious as to justify a finding of misconduct. Deliberate breach of the policy made by the Council will not automatically amount to misconduct – in such a case the Statutory Committee has to satisfy itself that the deliberate breach of policy was of such a quality as to constitute serious misconduct (see *R* v. *Statutory Committee of the Royal Pharmaceutical Society ex parte Boots the Chemists PLC, 1997*). In that case Boots deliberately flouted policy made by the Council in June 1993 to prohibit the introduction of collection and delivery services in areas where a community pharmacy already exists. The chairman of the Statutory Committee advised that Boots' conduct did not amount to misconduct in law. The High Court agreed and said that the legally unqualified majority of the committee should have followed the chairman's advice.

The Fitness to Practise Directorate

Parliament enacted the Pharmacists (Fitness to Practise) Act 1997 which established the Fitness to Practise Directorate of the RPSGB. The latter's function is to monitor and ensure compliance with the standards of conduct, performance and fitness to practise set by the RPSGB, and with obligations imposed on the profession of pharmacy by statute. Where a registered member of the Society fails to conduct a retail pharmacy business in compliance with those standards and legal obligations, the Fitness to Practise Directorate steps in accordingly and takes the necessary action to enforce those standards, and legal obligations are upheld.

Monitoring

Monitoring is performed by the Inspectorate, who regularly visit community pharmacies and who investigate any allegations or complaints made against persons registered with the Society or lawfully conducting a retail pharmacy business.

Compliance

Compliance is achieved by the provision of advice on the interpretation of the law and code of ethics, and by publication of the decisions of the Society's Fitness to Practice Committees.

The Directorate is also given power to impose conditions with which a pharmacist must comply if he continues to practise in circumstances where he is unwell. Investigations into a pharmacist's fitness to practise are initiated by the Directorate, which is required to inform the pharmacist involved and give him 28 days to respond. Following a hearing the Directorate's Infringements Committee is empowered to dismiss the allegation of unfitness to practise or, if it considers it to be well founded, to impose conditions on practice or suspend registration. Pharmacists who have been suspended or made subject to conditions of practice are able to request a review of the order against them. The Act also set up an appeal procedure.

The future

At the time of writing the RPSGB had consulted its members on a major reform of the profession's disciplinary machinery and the introduction of a requirement on pharmacists to undertake appropriate continuing professional development if they wish to retain the right to practice.

The catalyst for reform was provided by the NHS Plan published in July 2000, which requires health self-regulatory bodies such as the RPSGB to change so that they:

- are smaller, with much greater patient and public representation in their membership;
- have faster, more transparent procedures;
- develop meaningful accountability to the public and the Health Service.

These principles were expanded upon in the government consultation papers issued in August 2000 for the new Nursing and Midwifery Council (NMC) and the new Health Professions Council (HPC). A specific requirement contained within the proposals for new legislation for these professions is that a professional majority of more than one on either the Councils or their Committees is unacceptable to government.

The consultation papers provide for the key functions for the new Councils to be:

- establishing and keeping the register ("registration");
- establishing and reviewing standards of proficiency, and the training required, for admission to the register ("education");
- establishing and reviewing standards of conduct and ethics ("standards setting");
- establishing and reviewing arrangements to protect the public from those who are unfit to practice ("discipline and health");
- establishing and reviewing requirements for re-admission and renewal of registration ("competence based practising rights").

In any event, the RPSGB recognises that its powers and structures are outmoded and in need of reform, deriving principally from the Pharmacy Act 1954. The enactment of the Health Act 1999 enables professional regulatory bodies to amend their governing legislation by Order, and rising to the challenge in February 2001 the RPSGB distributed a paper to its members entitled "Reform of disciplinary machinery and the introduction of competence based practising rights" containing radical proposals to this effect.

The paper proposed the delegation of disciplinary functions by Council to two Committees. An Investigating Committee would replace the Council's existing Infringements Committee, and a Disciplinary Committee would replace the Statutory Committee. In all cases it is proposed that members of the Committee will have security of tenure to ensure that they are independent of influence. Lay members will be appointed after public advertisement and in consultation with the Privy Council.

The paper also addressed the need for the RPSGB's education division to explore ways to develop its continuing professional development pilot scheme in order to satisfy the government's broad requirements laid down in the NMC and HPC consultation documents.

A further consulation paper was published in 2003 entitled "Vision for Pharmacy in the New NHS". This summarised the progress made in the first 3 years of the programme and suggesting the next priorities for the profession. Further informa tion on these reports can be located on the RPSGB website.

Internet Pharmacy

The Internet offers an unprecedented medium unhindered by geographical barriers, and the opportunities to utilise its power for delivering and receiving information are almost boundless. However, in providing such freedom the Internet has created difficulties. In the medical context one major difficulty faced concerns the regulation of online prescribing.

The popularity of the drug Viagra (sildenafil citrate) provides a key example. Within days of the United States Food and Drug Administration's approval of Viagra the Internet was flooded with websites dedicated to the selling of the "lifestyle drug".

The Internet's exponential growth and the potential to accumulate major profits fuelled this growth. Such sites sell everything, from licensed drugs to "miracle cures" with astounding claims of efficacy.

Doctors from the United States were the first to grasp the opportunity, launching sites such as Confirmed.com. They were quickly followed by online pharmacies, both licensed and unlicensed including those purveying antidepressants and infertility pills.

Although many sites are convincing, the Internet is not discriminating in whom it allows to view them. A US case in which a child bought Viagra with the use of his parent's credit card has highlighted the ease of which purchases can be made and the lack of regulatory control surrounding drug prescription on the Internet. Further problems of the Internet include the ease with which patients can fail to provide a full clinical history or disguise their true intent, whilst it is difficult for a doctor to effectively evaluate the risks and benefits of prescription.

Internet prescribing of drugs on-line in the United Kingdom

The GMC has explicitly warned about prescribing medicinal products on the Internet, stating such activity fails to meet standards of good clinical practice and that it was unacceptable that any doctor should do so without first seeing the patient.

The British Medical Association (BMA) has also maintained a call for a ban on doctors prescribing medicinal products on-line. The main concern is that doctors cannot ascertain sufficient detail about a patient's condition simply by an exchange of email. Furthermore, there are concerns that patients may use the Internet to obtain medicinal products they do not need.

At present there are no regulations to protect patients. There are estimated to be over 20,000 sites on the Internet offering information about health, and an increasing number are offering advice directly to individual patients. In addition a number of GPs have launched websites in the United Kingdom to offer diagnoses and prescriptions to patients over the Internet.

Patients are normally protected from unscrupulous doctors by checking their registered status through the GMC. However, without stronger forms of authentication there is still a risk that an on-line doctor could falsely represent themselves as a GMC registered practitioner.

Pharmacists and legality of selling prescription drugs over the Internet

A ruling by the European Court of Justice in the case *of Deutsche Apothekerverband* v. *0800 DocMorris NV, 2005*, has provided some clear guidance to all EC pharmacists as to the legality of prescription drug sales on-line. The ECJ held that whilst European pharmacies are free to sell over-the-counter medicines on the Internet they cannot do the same for prescription drugs. The case was raised by a German court who had queried whether a national ban on all sales breached EU rules on the free movement of goods.

A German pharmacy trade body, the Deutsche Apothekerverband, had complained that Dutch on-line pharmacy 0800 DocMorris.com was selling prescription and non-prescription medicines, in languages including German, for consumers in Germany. The ECJ stated that where the ban related to medicinal products that had been authorised for sale on the German market, there was breach of the EU laws on the free movement of goods.

However, such a breach is only acceptable if it is justified by circumstances specified in EU law. In this case, said the Court, the breach could be justified by reason of being necessary for the "health and life of humans". Thus the ban could be justified with regard to authorised medicines only available on prescription, because "there may be risks attaching to the use of these medicinal products". Accordingly, "the need to be able to check effectively and responsibly the authenticity of doctors' prescriptions and to ensure that the medicine is handed over either to the customer himself, or to a person to whom its collection has been entrusted by the customer, is such as to justify a prohibition on mail-order sales". In addition the Court considered the provisions of the advertising law that prohibits the advertising of mail order. The Court ruled that where a prohibition of that kind applies to medicinal products that require authorisation but have not been authorised, or to medicinal products available only on prescription, the prohibition is in keeping with an existing prohibition in EU law.

NHS Prescription Fraud

Prescription fraud has proved a highly controversial topic within the NHS – with fraud estimated to have cost the NHS at least £117 million in 1997–1998. A concerted effort by the NHS Counter Fraud and Security Management Service has significantly reduced this figure following the introduction of fines and greater rigour in eligibility.

Pharmacists are required to ask people who get free prescriptions for proof. People entitled to free prescriptions include those under 18 and over 65, the unemployed, pregnant women, people on low incomes and those with certain health conditions such as diabetes. Thus between 1999 and 2004, counter fraud work cut pharmaceutical patient fraud by 60%, dental patient fraud by 25%, optical patient fraud by 23% and, in some areas, fraud by NHS professionals by 31–46%. Fraud detection rates have improved by more than 1400% and there is a 97% successful prosecution rate.

Pharmacists are offered a reward of £70 for every time they spot and report a false or fraudulent claim. Anyone caught making a false claim, or trying to make a false claim, face going to court and having a £100 fine. However, as with many other counter-fraud regimes it has been suggested that this greater rigour has discouraged genuinely eligible people from getting what they are entitled to, through excessive bureaucracy.

Forged prescriptions

It can be extremely difficult to detect a forged prescription, but every pharmacist should be alert to the possibility that any prescription calling for a misused product could be a forgery.

In many instances, the forger may make a fundamental error in writing the prescription or the pharmacist may get an instinctive feeling that the prescription is not genuine because of the way the patient behaves.

If the prescriber's signature is known, or is not known to be suffering from a condition which requires the medicinal product prescribed, the signature should be scrutinised and, if possible, checked against an example on another prescription known to be genuine. Large doses or quantities should be checked with the prescriber in order to detect alterations to previously valid prescriptions.

If the prescriber's signature is not known, the prescriber must be contacted and asked to confirm that the prescription is genuine. The prescriber's telephone number must be obtained from the telephone directory, or from directory inquiries, not from the headed notepaper, as forgers may use false letter headings.

A list of matters should alert a pharmacist and cause him to check further. These include the following:

- an unknown prescriber
- a new patient
- excessive quantities
- uncharacteristic prescribing or method of writing prescription by a known doctor before or after prescriber's signature.

These precautions should be applied to all prescriptions for medicinal products liable to abuse and not only for controlled drugs.

Chapter 26

Liability in Negligence

Dispensing mistakes

A pharmacist, like any other professional person, can make a mistake and, like doctors, the consequences of a pharmacist's mistake can be most serious. The customer may suffer serious personal injuries as a result of the mistake. It has been estimated that in the USA deaths due to medication errors exceed the number of fatal accidents on the roads. In the UK little research has been performed on dispensing errors in community pharmacy. Some research conducted in Glasgow in 1996 disclosed that dispensing errors occurred in 1% of prescriptions dispensed. Most of these errors related to dispensing the wrong medicine or strength of medicine (72%). Incorrect labelling accounted for 14% of errors.

The law concerning a pharmacist's civil liability for mistakes is considered in this section of the book. With the increase in professional negligence litigation, it is an area of law with which the contemporary community pharmacist needs to have some familiarity.

Breach of contract

Where a customer obtains medicinal products on the strength of an NHS prescription, even though he pays a prescription charge, the courts have held that the products are not supplied under a contract of sale, but rather by virtue of the pharmacist's statutory duty to supply the medicinal products (*Pfizer Corp.* v. *Ministry of Health (1965)*). Accordingly, if the customer is to recover any damages for a mistake in the dispensing process, he has to establish a case in negligence against the pharmacist at common law.

Negligence

A customer who wishes to recover damages for personal injuries has to prove four things:

(1) That the defendant owed him a duty of care.
(2) That the defendant was in breach of that duty.
(3) That he has suffered damage as a result of that breach.
(4) That the damage was reasonably foreseeable in all the circumstances.

Duty of care

A duty to take reasonable care arises when the defendant can reasonably foresee that the claimant (the one who complains) is likely to be injured by his conduct.

As Lord Atkin said in *Donoghue v. Stephenson (1932)*:

> You must take reasonable care to avoid acts or omissions which you can reasonably foresee would be likely to injure your neighbour. Who, then, in law is my neighbour? The answer seems to be ± persons who are so closely and directly affected by my act that I ought reasonably to have them in contemplation as being so affected when I am directing my mind to the acts or omissions which are called in question.

Breach of duty

It is always a question of fact whether the defendant has failed to show reasonable care in the particular circumstances of a case. The law lays down the general rules which determine the standard of care which has to be attained, and it is for the court to apply that legal standard of care to its findings of fact so as to find whether the defendant has attained that standard. The legal standard is not the standard of the defendant himself, but that of a person of ordinary prudence or a person using ordinary skill. In cases where a person has a particular skill, such as a pharmacist, the person is required to show the skill normally possessed by persons undertaking work of a similar nature. Thus in the case of a pharmacist, the pharmacist must exercise the standard of skill which is usual in his profession; he must exercise the same degree of care which a reasonably competent pharmacist would exercise in performing the same task.

Occasionally situations arise where the claimant is not able to establish exactly how the accident occurred. Nevertheless, the mere fact of the happening of the accident in certain circumstances may justify the inference that the defendant has probably been negligent and his negligence caused the injury. The maxim, known as *res ipsa loquitur* (i.e. "the thing speaks for itself"), is an evidentiary rule to the effect that the fact of the injury and the circumstances in which it was sustained, establish a prima facie case of negligence against the defendant, which he must then rebut in order to avoid a finding of liability.

Damage as a result of the breach

The claimant must show that the defendant's wrongdoing was a cause, though not necessarily the sole or dominant cause, of his injuries. In general, a defendant who commits a wrong takes his victim as he finds him. It is no answer to a claim for damages to say that the victim would have sustained no or less injury if he had not suffered from some pre-existing condition.

Foreseeable damage

There is a final hurdle which a claimant must surmount before he can recover damages for negligence. The type of injury which he has suffered must be reasonably foreseeable, in the sense that a reasonable man would have foreseen the type of injury as being likely to flow from the defendant's breach of duty.

Negligence causing death

All causes of action which accrue to the benefit of a claimant will survive for the benefit of his estate after his death under the provisions of the Law Reform (Miscellaneous Provisions) Act 1934. Additionally, where the breach of duty has caused death, the deceased's dependants may maintain an action and recover damages against the person liable in respect of the death under the Fatal Accidents Act 1976. The action must be brought by the deceased's personal representatives, and since only one action may be brought, claims must be included for all the dependants. In assessing damages under the Fatal Accidents Act, other than damages of £7,500 for bereavement, the court seeks to compensate the dependants for the loss which they have sustained as a result of the death.

Choice of defendant

In some cases the claimant may be faced with a choice of defendants. A typical situation arises where the claimant was a passenger in a motor car, which was in collision with another. If there is evidence to show that both drivers are to blame, it is normal practice to commence legal proceedings against both drivers. The same principles will apply where a patient has suffered injury caused by the breach of duty of a doctor and a pharmacist. Both may be sued together in one action. The basic rule is that each of the two tortfeasors will be liable for the whole damage resulting from their tortious act. However, where tortfeasors are jointly liable, the tortfeasors can ask the court to assess their respective liability in respect of the accident. This is done by one of the tortfeasors commencing proceedings against the other for contribution under the Civil Liability (Contribution) Act 1978.

Defences

The obvious defence, raised in most negligence actions, is the basic denial that the defendant has been guilty of any negligence and the further denial that, in the event of the claimant establishing any breach of duty against him, the injury resulted from the accident. The following specific defences tend to arise in practice in cases where pharmacists are involved.

Contributory negligence

Where the injury suffered is partly the result of the fault of the claimant, the recoverable damages are reduced by the court to the extent it thinks fit, having regard to the plaintiff's responsibility for the injuries: the Law Reform (Contributory Negligence) Act 1945. The court determines the percentage of contributory negligence. It will not deal in minute percentages, so the normal practice is to disregard responsibility evaluated at less than 10%.

Novus actus interveniens

(A new act intervening)

Situations sometimes arise where the sequence of events following on from the defendant's act or omission is interrupted. Once it is established that, in the ordinary course of events, the defendant's act or omission would not have resulted in the damage but for the intervening act (whether of some third party or of the claimant), the chain of causation is broken. In such an event the defendant will not be liable.

Volenti non fit injuria

(That to which a man consents cannot be considered an injury.)

To raise this defence it is necessary to show that the claimant agreed to run the risk involved; mere silence on the subject is not normally sufficient.

Limitation

In personal injury cases the claimant must normally commence his action within 3 years of the date when the cause of action accrued. The date when the cause of action accrued will be the date when the injury was sustained. There are, however, special cases. After sustaining personal injury a claimant may not have discovered the effects of the injury or the identity of the defendant until after the limitation period has expired. In this case a special period of limitation is prescribed. The period of limitation will be deemed to run for 3 years from the date when the claimant became possessed of full information about his case. The period begins to run when the claimant has knowledge of all of the following matters:

(1)   That his injury was significant.
(2)   That the injury was attributable in whole or in part to the acts or omissions complained of.
(3)   The identity of the defendant.

However, it is right to add that a party who has sustained injuries will be imputed with knowledge which he might reasonably have been expected to acquire either by his own observation or inquiry or by expert advice, which it might have been reasonable for him to seek. Finally, a court may direct that the limitation provisions should be disregarded in a personal injury case if in the view of the court it would be equitable for action to proceed, having regard to the degree of prejudice suffered by the claimant on account of the rules of limitation as well as the prejudice the defendant would suffer if the limitation period were disregarded.

Application of the law to pharmacists

Amongst other duties it is clear that a pharmacist is obliged as a supplier of medicinal products to take reasonable care to:

(1) Ensure that the correct medicinal products are supplied.
(2) Warn customers of the potential dangers or adverse effects of the medicinal products.
(3) Ensure that customers are instructed as to the correct dosage.

Failure to take reasonable care in the discharge of any of these tasks will render the pharmacist liable to legal proceedings for breach of professional duty. The application of these principles is demonstrated by a consideration of the following reported cases.

Dispensing the wrong medicine

Collins v. Hertfordshire County Council (1947)

The pharmacist at a pre-NHS hospital was asked to dispense "100 ml of 1% cocaine with adrenaline, for injection". The pharmacist did not question the order for an unheard-of dosage of a dangerous drug. He made up the cocaine and adrenaline as an injection and supplied it to the operating theatre. During an operation the cocaine preparation was injected and the patient died. In fact the final-year student doctor who had ordered cocaine had herself misheard the consultant surgeon who had actually ordered procaine. The hospital's standing instructions on ordering dangerous drugs had not been complied with by either the doctor or the pharmacist. The hospital authority was held liable for the pharmacist's failure to question the order, and for the student doctor's mistake.

Prendergast v. Sam and Dee Ltd, Kozary and Miller (1989)

A pharmacist misread a doctor's writing on a prescription. The doctor had prescribed Amoxil but the pharmacist read it as Daonil. He dispensed Daonil, and the patient, who was not a diabetic, suffered hypoglycemia and irreversible brain damage. The patient (Prendergast) sued the pharmacy company (Sam and Dee Ltd), the pharmacist (Kozary) and the doctor (Miller). The court found all three defendants liable. The doctor's writing was adjudged to fall below the standard of legibility required of him in the exercise of his duty to the patient. The court also held that although the writing was bad, the word could have been read as Daonil, and that certain aspects of the prescription should have alerted the pharmacist. On appeal the court specifically held that the chain of causation starting with the poor handwriting was not broken. The court held that the pharmacist had a duty to give some thought to the prescription he was dispensing and he should not dispense mechanically. If there is any doubt the pharmacist must contact the doctor for clarification. In this case if the pharmacist had been paying attention he would have realised that there was something wrong with the prescription, since the dosage and the small number of tablets were unusual for Daonil. Additionally, the claimant had paid for the prescription, yet drugs for diabetes (such as Daonil) were free under the NHS. The court apportioned damages between the defendants: 25% to the doctor, and 75% shared between the company and the pharmacist.

Dispensing the wrong dosage

Dwyer v. Roderick (1983)

This case is usually referred to as the Migril case. The facts can be summed up in three sentences.

(1) A doctor negligently directed the patient to take an overdose in the prescription.
(2) The pharmacist failed to spot the error.
(3) The pharmacist was held liable in negligence.

These facts illustrate the difficulties for pharmacists.

The owner of the pharmacy admitted negligence, and the court held that he was 45% liable for the damages of £100 000. The judge emphasized that the pharmacist:

(1) Owed a duty to the patient to ensure that drugs were correctly prescribed.
(2) Should have spotted the error.
(3) Should have queried the prescription with the doctor.

As a result of this case the RPSGB issued this Council Statement:

> Pharmacists are reminded that patients who are prescribed Migril tablets should take no more than four tablets for any single migraine attack and no more than six in any one week. Because there have been occasional reports of severe toxic effects from overdosage, the Council advises pharmacists to ensure that patients are aware of the maximum dosage.

Taking precautions

Community pharmacists would do well to take heed of the results of an Australian survey into the causes of dispensing errors. High prescription volumes, pharmacist fatigue, pharmacist overwork, interruptions to dispensing and similar or confusing drug names were put forward as the principal contributing factors to dispensing errors.

In the UK some recent research has shown that the tendency of manufacturers to use similar packs for different medicines or strengths of medicines is a significant contributory cause of dispensing errors. Indeed, a survey of 33 hospitals revealed that the most frequent sources of error were different strengths of product in almost indistinguishable boxes, and different medicines with similar names made by the same manufacturer. Sometimes medicine packs are distinguishable when viewed individually but look similar when stacked together in a dispensary.

Accordingly, in order to reduce the chances of making a mistake, community pharmacists would be well advised not to put similar packs together, to express strengths uniformly (e.g. either 60 mg in 2 ml or 30 mg/ml, but not both), and where possible to adopt uniform colours for different product strengths.

The future

As with medical negligence cases, the incidence of negligence claims against pharmacists will undoubtedly increase in future years. There are a number of situations which have not yet appeared in the reported cases. For example, a pharmacist will be liable if he dispenses medicinal products which are obsolete or damaged in such a way as to be dangerous, or where he fails to supply product leaflets intended by the manufacturer to be passed to the user. Recent research into the administration of carbamazepine (prescribed to epilepsy sufferers) has disclosed that dispensing errors occur, most often where the pharmacist confuses 200 mg and 400 mg modified release tablets. On occasions these errors led to profound medical, social and psychological consequences. The research concludes that inadvertent intoxication of epilepsy sufferers with carbamazepine is widespread as a result of dispensing errors, but that these errors could be avoided by changing the appearance of both the packaging and the tablets for different product strengths (see Research paper by Mack, Kuc, Grunewald, published in the *Pharmaceutical Journal*, 18 November 2000).

The RPSGB has given guidance in a fact sheet on how to deal with dispensing errors. Insurers prefer to settle these cases quietly, rather than run the risks of an adverse result with unwanted media attention and significantly increased legal costs.

Liability as an occupier of premises

The Occupiers' Liability Act

A community pharmacist may also find himself liable as an occupier if an accident occurs on his premises. The provisions of the Occupiers' Liability Act 1957 regulate the duty which an occupier of premises owes to his visitors in respect of dangers due to the state of the premises, or to things done, or omitted to be done on them. Where an act or omission creates a dangerous condition which later causes harm to a visitor, the Act applies. Typical examples would be where a chair for customers waiting for prescriptions collapses because it was in need of repair, or where the floor covering had become raised, thus constituting a danger to all customers who might enter the pharmacy.

An occupier

In order to be an occupier of premises, exclusive occupation is not needed. The test is whether a person has some degree of control associated with, or arising from his presence in, and use of, or activity in the premises.

A visitor

A visitor includes all persons to whom the occupier has given an invitation or permission to enter the premises.

The duty

The duty of the occupier is to take such care as in all the circumstances of the case is reasonable to see that the visitor will be reasonably safe in using the premises for the purposes for which he is invited or permitted by the occupier to be there.

Warning and knowledge of danger

In determining whether an occupier of premises has discharged the common duty of care, regard will be had to all the circumstances. For example, where the occupier warns a visitor of danger, and despite the warning damage is caused to the visitor, the warning itself does not absolve the occupier from liability, unless in all the circumstances it was enough to enable the visitor to be reasonably safe.

Access for disabled people

The Disability Discrimination Act 1995 has particular relevance to a community pharmacy, since the provisions of the Act will apply to many patients visiting a pharmacy. The Act imposes a duty on a service provider, which includes a community pharmacist, to make "reasonable adjustments" for disabled people to enable them to have better access to services.

With these considerations in mind, it is important for a community pharmacist to ensure that he does not have any practices or procedures which would make it difficult for a disabled person to make use of his services, that he provides auxiliary aids or services to enable disabled people to make use of his services, and that he provides a reasonable alternative method of making a service available where the physical features of the premises impede a disabled person in the use of the service.

Some community pharmacies operate from narrow retail units, where wheelchair access is often difficult if not impossible. Consideration must be given to constructing a ramp, or if this is not possible, to installing a bell at wheelchair height outside the pharmacy so that a disabled person can call for assistance. The layout of the pharmacy must also facilitate wheelchair access to the prescription dispensing area.

Before making any changes to the premises, a community pharmacist should contact the local disablement officer at the nearest Job Centre. In addition to advising on changes which could be made to comply with the provisions of the Act, the officer will know if there are any local funds available to assist with alterations made for this purpose.

The definition of a disabled person for the purposes of the Act is very wide. It embraces any person who has "a physical or medical impairment which has substantial and long-term adverse affects on his or her ability to carry out day-to-day activities".

Criminal liability for negligent conduct

In most situations, the malpractice action brought against a pharmacist, like all other health professionals, is unlikely to also give rise to liability in criminal law. Nevertheless there is the possibility that a criminal prosecution may be brought in certain situations. An example is the case of *R* v. *Ziad Khatab (2000)* in which a pharmacist was charged for manslaughter as a result of a grossly negligent dispensing error.

In the case of *R v. Seymour (1983)* the court required it to be established that the conduct of the defendant amounted to an "obvious and serious" risk of death. This approach was confirmed again in the House of Lords judgment in *R v. Adomoko (1994)* where an anaesthetist in the course of an eye operation failed to notice that the endotracheal tube used to assist the patient's breathing had become disconnected. After nine minutes, the patient suffered a heart attack and died.

In determining whether an act constitutes the offence of gross negligence manslaughter, the prosecution must establish the following:

- There was a duty of care owed by the accused to the deceased
- There was a breach of that duty of care by the accused
- Death of the accused was caused by breach of the duty of care by the accused and that the death caused was not too "remote" from the breach
- The breach of duty of care by the accused was so great as to be characterised as gross negligence and therefore a crime.

If no duty of care has been imposed by law, the prosecution has to consider whether the defendant accepted such a duty towards the deceased. Such considerations that need to be addressed concern:

- Nature and duration of relationship between accused and deceased; the longer and more involved the relationship, the greater the likelihood of a duty of care having been accepted.
- Action by the accused to prevent any other person from helping the deceased, where such assistance could have prevented death. This amounts to acceptance by the accused of a duty of care which must be performed to a reasonable standard.
- Whether the accused has claimed that they possess the skills necessary to perform an action competently, thereby leading others to allow them to carry it out.

The Law Commission has suggested various reforms in this area. It proposed that there should be a new offence of reckless killing. This would be committed if:

- A person by his or her conduct causes the death of another;
- He or she is aware of a risk that his or her conduct will cause death or serious injury;
- It is unreasonable for him or her to take that risk, having regard to all the circumstances as he or she knows or believes them to be.

Corporate manslaughter

In addition to the pharmacist in person, it is possible for his company to be prosecuted for gross negligence manslaughter. However, there are a number of difficulties which need to be addressed if a company is to be prosecuted successfully.

Identification of a controlling mind

For a company to be guilty of manslaughter, it is necessary to identify a "controlling mind", who is also personally guilty of manslaughter. This person must have acted "as the company", to the extent that his or her "is the mind of the company", and will therefore hold a senior position in the company. The individual or individuals will usually be prosecuted as well but there may be particular circumstances whereby they are not. Even when the individuals are not prosecuted, the prosecution must still be able to demonstrate that the named individual is guilty of the offence.

It is not possible to add up the negligence of several individuals to show that a company is grossly negligent. Even if a number of people, including directors, have acted negligently, the company is not guilty of manslaughter. A specific individual must be identified as the "controlling mind" for corporate manslaughter to be proven.

Once an individual controlling mind is established, all the other elements of gross negligence must be established. The prosecution must prove that the individual officer of the company had a duty of care towards the deceased; that there was a breach of that duty; that the breach directly caused the death; and that the breach was so great as to be classified as gross negligence.

Corporate Manslaughter Bill 2006

The Corporate Manslaughter Bill proposes a new offence of corporate killing, broadly corresponding to the individual offence of killing by gross carelessness. A company will be guilty of the new offence of corporate manslaughter where the way in which any of its activities are managed or organised by its senior managers causes a person's death through a gross breach of a duty of care.

The maximum penalty for a corporate manslaughter conviction will be an unlimited fine. There are no sentences of imprisonment. Although this is the same maximum penalty as under existing law, it is thought that the stigma attached to a corporate manslaughter conviction will be considerably greater than a conviction under existing law. In addition, where a company is convicted of corporate manslaughter the court may also impose an order requiring it to remedy the breaches which led to the death. Failure to comply with a remedial order is punishable by a further fine.

The Bill intends to make it easier for prosecutions to succeed against companies. This is primarily owing to the fact that under the proposed law the prosecution will no longer have to identify the controlling mind behind the organisation's activities. Instead, the prosecution will focus on the conduct of the senior management, both individually and collectively. In these circumstances, companies and their employees must do everything reasonably practicable to ensure the health, safety and welfare of everyone affected by their activities. In particular, appropriate safety management systems must be set up and followed, with adequate training, supervision, monitoring and auditing.

Although community pharmacists will already have proper systems and safeguards in place, there is some potential for the Corporate Manslaughter Bill to have an impact on hospital and community pharmacists. It is probably only a matter of time before a hospital or community pharmacist is prosecuted for gross negligence, together with his company or hospital the proposed Corporate Manslaughter Bill, following a dispensing error.

Chapter 27

Business Premises

When setting up a pharmacy, a pharmacist has to decide whether to buy shop premises or rent shop premises from a landlord. The purpose of this part of the book is to assist a pharmacist in making this decision, by explaining the basic difference between the ownership and rental of business premises and by describing the principal rights and obligations of leasehold ownership. Business premises, like residential dwellings, are either freehold or lease-hold.

Freehold premises

The owner of freehold premises owns them absolutely. In other words, the owner has freedom to make such use of them as he wishes. He may lease the premises to a tenant, and he may raise a mortgage or loan against the equity in the property. The only qualification to this freedom will be in the form of easements or restrictive covenants.

Easements

An easement is a continuing right or privilege enjoyed by someone other than the freeholder over the freeholder's land. For example, where A and B own adjacent premises, B may enjoy a right of way over A's land.

Restrictive covenants

A restrictive covenant is a restriction attaching to the premises which prevents the owner from carrying out specified activities. Such covenants are of particular importance to the purchaser of business premises as one of the most common forms prevents the carrying out of specified trades or activities on the premises. For example, if A owns two shop premises in the same road and sells one of them to B, a covenant may be included whereby B undertakes not to pursue a similar trade to A in the newly purchased premises. When B subsequently sells to C, the burden of the covenant will continue to attach to the premises.

In the normal course of events such covenants will become apparent before purchase during the normal searches carried out by the purchaser's solicitors. Failure to detect and warn about easements or covenants may render the solicitor liable to the purchaser in damages for negligence.

Pre-contractual enquiries

There are significant pitfalls to be avoided when a community pharmacist buys an existing retail pharmacy business, particularly where there are unresolved applications for a new contract, minor relocation and/or doctor dispensing rights. Unexpected changes in the way in which general medical services or pharmaceutical services are provided can impact significantly on the profitability of a retail pharmacy business which is the subject of the purchase. It is, therefore, imperative for the purchaser to discover the existence of any unresolved applications which might adversely effect the economic viability of the retail pharmacy business. This is not as easy as it sounds because a seller, whether a freehold seller or an assignor of leasehold premises, is under no legal obligation to disclose the existence of an unresolved application. There is no local register which can be consulted. Local health administrators may be prepared to reveal relevant information on request, but there is no duty on them to do so. Local health administrators are not obliged to do any more than make available for inspection a copy of the pharmaceutical list – see Regulation 22(1)(a) of the National Health Service (Pharmaceutical Services) Regulations 1992.

In these circumstances, it is absolutely vital for an intending purchaser and his solicitor to ask the right questions of the vendor/assignor. As well as asking both orally and in writing (by pre-contractual enquiries) about planning permission, the profitability of the retail pharmacy business and other matters of commercial interest which form the usual subjects of enquiry, an intending purchaser and his solicitor must ask the vendor/assignor whether there are any unresolved applications for a new pharmacy, minor relocation or doctor dispensing, whether any such applications have been made within the last 5 years, and whether the vendor/assignor has received notice (either formally or informally) that any such application is likely to be made. The intending purchaser must also probe the extent of the vendor/assignor's knowledge of any plans by a nearby doctors surgery to move premises. If the answer to any of these questions is "yes", the vendor/assignor must explore full details of the application or plans and obtain details of any determination which was reached. Any incorrect answer may give rise to an action in damages as a breach of warranty and/or as a negligent misrepresentation under *Section 2* of the Misrepresentation Act 1967.

The importance of making careful pre-contractual enquiries was demonstrated in the case of *Banks* v. *Cox (2000)* where during the sale of a nursing home the purchaser asked the vendor whether there had been any material change in the nature or conduct of the business. The Court held that the vendor was guilty of fraudulent misrepresentation when he failed to bring to the purchaser's attention a change in social services policy which seriously affected the profitability of the business.

Leasehold premises

Instead of purchasing a freehold interest, a pharmacist may acquire a leasehold interest in business premises. A lease is, like a freehold, an interest in land. The leaseholder is in effect the owner of the leasehold premises for the duration of the lease. A business lease should be negotiated by a solicitor and contained in written form; however, more informal agreements do sometimes occur. Whether the lease is contained in a formal document or not, there are certain preconditions which must exist to create a lease, as opposed to a mere licence, which is no more than permission, revokable at will, to be present on the premises. For a lease to exist, the agreement must be for a fixed term at a rent and grant exclusive possession of the premises.

Fixed term

A lease does not have to be for a term of years, but must be expressed for a fixed, ascertainable duration. Usually the lease will be for a definite period of time terminating on a specific date. A periodic tenancy may also be created where the lease is renewable at short intervals, e.g. monthly, quarterly or yearly. As long as the intervals are expressly specified, a lease is capable of being created.

Exclusive possession

Exclusive possession means that the tenant has the sole right to occupy the premises. A possible qualification to this may be a clause in the lease which confers on the landlord a right to re-enter the premises from time to time in order to inspect them or to carry out repairs. A grant of anything less than exclusive possession is incapable of creating a tenancy.

Rent

The term "rent" is more or less self-explanatory. Most leases will contain specific clauses dealing with the amount of rent payable and the dates upon which it should be paid. It is very unusual for rent to take a form other than money, but it is possible for it to take the form of the provision of services. If rent is not payable, it is highly unlikely that anything other than a mere licence has been created.

Formalities

In order to create a legal lease which exceeds three years in duration, it is necessary for the lease agreement to be contained in a deed (*Section 52* of the Law of Property Act 1925). The document creating the lease will set out the names of the parties and the period for which the lease is to run. A rent will be specified and each party will undertake in various clauses to abide by certain obligations. For example, the tenant may undertake to keep the premises in a good state of repair. There will usually be a clause by which the landlord is permitted to re-enter the premises should the tenant fail to pay the rent, or if he is in breach of certain of his obligations. If for some reason a lease has not been created by deed, it may be recognised by a court if it can be ascertained that the parties intended to create a lease, and that acts consistent with that intention have been carried out by the parties.

Terms of a business lease

A lease will, by its clauses, impose obligations on both parties. It will create rights for the benefit of one party in the event of a breach of an obligation by the other.

A distinction exists between terms which are known as conditions, and those which are known as covenants.

Conditions

Conditions are terms which have to be fulfilled for the lease to come into existence, or for it to continue. For example, it may be a condition of the lease that the premises are to be used exclusively for the purposes of carrying on business as a pharmacy. Should the tenant cease to comply with this condition, the landlord will have the right to re-enter the premises whether or not that right is expressly reserved in the lease.

Covenants

A covenant is an agreement between the parties whereby one party promises to fulfil certain obligations. Examples include covenants:

- to pay rent
- to maintain the premises in a certain condition
- to insure the premises
- not to sub-let.

A breach of covenant may give rise to certain legal remedies such as damages or injunction. A breach on the part of the tenant will not automatically entitle the landlord to re-enter unless this has been expressly provided for.

If an enforceable lease has been entered into which does not contain covenants, a court will imply the usual covenants. These may include covenants on the part of the tenant:

- to pay rent
- to repair the premises at the end of the term
- to pay rates
- to deliver the premises up to the landlord at the end of the term.

The landlord will be obliged to grant quiet enjoyment of the premises to the tenant, and will be entitled to re-enter the premises for non-payment of rent.

Specific covenants

The covenants which commonly give rise to the greatest potential for difficulty or dispute during the currency of the lease are covenants:

- not to assign or sub-let
- not to change the use made of the premises
- not to alter or improve the premises
- to repair and to insure the premises.

Each of these merits some closer attention.

Covenants limiting the right to assign or sub-let

If the landlord wishes to restrict the tenant's right to sub-let or assign premises (i.e. to prevent the tenant from creating a sub-lease or vesting the benefit of a lease in a third party), he must do so by express words in the lease. Such a covenant will not be implied. If the words of the covenant are unconditional and prevent any sub-letting or assignment whatsoever, then the tenant is bound by the covenant absolutely.

However, it is common for a clause to be inserted whereby assigning or sub-letting is permitted subject to the landlord's consent. Where this is the case, *Section 19(1)* of the Landlord and Tenant Act 1927 then inserts into the covenant a proviso that such consent will not be withheld unreasonably. The question of when it is reasonable for a landlord to refuse consent is discussed below, but the effect of an unreasonable refusal is the removal of the covenant, so that assignment or sub-letting can take place without consent. The usual course for the tenant to take when faced with an unreasonable refusal is to seek a declaration in the county court (under *Section 53* of the Landlord and Tenant Act 1954) that the landlord's refusal was unreasonable. The tenant formerly bore the burden of proving unreasonableness but this has now been reversed by the Landlord and Tenant Act 1988, *Section 1* (*Midland Bank PLC v. Chart Enterprises Inc. (1990)*).

Under the Landlord and Tenant Act 1988, *Section 1*, a landlord who is asked to give his consent to assignment or sub-letting must give his consent or justify his refusal as reasonable. Failure to do so may render the landlord liable in damages or to an injunction.

A landlord can circumvent the application of *Section 19* of the Landlord and Tenant Act 1927 by either: including an express prohibition on any sub-letting or assigning; or by including a condition that if the tenant wishes to assign or sub-let, he must first offer to surrender the lease to the landlord. The landlord may then take possession of the premises if he does not wish to allow the assignment or sub-letting.

Unreasonable refusal

Where a tenant makes a written application for consent to assign or sublet the landlord must within a reasonable time give written notice of the reasons for refusing consent (Landlord and Tenant Act 1988, *Section 1(3)(b)(ii)*). The landlord will not be held to have acted unreasonably if he has acted as a reasonable person might do. A refusal of consent will be unreasonable if the grounds for refusal do not relate to the personality or credit-worthiness of the proposed assignee or sub-tenant, or to the effect of the proposed assignment or sub-lease on the use or occupation of the premises (*Houlder Bros & Co. v. Gibbs (1925)*).

Motives

The landlord is entitled to be selfish in his reasons, except where the reason for his refusal is to achieve some purpose totally unconnected with the lease, or where there is such disproportion between the benefit to the landlord and the detriment to the tenant brought about by the refusal, that it would be unreasonable for the landlord to withhold his consent. Where the assignee has an ulterior motive in obtaining the benefit of the lease, e.g. in using the nuisance value of the lease to force his way into a new development, refusal may be reasonable. It is unreasonable for a landlord to refuse consent on the grounds of race, sex or disability: Race Relations Act 1976, *Section 24*; Sex Discrimination Act 1975, *Section 31*; Disability Discrimination Act 1995, *Section 22*.

Where the covenant provides that the landlord's consent is required for subletting or assigning, money may not be requested as a condition of consent being granted (unless the lease expressly provides for such a payment), but a reasonable amount may be requested to cover expenses.

In some cases, the covenant restricting assignment and sub-letting will clearly evidence the purpose for which the covenant was made. In such a case the words of the covenant will be strictly construed. An assignment or sub-letting will not be permitted where to do so would defeat the original purpose of the covenant. It will usually be unreasonable for the landlord to refuse his consent on the grounds that he anticipates that the assignee or sub-tenant will breach a covenant restricting the use which can be made of the premises, as his right to enforce the covenant will remain unaffected.

Covenants concerning change of use

Many legal documents substitute the term "user" for "use". The above heading will appear as "Covenants concerning change of user".

Many business leases contain a covenant preventing the tenant from changing the use made of the premises during the period of the tenancy. Such a covenant will either be absolute or conditional upon the consent of the landlord.

Where the landlord's consent is required for a change of use, *Section 19(3)* of the Landlord and Tenant Act 1927 prevents the granting of consent from being conditional upon the payment of money by the tenant. The landlord may, however, be entitled to compensation for any loss as a result of the change of use.

Unlike *Section 19(1)* which imposes a requirement of reasonableness on the landlord's granting of consent, *Section 19(3)* makes no such provision. Often the covenant may include words to the effect that the landlord may not refuse his consent unreasonably. In determining whether consent has been unreasonably withheld, similar considerations apply as to the requirement of reasonableness in consenting to sub-letting or assignment (see above). An example of unreasonable refusal can be found in the case of *Anglia Building Society* v. *Sheffield County Council (1983)* in which the refusal was held to be unreasonable where it was used merely as an attempt to secure an advantage for the landlord wholly unconnected with the lease, and wholly outside the intention of the parties. The correct procedure for challenging the reasonableness of the landlord's decision is to seek a declaration in the county court under *Section 53* of the Landlord and Tenant Act 1954. If the refusal is declared unreasonable, the covenant becomes of no effect, and the tenant can change the use he makes of the premises as desired.

Landlord's remedies for tenant's breach of user covenant

Where the tenant breaches the change of user covenant, the landlord has a remedy in damages; and where the covenant contains a proviso for re-entry, the lease may be forfeited. The court may also grant an interlocutory injunction preventing the change of use pending a full trial of the issue. It should be remembered that the change of use will be subject to any restrictive covenants attaching to the freehold of the premises, and to planning regulations. Any change of use should therefore always be carried out in consultation with the landlord.

Covenants against alterations or improvements

A lease may contain covenants not to carry out any alterations or improvements to the premises. These may be either absolute prohibitions, or qualified by the requirement of the landlord's consent. If the covenant is absolute, the tenant's hands are tied. Where the landlord's consent is required, *Section 19(2)* of the Landlord and Tenant Act 1927 provides that any refusal must be reasonable if the alterations amount to improvements. The section also provides that the landlord: may require a sum of money for any diminution in the value of the premises, or of any neighbouring premises belonging to the landlord; or may require the tenant to reinstate the premises to its original state at the conclusion of the tenancy.

The court will decide whether an alteration amounts to an improvement from the tenant's point of view (*Lambert* v. *F.W. Woolworth and Co. Ltd (1938)*). It was also said in that case that many considerations, aesthetic, historic or even personal, may be relied upon as yielding reasonable grounds for refusing consent.

A tenant who breaches a covenant against alteration or improvement may be liable in damages and to forfeiture should the landlord succeed in proving that his consent was not unreasonably withheld. Therefore, as with activities encroaching on all types of covenants, the tenant should negotiate with the landlord, and as a last resort seek a declaration from the county court.

Repairing covenants

Covenants obliging either party to repair the premises will either be express or implied. In commercial leases such covenants will usually be expressed in the lease. Should no such covenants be contained in the lease, obligations may be implied by common law.

The only obligation imposed on the tenant at common law is to occupy the premises in a tenant-like manner, i.e. to take reasonable care of the premises and to make good any damage which is caused by the tenant or his employees or visitors. This does not extend to making good minor damage caused by fair wear and tear. A landlord is obliged to maintain his own premises ancillary to the leased premises where maintenance of his premises is necessary for the enjoyment of the leased premises. For example, where the tenant has leased a shop on the ground floor of the premises, the remainder of which is owned by the landlord, the landlord will be obliged to maintain the roof and common parts of the building unless the lease expressly provides otherwise.

The landlord may also be obliged to carry out such repairs as are necessary to give business efficacy to the agreement. For example, where the tenant has covenanted to maintain and repair the interior, the landlord may be required to ensure the good repair of the exterior.

Express covenants to repair

Express covenants to repair are usually expressed as obligations to keep the premises in good, habitable or tenantable repair. The old case of *Proudfoot* v. *Hart (1890)* provides general guidance that this means:

> such repair as, having regard to the age, character and locality of the premises, would make it reasonably fit for the occupation of a reasonably minded tenant of the class who would be likely to take it at the time when the lease was granted.

Covenants to repair do not create an obligation to renew or improve the premises

The line between repair and improvement is a difficult one to draw, but as a rule of thumb, the duty can be no higher than restoring the premises to the condition in which they were originally found. The question of what amounts to simple repair is a question to be decided in the specific circumstances. For example, repair will not normally include the duty to cure inherent defects in the premises, e.g. replacing defective guttering. However, in some circumstances, the secondary damage can only be repaired by repairing the primary cause. The repair of the primary cause may be construed as an improvement, but may nevertheless be covered by the repairing covenant. The tenant is not obliged to repair a structural defect in the building which pre-dates the commencement of the lease (*Quick* v. *Taff Ely Borough Council (1985)*). If, however, a pre-existing defect causes secondary damage, e.g. a leaking roof causing damp penetration, secondary damage caused during the period of the lease will have to be repaired by the tenant.

Special care should be taken prior to the signing of the lease to ensure that the tenant is not to be held liable for the re-building of premises destroyed by fire or flood, etc. It is common for the liability for rebuilding to be expressly attached to the landlord in the lease.

Landlord's remedies for breach of repairing covenant

If a tenant is in breach of his covenant to repair, the landlord has the remedies of damages and forfeiture. The measure of damages is the difference between the value of the unrepaired premises, and the value of the premises had the repairs been executed. However, if it is the landlord's intention to demolish the premises at the end of the tenancy, there will be no justification for such an award of damages.

Forfeiture

If a landlord seeks to obtain forfeiture of the premises consequent upon a breach of a repairing covenant, he must serve a notice under *Section 146* of the Law of Property Act 1925 containing details of the breach, requiring the breach to be remedied, and requiring the payment of compensation. In the case of premises leased for at least 7 years with at least 3 years left to run, special procedures are provided by the Leasehold Property (Repairs) Act 1938. When the landlord serves a notice under *Section 146* of the Law of Property Act 1925, he must inform the tenant of his right to serve a counter-notice under the 1938 Act. If a counter-notice is served within 28 days, the landlord's action cannot proceed without the leave of the court. Leave will only be granted if one of the following five circumstances exists:

(1) The value of the landlord's interest in the premises has been, or is likely to be, substantially diminished if the repairs are not carried out.
(2) The repair is necessary to comply with an order of any authority or local bye-law.
(3) Where the tenant does not occupy the premises, the repair is necessary in the interests of another occupier.
(4) An immediate repair will avoid further deterioration leading to more expensive repairs.
(5) There are special circumstances making leave to proceed just and equitable.

The landlord must prove both the breach of covenant and the ground or grounds relied on, on the balance of probabilities, *Associated British Ports* v. *C. H. Bailey (1990)*.

Right of entry to repair

Under some leases the landlord may have a right to enter the premises to carry out repairs, and to recover the cost of repairs as a debt. It was traditionally thought that a landlord cannot force the tenant to carry out repairs (i.e. that the contractual remedy of specific performance is not available). It has now been held that specific performance may in principle be available where damages are not adequate compensation for the landlord, *Rainbow Estates* v. *Tokenhold (1998)*.

Tenant's remedies for breach of repairing covenant

The tenant of business premises may sue the landlord for damages if the landlord is in breach of a repairing covenant. In the past, damages have been awarded for discomfort, loss of enjoyment of the premises, and bouts of ill-health caused by the poor state of repair. There have also been some indications in the decided cases that the cost of alternative accommodation is recoverable. The landlord of business premises cannot be forced to repair, i.e. the remedy of specific performance is not available to the tenant.

Cost of repairs set off against rent

The case of *Lee Parker* v. *Izzet (1971)* decided that a tenant may deduct the cost of repairs from future rent. However, to avoid complications over whether the amounts spent on repair are reasonable, it is advisable for a tenant to obtain a county court declaration that the landlord is in breach of his covenant.

Insurance covenants

A commercial lease will make express provision for the insurance of the building. Often the tenant will be required to pay the insurance premiums and to refrain from acts which will suspend the cover.

Destruction of a building

A clause will usually be inserted to oblige the landlord to use insurance monies to rebuild the premises should they be destroyed during the period of the lease. In the absence of such a covenant, the landlord will not be obliged to rebuild the premises. Where a building has been destroyed and the landlord does not intend to rebuild, a dispute may arise as to which of the parties is entitled to the insurance monies and in what proportions. Following the case of *Beacon Carpets Limited* v. *Kirkby (1984)* the most likely outcome is that the monies will be divided between the parties in proportion to their interest in the building.

Rent

Commercial leases will invariably contain express terms setting out:

- the amount of rent to be paid
- the times at which it is to be paid
- the consequences of non-payment (usually forfeiture)
- provision for a review of the amount of rent payable at a set date or dates during the tenancy.

The rent is payable for the land upon which the premises stand, and not for the premises themselves. Therefore, should the building be destroyed during the period of the lease, rent continues to be payable.

Rent on assignment or sub-letting

Until the Landlord and Tenant (Covenants) Act 1995, an original tenant used to be liable to the landlord for rent under the terms of the lease, even where he had assigned or sub-let the lease with the landlord's permission. The 1995 Act was passed to alleviate the considerable hardship which this rule imposed on original tenants, requiring them in effect to guarantee payment of rent for the duration of the term of the lease, even after their interest in the lease had been assigned to a third party.

The effect of the Act in easing the position of tenants is to some extent mitigated by allowing landlords to require tenants to enter into "authorised guarantee agreements" which guarantee payments by the immediate person to whom the tenant may in future assign the lease, a transaction over which the tenant does, after all, have some control. The legal status of these guarantees, known as "AGAs", is presently uncertain and any pharmacist who is asked to provide an authorised guarantee should obtain legal advice before doing so. A landlord can assign his interest (the "reversion") in the premises to a third party. If so, the rent becomes payable to the assignee, but only if the landlord has issued a notice to the tenant complying with *Section 151(1)* of the Law of Property Act 1925.

Guarantors

If payment of rent is secured by guarantors under the terms of the lease, they will be fully liable for payment of unpaid rent should the tenant fall into arrear. The guarantors are then left to pursue the tenant for the sums in which they have been held liable. Where the tenant is a small private company it is common for landlords to require the directors or main shareholders (who are usually the same) to give guarantees in their personal capacity. This is to protect the landlord in the event of the company going into liquidation but means the directors/shareholders carry considerable personal risk.

Rent review

A commercial lease will usually contain a clause stating that at a fixed date or dates during the lease the rent will be revised by an independent third party, usually a surveyor. The lease may provide that the landlord and tenant should agree on the appointment of a surveyor jointly, or it may provide that a third party, e.g. the President of the Royal Institution of Chartered Surveyors, should make the appointment.

The review clause will specify that the rent is to be revised according to the current market rent. The decision of the surveyor is usually expressed to be final, and a clause is often inserted whereby even if the surveyor determines that a reasonable market rent would be less than that already being paid, rent will nevertheless continue to be paid at the existing rate.

The surveyor is under a duty to carry out the rent review according to his professional standards. All relevant factors will be taken into account such as the rent being paid for similar premises in the same area, the condition of the premises and the effect of, for example, the existence of a covenant restricting change of user. For obvious reasons, it is vitally important that the tenant makes himself aware of the rent review procedure at the outset.

Consequences of non-payment of rent

The usual remedy for non-payment of rent is forfeiture. All formal leases will inevitably include a clause providing for the surrender of the premises if the rent should cease to be paid for a specified period after the due date. The usual procedure is for the landlord to make a formal demand for unpaid rent before commencing forfeiture proceedings, although many leases will dispense with this requirement.

Once he has commenced forfeiture proceedings, if the landlord then does any act which indicates that he accepts the continuation of the tenancy, he loses the right to forfeiture. Accepting payment of arrears would constitute such an act. However, the landlord still has the right to receive rent for the continuing occupation. Such sums are known as "mesne profits" (pronounced "meen"), and are assessed at current market rates.

Relief against forfeiture

In High Court proceedings the tenant has a right to relief against forfeiture of the lease where he is no more than 6 months in arrears and if he pays all outstanding sums and costs into court before judgment is given. Thereafter there is a mere equitable right to relief upon payment of all arrears and costs at any time up to 6 months from the date of the landlord's re-entry. As the right is only equitable, it will be granted only where the High Court considers it fair to do so in all the circumstances.

In county court proceedings, the tenant has the automatic right to relief against forfeiture if all arrears and costs are paid up to 5 days before the date set for the possession hearing.

Under *Section 138* of the County Courts Act 1984, the court has a discretion to order relief against forfeiture if all costs and arrears are paid within 4 weeks after the granting of the order for possession. By *Section 55* of the Administration of Justice Act 1985, the High Court may grant relief against forfeiture ordered by the County Court for up to 6 months following the date of the order.

Renewal of tenancies

The procedure for the renewal of business tenancies and compensation for improvements carried out by a tenant during the currency of the lease is governed by Part II of the Landlord and Tenant Act 1954, and by Part I of the Landlord and Tenant Act 1927. These statutes create mechanisms which come into play at the end of a tenancy, and which have as their object the resolution of matters between landlord and tenant by means of mutual agreement rather than resort to the courts.

The legislation creates a framework of procedural steps which must be complied with if a business tenancy is to be terminated, and provides for the continuation of the tenancy on its existing terms should these steps not have been taken. The legislation also creates a right to request a renewal of the tenancy for a period of up to 14 years.

Tenancies covered by the legislation

Section 23 of the 1954 Act states that the Act covers:

> any tenancy where the property comprised in the tenancy is or includes premises which are occupied by the tenant and are so occupied for the purposes of a business carried on by him or for those and other purposes.

These words are to a large extent self-evident. Formally agreed business leases in documentary form will invariably be covered if the business is not being carried out in breach of a user clause.

Under *Section 43(3)(a)*, the Act does not normally apply to tenancies granted for a period of less than 6 months where there is no provision for renewing the term. However, if in that case the tenant has been in occupation for over 12 months he is deemed to have an established business which will be protected by the Act. The only other notable exceptions are leases where the landlord is a government department, local authority, a statutory undertaking or a development corporation, or where the landlord has specified that the use of the premises will change on a specified date.

Contracting out of the 1954 Act

The parties to the lease may contract out of the 1954 Act, and thereby avoid the protection afforded by it, or by following the procedures set out in *Section 38A* of the Landlord and Tenant Act 1954. Application to the County Court may be either before the commencement of the lease or at any time during the currency of the lease, under *Section 38*. Contracting out can only be achieved through agreement: neither party can exclude the protection of the Act unilaterally.

The procedure for renewal

Section 24(1) of the 1954 Act provides that the lease will continue after its expiry upon the same terms as during the currency of the lease, until either party issues a notice to renew the tenancy.

The renewal procedure may be initiated by either the landlord or the tenant issuing a notice in the prescribed form. A tenant may make a request for a new tenancy under *Section 26*. In order to issue such a notice, the tenant must have held the lease for at least 1 year and must request a starting date for a new tenancy between 6 and 12 months from the date of service of the notice. The notice must also refer to the property to be comprised in the new lease and to the terms and rent proposed.

The tenant cannot serve a notice under *Section 26*:

(1) if the landlord has already served a notice under *Section 25* (see below); or
(2) if the tenant has already given notice to quit; or
(3) if he has given notice under *Section 27* that he will be surrendering the lease at the end of the fixed term.

Under *Section 25* the landlord may serve a notice to propose a new tenancy (usually with modified rent), or to state grounds of objection to a new tenancy under *Section 30*. The landlord's notice cannot take effect until a specified date between 6 and 12 months from the date of service, and, in any event, not before the expiry date of a fixed term lease. The notice must contain the proposed terms of the new lease or, if continuation is objected to, the grounds of objection must be set out. The tenant must serve a counter-notice within 2 months of the service of the landlord's notice stating whether he intends to give up possession. In theory, the notice procedure is intended to stimulate negotiations between the landlord and the tenant and to encourage settlement between the parties. Failure of either side to respond to a notice issued by the other within the prescribed 2-month period will result in an agreement being presumed in the terms of the notice. Following the Regulatory Reform (Business Tenancies) (England and Wales) Order 2003, SI 2003/3096 either party may now apply to the court for renewal of the tenancy (provided the other has not already done so). The tenant can apply any time after the service of a *Section 25* notice, but neither party can apply until 2 months has elapsed since the serving of a *Section 26* notice.

Within 6 months of the issue of a *Section 25* notice, either party may apply under *Section 24A* of the Act for an interim rent to be determined by the court. If the renewal of the lease is unopposed the interim rent is likely to be based on market rent; if the renewal is opposed the interim rent is based on what it would be reasonable for the tenant to pay.

The landlord's grounds of opposition

Under *Section 30* the landlord has seven grounds of opposition to the grant of a renewed tenancy.

(1) Failure of the tenant to comply with repairing obligations under the lease resulting in the property being in a state of disrepair. The extent of the disrepair and the requirements of the repairing covenant will be the major factors the court will have to consider in exercising its discretion under this head.

(2) Persistent delay by the tenant in paying rent when it has become due.

(3) Other substantial breaches of covenant by the tenant, or "any other reason connected with the tenant's use or management of the holding". There is considerable room for judicial discretion under this head, but substantial and/or frequent breaches of covenant will have to be proved by the landlord.

(4) The offer by the landlord of suitable alternative premises on terms which are reasonable having regard to the terms of the current tenancy, and to all other relevant circumstances, e.g. the suitability of the proposed new premises for the tenant's business including the tenant's need to preserve goodwill.

(5) Where the current tenancy is a sub-letting of part of premises in which the landlord has an interest in the freehold reversion at the conclusion of the superior tenancy, and the landlord could get a much better return by letting the premises as a whole.

(6) Where on the termination of the tenancy the landlord intends to demolish or reconstruct the whole or a substantial part of the premises, and the proposed works can only be carried out by obtaining possession. In order for the landlord to succeed under this head he must be able to prove his intent at the date of the hearing. This is usually done by pointing to some actual steps which have been taken towards carrying out the intention. In order for the requirement of reconstruction to be proved, it must be proved that the demolition of at least part of the premises will be necessitated – *Cadle* v. *Jacmarch (1957)*.

The tenant has two defences, provided by *Section 31A*, to the assertion that possession is required to execute the work:

(a) That a new lease could be granted, but containing a clause permitting the landlord to enter to execute the works. This will only succeed if it can be shown that the tenant's business will not be substantially interfered with or for a substantial time, and that the works can be carried out with the tenant remaining; or

(b) That the tenant could be granted a new lease in an economically severable part of the premises, and that the granting of such a lease would not prevent the landlord from carrying out the works.

(7) That the landlord intends to use the premises or part of them for his own business or residence at the end of the tenancy. This ground of objection requires the landlord to prove his intent, and to show that he is the one who will occupy the premises. It is not sufficient for him to intend to let it to others.

Where the landlord succeeds in proving one of the grounds for objection, he will be awarded possession after the expiry of a minimum period of 3 months.

Under *Section 31(2)*, if the court decides that one of the grounds (4), (5) or (6) above are not proved at the date of the hearing, but would be in up to 12 months time, the grant of a new tenancy may nevertheless be refused and an order made specifying the date on which the court would have been satisfied of the grounds. In this event the existing tenancy subsists until that date and the tenant can apply to the court within 14 days under *Section 31(2)* to amend the date.

The grant of a new tenancy

Where no objection is raised by the landlord or where his objection fails, the tenant may be granted a new tenancy. Under *Section 32*, the tenant has a prima facie right to a tenancy only of the premises to which the original lease applied. If this raises matters of dispute, they can be resolved by the court.

The court is in theory entitled to award a new tenancy of anything up to 15 years' duration, but in practice tends only to grant leases of similar length to that which previously subsisted.

Rent under the new tenancy may be fixed by the court where the landlord and tenant fail to agree. It will be fixed at a level at which "having regard to the terms of the tenancy, the holding might be expected to be let on the open market by a willing lessor". However, the court will not take into account the following:

(1) The tenant's previous occupation.
(2) Any goodwill attaching to the premises generated by the tenant's business.
(3) Improvements carried out by the tenant other than those required by covenant, provided that the tenancy has always been protected by the Act, that the improvements were carried out within 21 years of the renewal, and that the tenant did not surrender the premises at the end of the tenancy in which the improvements were carried out.
(4) The value attributable to a liquor licence on licensed premises.

Under *Section 35*, the court has a very wide discretion to determine other terms of a new lease which the landlord and tenant have failed to agree, but there will be a strong presumption in favour of the terms of the original lease. This presumption can be rebutted if there is good reason, but such reasons would have to be very strong, e.g. certain terms will need to be included in order to give commercial efficacy to the agreement.

Tenant's compensation at the end of a tenancy

At the conclusion of a tenancy, whether by surrender or by court order, the tenant may be able to recover compensation for improvements made during the lease. Under *Section 37* of the 1954 Act the right to compensation arises where the tenant has been unsuccessful in obtaining a renewed tenancy due to a successful objection by the landlord on one of the grounds numbered (4), (5) and (6) in the list in the section above entitled "The landlord's grounds of opposition" (i.e. the grounds in *Section 30*), providing that the landlord has not offered suitable alternative accommodation.

The right to compensation cannot be excluded where the tenant has been in occupation for at least 5 years (*Section 38*). However, if the tenant is a successor to a business which has been carried on the premises for at least 5 years, the right will remain even if the successor has been in occupation for less than 5 years.

The parties may contract out of the compensation provisions at any time before the commencement or during the currency of the lease, as part of an application to the court to contract out of the protection afforded by the Act generally.

The amount of compensation payable is dependent upon the length of time the tenant has been in occupation. *Section 37* provides that tenants who have been in occupation for more than 14 years will receive a sum of twice the rateable value of the premises times the "multiplier" (which in most cases is currently one). Tenants who have been in occupation for less than 14 years will receive the rateable value times the multiplier.

Compensation for improvements

At the conclusion of a tenancy the tenant is able to claim compensation for loss of authorised improvements carried out by the tenant under *Section 1* of the Landlord and Tenant Act 1927.

The availability of compensation will not be affected by the reason for the termination of the tenancy. An application to the court for compensation must be made within 3 months of the service of the landlord's counter-notice if the tenant has terminated the tenancy by applying for a renewal; between 3 and 6 months before the termination of the tenancy if it is to terminate by effluxion of time; or within 3 months of a court order for forfeiture or re-entry.

In order to claim compensation the following requirements must all be met:

(1) The premises must have been used for business purposes.
(2) The improvements must have been executed by the tenant.
(3) The improvements must not have been executed pursuant to an obligation under the lease.
(4) The landlord must agree, or the court must have issued a certificate stating that the improvements add to the value of the premises without devaluing neighbouring property of the landlord.
(5) A formal claim for compensation must be made to the court.

Level of compensation

Section 1 of the 1927 Act provides that the level of compensation will be calculated either on the basis of the additional value to the premises by the improvements, or on the basis of the cost of carrying out the improvements at the end of the tenancy, minus an appropriate sum representing the cost of putting the improvements into a good state of repair. The court has a discretion to settle any differences arising and finally to settle the compensation sums.

Misrepresentation

Where the tenant can show that the court's refusal to grant a new tenancy was based on a misrepresentation by the landlord, "the court may order the landlord to pay to the tenant such sum as appears sufficient as compensation for damage or loss sustained by the tenant as a result of the order or refusal" (*Section 55* of the 1954 Act). For example, where the landlord has successfully opposed an application for a renewed tenancy on the basis that he intends to use the premises for his own business, if he subsequently lets the premises to another party, the former tenant may apply for compensation to the court which ordered possession. However, these provisions do not apply to cases where the landlord or tenant gave notice after 1 June 2004.

Compulsory acquisition

If the premises are acquired compulsorily, in assessing the compensation payable, the local authority is obliged, by *Section 47* of the Land Compensation Act 1973, to assess the potential loss that may be suffered by the tenant as a result of his loss of rights to renew the tenancy of the lease.

Planning law

Changes of use and alterations of premises

A change in the use of a business premises may arise by a simple alteration in the nature of the use, or through alterations and additions which modify the use. A change of use may also arise through a material intensification in the present use, or by subtly altering the present use to a point where the changes amount to development.

Planning permission will be required for the construction of new business premises with the exception of some minor extensions, repairs and maintenance, internal alterations, small works outside the building (such as installing an alarm box) and putting up walls, fences, etc. within height limits. Unlike domestic properties the range of permitted development rights available to commercial properties are more limited.

Changes of use are not always a clear-cut issue and should be treated with care. There are certain types of change of use, which do not require planning permission. For example, a change of use from one type of shop to another does not (normally) require planning permission. These are set out in the Town and Country Planning (Use Classes) Order 1987.

Certain changes are permissible between and within the use classes without the need for planning permission, subject to satisfying the appropriate criteria. Shops can alter their use to another type of shop without planning permission. Therefore a newsagents could be changed to a chemist shop without permission.

In addition, changes between certain types of use may be made without permission. For example, one can alter a storage use to a business use, but not the other way round. These changes are permitted by virtue of the Town and Country Planning (Use Classes) Order 1987.

Other uses are considered *sui generis*; that is, they are uses on their own unrelated to other uses. Examples would include a change of use from a domestic garage to a business workshop or a house to a hotel.

There may be circumstances where the intention is to make a minor alteration to the use of land or premises and this opens up the question of whether the change is so substantial as to require planning permission.

Any change of use must be a "material change of use" in order to require consent. Defining what is and what is not a material change is often difficult and open to interpretation. Inevitably the courts have provided guidance over the years in deciding cases, but given the diversity of potential uses the issue remains open to debate.

Additional or supplementary uses may also create a situation where planning permission is required. A builders yard used for the storage only of building materials, which then becomes used for the parking of vehicles may require planning permission, depending upon the circumstances of the case.

The limitations on use imposed by the planning permission over the land or buildings and any conditions that may be attached should not be overlooked. The wording of planning permissions is often critical. For example, "use of building for B8 storage" is substantially different from "use of building for the storage of farm implements only".

Extensions

Extensions to shops and offices will require planning permission. Planning permission will be required if:

- The allowable increase in volume has already been used for previous extensions.
- The extension will affect the external appearance of the building.
- The extension is to be within 5 m of the property boundary.
- The extension will be on land required for parking or vehicle turning.

Chapter 28

Business Associations

When setting up in business there are several different ways in which a pharmacist may operate. He may set up either as a sole trader, in partnership with some other party, as a limited liability partnership, or as a corporate body. Each manner of operation has certain advantages and disadvantages. These are considered in this section of the book, with particular reference being made to the limited company.

The sole trader

The sole trader carries on business in either his own name or one created for the business. He bears the burden of full personal responsibility for the business and all its liabilities. Unlike a limited company, in which the company and its managing director are separate legal entities, the sole trader and his business are one and the same thing: the sole trader is liable for all the debts of the business, and his personal property is therefore put at risk.

Trading as a sole trader is therefore advisable only for those who do not expect to incur business debts or liabilities on any large scale. In setting up a pharmacy, a sizeable outlay will be made in the purchase of business premises and stock, and the potential personal liability will be considerable.

Partnership

Partnerships are comparatively common, and so require considerably more explanation. A partnership arises where two or more persons carry on a business in common with a view to making a profit. A partnership is called a firm, but the partnership has no legal entity of its own and the liability of the partners is personal.

The law relating to partnerships is to be found mostly in the Partnership Act 1890. This statute lays down the rules for determining the existence of a partnership, the relationship between partners and third parties, the relationship between partners, and the rules governing termination of partnerships. All references to statutory sections below are to the Partnership Act unless otherwise indicated.

Partners and third parties

Every partner is an agent of the firm, and accordingly any acts done as a partner, including the incurring of extensive liabilities, will bind all the other partners. The relationship between partners therefore has to be based upon a high degree of trust. The exception to this rule is where a partner pledges the credit of the firm for his own personal debts. In this event the firm will not be bound. The partners' liabilities for the firm are joint and several. Thus each partner is potentially liable for the whole of the firm's liabilities, subject to the partners' rights of indemnity against each other. However, the right of indemnity may be of little use where only one of the partners in a firm has sufficient funds to pay a judgment debt to a creditor; he will have to pay the creditor and take his chance against the other partners.

By *Sections 10, 11*, and *12* of the Act, partners are rendered liable for wrongful acts and omissions of other partners acting in the ordinary course of business or with the consent of the other partners, and for misapplication of money or property received for the firm or in the firm's custody. However, a partner is not liable for any liabilities incurred by the firm while he is not a partner. Furthermore, by *Section 14*, any person who is not a partner of the firm, but who holds himself out as being a partner, is liable to the representee as if he were a partner.

Relations between partners

Formally created partnerships are usually governed by a partnership deed which will set out the rights and obligations of the partners in the firm. There is no express requirement for a partnership deed, but it lends certainty. By *Section 19* of the Act, partners may vary the terms of their partnership by mutual consent, or such variation may be implied from a course of dealing.

Fiduciary duty

The basic duty of a partner towards the others is one of good faith, i.e. to act honestly and for the benefit of the partnership as a whole. In modern times this is known as a fiduciary duty. There are three statutory aspects to this duty.

(1) *Section 28* provides that "partners are bound to render a true account of all things affecting the partnership to any partner or his legal representative". This means that partners are bound to inform each other of all material facts in relation to partnership business.

(2) *Section 29* provides that "every partner must account to the firm for any benefit derived by him without the consent of the other partners from any transaction concerning the partnership, or from any use made by him of the partnership name or business connection". An example of the operation of this section is where a partner makes a secret profit which he fails to disclose to the others. When it is discovered, the others may take out an action for account which may result in the secret profit being re-distributed amongst the partners.

(3) *Section 30* provides that "if a partner, without the consent of the other partners, carries on any business of the same nature as and competing with that of the firm, he must account for and pay over to the firm all profits made by him in that business". This section is quite clear; the key question is whether the other business is in competition with the firm. If competition is established, liability is established.

Partnership property

Additionally, *Section 20* provides that all property originally brought into the partnership or acquired on account of the firm for the purposes and in the course of partnership business constitutes partnership property and must be held and applied as such in accordance with the partnership agreement. Thus all partnership property is held jointly by all the partners for their mutual benefit. Unless the contrary intention appears in the partnership agreement, the following provisions, created by the Act, apply.

Section 21 provides simply that unless it has been agreed otherwise, property bought with the firm's money is deemed to have been bought on behalf of the firm and will therefore be held for the benefit of all the partners.

Section 24 provides that:

(1) Partners are entitled to take part in the management of the business, but are not entitled to remuneration for so doing. The idea is that each partner will receive his reward by a straightforward share of the profits, and possibly interest on his original capital investment.
(2) Partners are entitled to indemnity from the firm in respect of liabilities incurred in the proper conduct of the business or in its preservation. Partners are therefore entitled to reimbursement for expenses, etc., incurred whilst carrying out partnership business.
(3) Partners are entitled to equal shares in the capital and profits of the firm, and are liable to contribute equally towards losses.
(4) Partners are entitled to interest on money advanced to the firm, but not on capital until the profits have been ascertained. In practice this provision makes little difference, as interest is frequently payable on capital, but it creates the automatic right to interest on money lent to the firm, subject to contrary agreement.

Taxation

A joint assessment to tax is made in the partnership name (Income and Corporation Taxes Act 1988). However, each partner may make a separate claim for allowances and deductions, his income from the partnership being deemed to be the share to which he is entitled in the partnership profits.

Termination of partnership

Where the partnership is for an indefinite duration, it may be dissolved by one partner giving notice to the others (*Section 32* of the Partnership Act 1890). A partnership may also be dissolved by the court on the application of a partner:

(1) Where one of the partners becomes permanently incapable of performing his part of the partnership contract.
(2) Where one of the partners has been guilty of conduct calculated to prejudice the carrying on of the business.
(3) Where the business of the partnership can only be carried on at a loss.
(4) Where circumstances arise which make it just and equitable that the partnership is dissolved.

A partnership may also be rescinded like any other contract for fraud or misrepresentation. In this eventuality, *Section 41* gives the partner who has been the victim of the misrepresentation or fraud at the hands of another partner the right to an indemnity for his loss and rights over partnership property to cover his loss.

On dissolution, the property of the partnership is applied first in the payment of the firm's debts and liabilities, then in the payment of what is due to each partner, first for advances and then for capital. Any surplus is divided among the partners in the proportion in which profits are divisible (according to the terms of the partnership agreement). Losses are paid out of profits if there are any, and if not, out of capital. If the residual capital is insufficient, losses are paid personally by the partners in the proportion in which they were entitled to profits.

Limited partnership

The limited partnership is a hybrid form where the firm has at least one general partner with unlimited liability, and one or more limited partners who contribute money or property to the partnership and are liable only to the extent of their contribution. This form of partnership is governed by the Limited Partnership Act 1907.

The main reason for instituting a limited partnership is to attract capital into the business. Hence the provisions in the Limited Partnership Act mean: that the limited partner is prohibited on pain of unlimited liability from taking part in the management of the business and cannot bind the firm; his death or bankruptcy does not dissolve the partnership; his consent to the introduction of a new partner is not necessary; he has no power to dissolve the partnership; the charging of his share (i.e. the raising of money against it) is not a ground for dissolution; and he can take no part in the winding-up of partnership affairs unless the court directs. Furthermore the limited partner is unable to withdraw any part of his contribution during the continuance of the partnership. Precisely because the position of the limited partner is so precarious, i.e. he has no right to determine what use is made of his investment in the partnership, there are very few limited partnerships in existence. The modern simplification of the process of creating a limited company has almost entirely replaced the limited partnership.

Disadvantages of partnerships

The major disadvantage of partnership is the unlimited liability of members. The creation of a limited company avoids this problem and is far more attractive to those wishing to set up in a business which is going to incur any level of indebtedness, or in which extensive commercial risks will be taken. The many small businesses which make the transition to company status enjoy comparative security and have a prescribed structure within which to conduct the firm's affairs.

Limited liability partnership

From 6 April 2001 pharmacists have been able to utilise a new trading entity introduced by the Limited Liability Partnerships Act 2000. This new entity may be formed by two or more persons "associated for carrying on a lawful business with a view to profit", and unlike a partnership, the entity will have a legal personality in its own right. The partners in a limited liability partnership may be individuals or companies, and since the entity will have its own legal identity the partners will not have any contractual liability to the partnership's creditors. It is unclear at the present time whether circumstances may arise where the corporate veil will be lifted in a case where an individual acts negligently.

The internal arrangements between the partners will closely resemble the position in a conventional partnership. Relations between the partners will be regulated by agreement, and where there is no agreement, the provisions in the Partnership Act 1890 will apply. However, the limited liability partnership will have to file an annual return, with audited accounts, and many of the provisions of the Companies Acts will apply. Partners will be taxed individually, and the creation of a limited liability partnership will be tax neutral.

There is no restriction on the type of business that can trade as a limited liability partnership. It is expected that the main users of limited liability partnerships will be firms of accountants and solicitors, but there is no reason why others, such as pharmacists, should not conduct their professional activities using this entity.

At the present time it is difficult to tell whether this new entity will prove popular with pharmacists as a vehicle for professional practice. It is quite possible that the more familiar limited company will continue to be a more attractive proposition when the competing advantages and disadvantages are taken into account.

The limited company

There are three types of limited company, the most significant of which for present purposes is the private limited company. The others are the public limited company and the company limited by guarantee.

Public limited companies (plcs) are usually quite large operations. They must have an allotted share capital of at least £50,000 (one quarter of which must be paid up), and the company may offer their shares or debentures (explained below) for sale to the public. Many public limited companies are quoted on the Stock Exchange, and their shares may be bought and sold through stockbrokers. Their basic structure, however, is similar to that of the private limited company (explained below).

Companies limited by guarantee are usually non-profit making companies formed for purposes ranging from the charitable, religious or educational, to the merely administrative, such as companies set up to manage a block of flats on behalf of the residents. This form of company is used chiefly as a method of incorporating groups of persons with common interest who do not have profit as the main motive.

Advantages of creating a limited company

There are a number of advantages in trading as a private limited company which can be summarized as follows.

(1)　The liability of the members is limited to the value of their shares.
(2)　The company has a legal personality of its own separate from its members.
(3)　The name of the company is prevented from being used by other companies.
(4)　There are certain advantages in borrowing money (see below).

(5) The interests and responsibilities of the persons engaged in the business are clearly defined, including the management responsibilities of the firm.

(6) The company has a continuing existence of its own independent of its members.

(7) In some circumstances there are taxation advantages.

(8) Whereas in the case of a sole trader maximum pension contributions are limited on a sliding scale depending upon age to a percentage of income between 17.5 and 40%, there are greater possibilities for the directors of a company.

(9) The appointment, retirement or removal of directors is carried out in the prescribed manner.

(10) Employees may gain the opportunity of acquiring shares in the company, and outside investors may become shareholders.

The company's legal personality

An incorporated company has a separate legal personality which enables it to carry transactions and other functions in its own right. For example, the company may enter into contracts, purchase or lease property, sue or be sued in the company name.

A company is the beneficial owner of its own property, i.e. it does not hold it as trustee for its members, and they have no legal or equitable interest in it. A company's transactions are carried out solely in the company's name. A shareholder cannot enforce a contract made by his company; he is neither a party to the contract nor entitled to the benefit of it. Likewise, a shareholder cannot be sued on contracts made by his company, nor can a court compel a shareholder to vote at a company's general meeting in such a way as to ensure that the company fulfils its contractual obligations, or prohibit him from voting in any other way.

A member of a company cannot sue in respect of civil wrongs (known technically as "torts") committed against the company, and cannot be sued for such wrongs committed by it. Even where it is proved that the company has committed a tort, the directors will only be liable where it can be shown that they actually participated in its commission.

Exceptions to the rule of separate legal identity

There are several exceptions to the rule that companies have a separate legal personality.

First, if a company continues trading without having at least two members for a period of more than 6 months, the person who is the remaining member during any period after the 6 months has elapsed is liable jointly and severally with the company for its debts contracted during that period (*Section 24* of the Companies Act 1985). Liability does not arise until the period of 6 months has elapsed, and relates only to debts incurred after the expiration of that period. Liability can therefore be avoided by the single shareholder transferring some of his shares to a third party before the time expires. Furthermore, the remaining member will only be held personally liable for debts incurred at a time when he was a member of the company.

Secondly, if a person is involved in the management of a company while he is an undischarged bankrupt, or while a court order preventing him from being a company director remains in force, he will be personally liable for the debts of the company incurred while he is a director or is concerned in its management. A person who knowingly acts on the instructions of an undischarged bankrupt or of a person who is disqualified by court order from being a director is also liable for company debts.

Thirdly, under the 1986 Insolvency Act, it is an offence for a person who has been a director of a company in the 12 months before it went into liquidation, to be a director of, or to be concerned directly or indirectly in the promotion, formation or management of another company with the same or similar name without leave of the court. A person committing this offence, or a person knowingly acting on the instructions of such a person, will be liable for the debts and liabilities of the company incurred during the period in which instructions were carried out for a person committing the offence.

Fourthly, if, when a company is wound up, it appears that it has been trading with intent to defraud its creditors or the creditors of another person, or for any other fraudulent purpose, the court may, on the application of the liquidator, order that any persons who are knowingly trading in that way are to be personally liable to such extent as the court thinks fit. A person who participates in fraudulent trading is guilty of a criminal offence, and a prosecution may be brought whether the company is being wound up or not.

Fifthly, if in the winding-up of a company which has gone into insolvent liquidation, it appears that a person who was a director at the time before the commencement of the winding-up knew or ought to have concluded that there was no reasonable prospect that the company would avoid such a liquidation, on the liquidator's application the court may order that person to contribute such amount to the assets of the company as it thinks fit. Such an order can be made where the director cannot be proved knowingly and fraudulently to have carried on the business, but where by the exercise of proper skill and care he must have concluded that liquidation could not be avoided.

Sixthly, in a minute number of cases the court may disregard the separate legal identity of a company where there is an overriding public interest in doing so, e.g. where in war time all the directors of a company are enemy aliens.

Seventhly, in a small number of cases the courts have disregarded the separate legal identity of a company where it had been formed solely for the evasion of a legal liability. For example, in *Gilford Motor Co v. Horne (1933)*, a former company employee sought to evade the effect of a "no competition" clause in his contract with his former employer by setting up a company in direct competition. The court decided that the company was a "mere cloak or sham" employed solely to evade the effect of the clause, and an injunction was issued preventing the company from carrying on business in competition.

Eighthly, in some cases the courts have ignored the separate legal personality of a company where it appears that the company was acting as an agent for its shareholders, or that the company held its property as trustee for its shareholders. This is very rare and will usually occur only where the strict application of the principle of separate personality would work an injustice. This result may occur where, for example, the directors of a subsidiary company are also all directors of the parent holding company, and where the two companies carry on the same business and use the same accounting facilities. In such circumstances the court may discount the separate legal personality of the subsidiary and treat it merely as an agent of the holding company.

Limited liability

The concept of limited liability means that the liability of a company's shareholders is limited to the value of their shares (including any amount unpaid towards the value of the shares). In most private companies shares are fully paid up, so investors stand only to lose their investment plus any loan made to the company. Other potential liabilities may be personal guarantees for company borrowings or liabilities, e.g. bank overdrafts or guarantees of rent payments under business leases. In practice banks lending money to a small private company and landlords of business leases will inevitably require such personal guarantees so for these debts the concept of limited liability is a fiction.

If a company is unable to pay its debts, its creditors may petition the court to wind it up under the provisions of the Insolvency Act 1986. If the court orders the company to be wound up, a liquidator is appointed to realise the company's assets. If he fails to realise sufficient to meet liabilities through the sale of company assets, then the value of the shares in the company will be called up.

As a shareholder is not liable to pay the company's debts himself, a creditor of the company cannot sue him. A creditor can only obtain unpaid capital by petitioning the court to wind the company up, and awaiting such payment as can be met by the liquidator. The liquidator discharges the company's debts rateably, thereby ensuring that one creditor does not get preferred treatment merely by being the first to sue. (The protection afforded by limited liability is of course subject to the exceptions to the principle of separate legal identity discussed above.)

The protection of company names

Protection is given to company names by the Companies Act 1985. Under the Act the Registrar of Companies is not permitted to register a company in a name which is already in use. The Department of Trade and Industry is also empowered under the Act to require a company to change its name within a year of incorporation if it is the same as or too similar to a name already on the register.

A certain amount of protection is afforded to partnership names under the Business Names Act 1985, but sole traders enjoy no such protection. However, if another business uses the name of a sole trader and members of the public can be shown to be unable to distinguish between the two concerns, the first user of the name may take out a "passing off" action against the other for the damage done to his business. Such litigation is, however, costly and always carries substantial risk.

Financing the company – shares and loan capital

Shares
Most small companies have only one type of share known as ordinary shares. They are issued in order to provide permanent capital for the company, and will normally carry with them voting rights and an entitlement to a share of the company's profits or dividends.

The larger the company, usually the larger the number of shareholders. In companies where there are many shareholders, there may be different classes of shares. The most common form of shares other than ordinary shares are preference shares.

The holder of preference shares is entitled to a dividend of a fixed amount before any dividend is paid to the holders of ordinary shares. The terms of issue of preference shares often provide that the holder is also entitled to a priority in the repayment of share capital in the event of a winding-up.

The preference shareholder is in a more secure position than the ordinary shareholder as he is entitled to fixed dividends, usually calculated as a percentage of the value of the shares. The ordinary shareholder, however, has the opportunity of greater return as the level of dividend is not restricted to a fixed amount and will fluctuate in accordance with the company's profitability. Furthermore, in a winding-up, when preference shareholders have been repaid the nominal value of their shares, unless they have an express entitlement to a share in any surplus, the whole of the remaining assets of the company will be distributed among the ordinary shareholders in proportion to their holding. Ordinary shareholders hold most of the power at general meetings, and it will be they who will control company affairs and appoint directors. Thus the ordinary shareholder has more rights in determining the way in which a company conducts itself, but the nature of the investment carries a greater risk.

Loan capital

Loan capital is an expression used to describe the long term indebtedness of the company secured by mortgages, debenture stock and loan stock. All companies have an implied power to borrow and to give security for loans made to them. Unless the company's Memorandum of Association (explained below) provides otherwise, the amount a company may borrow is unlimited.

One way in which a company may raise capital is to issue debentures. Debentures are similar to shares in that they have a nominal value. They are usually redeemable at a fixed future date, and their nominal value is the amount payable to the holder on redemption (unless by the terms of issue a premium is also payable on redemption). Debentures usually carry a fixed rate of interest on the amount invested in the company, and are usually secured by a fixed or floating charge over the company's assets. Thus in theory they represent a relatively safe form of investment. The debenture is therefore akin to an "IOU" issued by a company to an investor, with pre-arranged terms concerning interest and repayment. As with preference shares, debentures enjoy priority in the repayment of interest and repayment of capital in the event of the company being wound up. However they do not carry voting rights, and holders do not participate in the running of the company.

Bank loans and overdrafts

Loans by banks are usually secured by a fixed or floating charge over company assets, and by personal guarantees given by directors. Even if assets are subject to a floating charge they may be dealt with freely, as the charge is not fixed to any asset or assets in particular until it becomes operational, i.e. until repayments are not made and the bank seeks to realise company assets to meet the debt. Loans subject to a fixed charge are secured against specific company assets, usually business premises and/or stock.

The creation and structure of a private limited company

The company name

When setting up a company, certain rules apply to the use of a company name.

(1) The new name must not be in the name of a company already on the register.
(2) Certain insensitive words cannot be used without the consent of the Secretary of State for Trade and Industry or some other relevant body. For example, under *Section 78* of the MA 1968, the name "chemist", "druggist" or "pharmacy" cannot be used unless it will apply to a registered pharmacy.
(3) The name must not give the impression of a connection with the government or local authority.
(4) The words "limited", "unlimited" or "public limited company" must not be used except at the end of a name.
(5) The name must not be offensive.
(6) Unless exempted, the word "limited" must be used at the end.

The Secretary of State is empowered to direct a company to change its name where:

(1) The chosen name is too like a name already on the register.
(2) If within 5 years of incorporation he believes that false information was provided for the purpose of registration.
(3) If at the time the name by which it is registered gives so misleading an identification of the nature of its activities as to be likely to cause harm to the public.

It is imperative that once a company has been named, it continues to use exactly the same name, even down to the use of upper- and lower-case letters.

Formalities

To incorporate a company, various documents must be completed and lodged at the Companies House.

(1) Memorandum of Association (discussed below).
(2) Articles of Association (discussed below).
(3) Statement of the particulars of the first director(s) and company secretary, together with their signed consents to acting in these capacities, and the address of the registered office.
(4) Statement of particulars of shares to be issued on incorporation signed by a director or by the secretary.
(5) Declaration of compliance with the Companies Act. This form may be made and signed either by a solicitor engaged in the formation, or by a director or by the secretary. The declaration must be made before a Commissioner for Oaths, Notary Public, Justice of the Peace, or solicitor having the powers conferred on a Commissioner for Oaths, and such person must also state where the declaration was made, sign and date the form.

The Memorandum and Articles of Association must be signed by at least two subscribers, who must write opposite their names the number of shares they agree to take. The names and addresses of the subscribers must be given and their signatures attested by one or more witness(es). The completed documents must then be lodged at the Companies Registry together with the appropriate capital duty at 1% of the capital subscribed for, and the official registration fee. The Registrar examines the documents, and if they are correct a certificate of incorporation is issued. The issuing of the certificate may take several weeks, but once it is issued the company's subscribers may begin to act as a body corporate.

Memorandum and Articles of Association

The company's constitution is set out in two documents known as the Memorandum and Articles of Association. The Memorandum lays down the company's powers and its relationship with the outside world, and the Articles regulate dealings between the company and its members, directors and other officers.

The Memorandum

The Memorandum of Association consists of clauses containing the following information:

(1)   The name of the company.

(2)   The location of the registered office, i.e. whether it is in England, England and Wales, Wales, or Scotland. It need not be more specific. Documents of companies whose registered office is to be situated in Scotland must be lodged at the Companies Registration Office in Edinburgh. These will be classified as Scottish companies. A company must at all times have a registered office at a particular address to which all communications and notices may be addressed.

(3)   The objects of the company. It is invariably the longest clause and requires careful thought. The objects will set out the company's purpose and will set out the kind of activities in which the company seeks to be engaged. The clause will be subdivided as follows:

(a)   The first sub-clause will set out the nature of the company's main business. It must be comprehensive and must detail all potential areas of business. If required, it can be amended at a later date by means of specific resolution.

(b)   The second sub-clause usually covers any other business which in the opinion of the directors may be advantageously or conveniently carried on in conjunction with the main business of the company.

(c)   The subsequent sub-clauses will cover general objects common to most businesses. These may include, for example, powers to lease, sell and purchase property; to purchase/lease equipment or machinery; to mortgage, charge or let out loans against company property; to issue and purchase shares; to issue debentures; to purchase shares in other companies; to sell the company; to draw bills of exchange and negotiable instruments; to distribute property amongst members; and to do all such things as may be necessary towards the attainment of the company's main objective. This list is by no means exhaustive, and will vary considerably between undertakings.

Since the European Communities Act 1972, all transactions carried out by the directors in the company's name are binding as against the company even though they are apparently outside the scope of the Memorandum of Association. However, the shareholders may in this event take out an action for misfeasance against the directors.

(4)   The limited liability of the members.

(5)   The amount of share capital with which the company proposes to be registered and the nominal value of each of the shares into which the share capital is to be divided. The division of shares into different classes, the proportion of shares in each class and the rights conferred on the holders of each class of shares are sometimes stated, but this is very rarely done in practice as it is then more difficult to vary the rights at a later date. These matters are usually dealt with in the Articles so that any alteration can be effected by passing a special resolution.

(6)   Further additional clauses may be included, usually of a kind found in the Articles of Association. The advantage of inserting additional matters in the Memorandum is that they can be protected against subsequent alteration, whereas if they were in the Articles of Association, they could be altered by a special resolution passed by a general meeting of the company despite any provision to the contrary in the Memorandum or Articles.

(7)   The Memorandum of Association concludes with an association clause by which two or more subscribers state that they are desirous of being formed into a company in pursuance of the Memorandum, and if the company has share capital, that they agree to take the number of shares set opposite their names.

The Articles

The Articles of Association regulate the internal affairs of the company. These regulations govern the relationship between the company and its shareholders and the relationship of the shareholders between themselves. A table (known as "Table A") of model articles is found in the Companies Act 1985. It is normal practice to adopt articles which include Table A and to make modifications. The following is a non-exhaustive list of categories of provisions usually found in Articles of Association.

(a)   *Classes of shares.* Where there is more than one type of share, the rights attaching to the owners of each class will be set out. For example, the priority of preference shareholders in the payment of dividends, the rules governing the apportionment of capital and the voting rights attaching to the holders of different classes will be set out. The Articles may also state the way in which these rights may be altered, or the classes of shares created.

(b)   *Share issue restriction. Sections 89–96* of the Companies Act 1985 accords existing shareholders the right of first refusal to any new shares issued. Existing shareholders must be offered the new shares in proportion to their current holding and must be notified in writing. These statutory rights may be altered or excluded by the Articles of Association. For example, directors may be given discretion over share issues. If this is the case, the directors' authority must be renewed every 5 years.

(c)   *Share transfer.* The Articles will often give the directors the discretion not to register a transfer of shares. In a small business with only a few shareholders, the right of pre-emption is usually given to existing shareholders when one member decides to sell his shares. The Articles will contain detailed procedural provisions regulating this process.

(d)   *Company's purchase of its own shares.* In a private limited company, the Articles may provide that a company has authority to purchase its own shares. However, advice should always be taken as to the taxation implications of such a course.

(e)   *Regulation 64 of Table A.* This states that a company must have at least two directors, but is not restricted to a maximum number. A private company is legally obliged to have only one but the sole director cannot be the company secretary. As the initial directors will already have been appointed before incorporation, the Articles can only provide the procedure for appointing subsequent directors.

   Often the Articles of a small firm name directors as permanent directors. This is achieved either through private agreement within the company (which can be overturned by a resolution at a company meeting), or more securely by attaching enhanced voting rights to the directors' shares, thus enabling them to vote out any resolution tabled for their removal.

(f)   *Power of directors and remuneration.* The power to run a company is normally vested in the directors who will exercise this function through resolutions passed at duly convened board meetings. In practice in small companies, however, decisions are taken on a daily basis by all directors.

   The Articles usually contain a provision to vest in the directors the power to deal in company property, to mortgage company property, and to issue securities. It is possible, if required, to limit the total amount of debt the directors may incur on behalf of the company at any one time without the prior consent of the shareholders. Provision for directors' remuneration and expenses is made in the Articles; however, a contract of employment is usually drawn up separately to cover the directors' entitlements to salary, share of profits and expenses.

(g)   *Miscellaneous provisions.* Further provisions in the Articles will deal variously with matters such as allocation of shares following the death of a shareholder; the procedures for calling and conducting general meetings; voting rights at company meetings; appointment and removal of directors and the company secretary; use of the company seal; payment of dividends on shares; and provisions governing the winding-up of the company.

Formal requirements for running a company

Every company must have a registered office, the location of which determines the tax office which will deal with the company's tax matters. Outside the registered office and every office or place of business of the company, the company's name must be permanently displayed. The registered office does not have to be the company's place of business; sometimes a company will nominate its solicitors or accountants to act in this capacity and give their address.

Company stationery

The company name must appear on all stationery including letters, cheques, invoices (which must also state the company VAT number), and receipts. Business letters must also show the address of the registered office, the place of registration and the registered number of the company.

Accounts

A company must decide a date on which all its accounts for the preceding year will be presented (the accounting reference period). The Registrar of Companies must be notified of this date, on form G224, within 6 months of incorporation. The Companies Act 1985 imposes the requirement that accounts must be kept which are capable of showing with reasonable accuracy the financial position of the company at any given time. Accounts must show:

(1)   All moneys paid and received by the company and the details of the transactions.
(2)   The current assets and liabilities of the company.
(3)   The level of stock held at the end of each financial year.
(4)   Details of creditors and debtors.

Accounts must be laid before a general meeting of members within 10 months of the accounting reference period. The company auditor should be appointed before the first Annual General Meeting and must be a chartered or certified accountant, or a person authorised as an auditor by the Department of Trade and Industry. The auditor of a small company is often its accountant, but the liability to prepare accounts and make tax returns vests in the directors. The duty of the auditor is to inform the members of the accuracy of the company's accounts.

Company seal and statutory books

A formal register must be kept giving details of shares and shareholders; directors and the company secretary; directors' interests; and mortgages and charges. All share issues and issues and transfers must be documented in the register. A numbered share certificate will then be issued by the company secretary and pressed with the company seal. A minute book and a book of share certificates must also be maintained. A company must have a seal with its name engraved upon it. The seal must be used on formal company documents which would be made by deed if executed by an individual, e.g. mortgage documents, share certificates, debentures.

Meetings

The conduct of the business of the company is determined in meetings of directors and company members. The procedure for calling and conducting meetings is contained in the Articles of Association.

The meetings held by directors or "board meetings" deal with the day-to-day conduct of the company's affairs. At the very first board meeting the directors should ensure that the formalities outlined above have been complied with or are under way.

At general meetings the members of the company exercise their power over company affairs by passing resolutions. An Annual General Meeting (AGM) must be held within 18 months of incorporation and every year thereafter. Members must have 21 days' notice of an AGM. The main functions carried out at AGMs are:

(1) The receipt of the company accounts and chairman's report.
(2) The proposal of a dividend on shares.
(3) The re-election of directors and other officers and the re-election of auditors.

Extraordinary general meetings (EGMs) may be called at 14 days' notice to deal with urgent business that cannot wait until the AGM to be dealt with. The procedure for proposing and voting on resolutions is similar to that used in AGMs.

Mortgages, debentures and charges

Every charge or mortgage created or debenture issued must be registered with the Registrar of Companies within 21 days of its commencement. Failure to register will result in the imposition of a fine.

The Registrar will issue a certificate of registration for every debenture issued, which must be endorsed on each debenture. When a charge has been satisfied a memorandum of satisfaction should be lodged with the Registrar.

Annual return

Every company must deliver to the registrar of companies successive annual returns each of which is made up to a date not later than the date which is from time to time the company's "return date", that is either the anniversary of the company's incorporation; or if the company's last return delivered was made up to a different date, the anniversary of that date. This document states the address of the registered office; details of the company's shares and shareholders; details of the company's debts; a list of all members and changes in members since the last return and details of the directors and secretary. The return must be signed by a director and the company secretary and be submitted together with the correct registration fee. If a company fails to deliver an annual return before the end of the period of 28 days after a return date, the company is guilty of an offence and liable on summary conviction to a fine not exceeding the statutory maximum and, on conviction after continued contravention, to a daily default fine not exceeding one-tenth of the statutory maximum (see *Section 24* (1426) Companies Act 1985).

Taxation

Corporation tax is charged on the profits of a company's accounting period and is payable 9 months after the expiration of that period (1 April to 31 March). Therefore, if a company's accounting period straddles financial years for which different rates of corporation tax have been fixed, profits will be apportioned to the period falling either side of the end of the year. Tax returns are made quarterly and additionally on the annual accounting date if that does not coincide with a quarterly accounting date. By careful consideration of the first accounting reference period, the first payment of tax can be considerably lessened and cash flow improved for the first year. Professional advice should be taken in this respect.

VAT is dealt with separately and collected by HM Customs and Excise. VAT returns must be made quarterly on prescribed dates. Strict rules govern the keeping of VAT accounts and hefty fines are levied for late payment. VAT matters are invariably dealt with by the company accountant.

The imputation system

Where a company proposes to issue a dividend to shareholders, advance corporation tax is payable on the amount of the dividend. Payment of advance corporation tax must be made at the quarterly return date or on the annual accounting date. The amount of advance corporation tax paid will then be deducted from the overall tax liability for that period.

Notification of changes after incorporation

The Registrar of Companies must be notified of any of the following changes taking place after incorporation.

(1) Change of directors or secretary – notification within 14 days on form 288 by new director/s and company secretary:

- For appointments use form 288(a)
- For resignations use form 288(b)
- For change of personal details use form 288(c).

(2) Change of registered office – notification on form 287 within 14 days signed by a director and the company secretary.

(3) Increase in company capital – notification within 15 days on form 123.

(4) Change in allotment of shares – notification within 1 month on form PUC(2) where the change has taken place for cash consideration, or on form PUC(3) where there has been no cash consideration. This form must be accompanied by the written contract together with the prescribed details on form 88(3).

(5) Change of company name together with a copy of the special resolution authorising the change.

(6) Changes in the Memorandum or Articles of Association together with the authorizing special resolution within 15 days.

Winding-up

A company can be wound up or dissolved by the members themselves or by the court. There are three routes to winding-up or liquidation.

(1) voluntary winding-up by the members
(2) voluntary winding-up by the creditors
(3) compulsory winding-up by the court.

The first two forms do not involve the intervention of the court. They are so named because it is either the members or the creditors who take the initiative in winding-up.

This will either be done because the purposes for which the company was formed have been completed or exhausted, or because the company has run into financial trouble from which it cannot reasonably be expected to recover.

Upon liquidation the powers of the directors cease and the management of the company is taken over by a liquidator. The liquidator may be appointed by the members, creditors or court. The liquidator must use his best endeavours to satisfy as much of the company's indebtedness as possible, and must draw up accounts demonstrating what funds and/or assets are available for the satisfaction of the creditors.

The liquidator owes fiduciary duties to the company whose agent he is, i.e. he owes a duty to the company to do the best financially for it as he can. In a compulsory liquidation, he may be empowered to engage in litigation in the company's name, carry on such of the company's business as may be necessary and pay the company's debts or enter into such compromises or arrangements with creditors as are necessary. If there are sufficient funds within the company to satisfy all the creditors, the remainder will be divided among the shareholders according to their entitlements as laid out in the Articles of Association.

Striking-off the register

A company may be struck off the register where it appears to the Registrar that it has ceased trading. This inference will be raised where no annual return is filed. The directors of a company which has ceased trading and which has no assets or liabilities may initiate the striking-off of their own motion in order to avoid the possible expense of a voluntary liquidation using form 652A with a £10.00 filing fee. However, striking-off of a company is only applicable to a private company if, in the past 3 months, it has not:

- traded or otherwise carried on business;
- changed its name;
- disposed of value of property or rights that immediately before ceasing to be in business or trade, it held for disposal or gain in the normal course of that business or trade; or
- engaged in any other activity except one necessary or expedient for making a striking-off application, settling the company's affairs or meeting a statutory requirement.

Chapter 29

The Sale of Goods

The range of transactions which can be described as a sale of goods is enormous, and includes sales of goods worth from a few pence to millions of pounds. Yet the basic legal framework governing the diverse range of transactions is the same.

This area of law affects the pharmacist in his dual role as purchaser and seller of medicinal and other products. As a purchaser, the pharmacist will come into daily contact with this area of the law when he purchases medicines and other products from his wholesaler suppliers. The same law will regulate the pharmacist's onward sale of these products to the customer. The object of this section of the book is to provide a synopsis of the relevant law, much of which is to be found in the Sale of Goods Act 1979.

Unless otherwise stated, references to statutory sections in this chapter will refer to the Sale of Goods Act 1979.

Contract for the sale of goods

The basic definition of a sale of goods is found in *Section 2(1)*, which defines it as a "contract whereby the seller transfers or agrees to transfer the property in goods to the buyer for a money consideration, called the price". "Property in goods" is a way of describing what is commonly called ownership, but a sale of goods can include an agreement to sell whereby the ownership of the goods passes at a later date. "Money consideration" generally means that the buyer must pay in money. A combination of money and goods in exchange, for example a trade-in on a new car, comes within this definition, but a pure exchange of goods does not.

Contracts for labour and materials supplied and contracts of hire purchase do not fall within the law on sale of goods. In the former, the principal object of the contract is the provision of services. In the latter, the hirer (the buyer) does not acquire the ownership, but merely an option to purchase when all the instalments are paid. There is statutory protection for the customer in these circumstances outside the sale of goods law.

Formation of the contract

The precise moment when the contract is formed is critical, in that before the contract is formed either party is free to withdraw. The contract is made when an offer made by one party is accepted by the other. An offer is an offer to buy. The display of goods for sale in a shop, for example, is merely an invitation to make offers. The customer makes the offer when he produces the goods to the cashier, and it is accepted when the cashier accepts payment.

The Carbolic Smoke Ball

One of the principal cases in the law of contract concerned a proprietor of a medicinal product. In *Carlill v. Carbolic Smoke Ball Co. (1893)*, the defendants, who were the owners of a medicinal product called "The Carbolic Smoke Ball", issued an advertisement in which they offered to pay £100 to any person who succumbed to influenza after having used one of their smoke balls in a specified manner and for a specified period. They added that they had deposited a sum of £1000 with their bankers to show their sincerity. The plaintiff, on the faith of the advertisement, bought and used the ball as prescribed, but succeeded in catching influenza. She sued for the £100. The defendants argued that the advertisement was a mere "puff", never intended to create a binding obligation, that there was no offer to any particular person, and that, even if there were, the plaintiff had failed to notify her acceptance. The Court of Appeal rejected these arguments. Although the offer was made to the world, the contract was made with that limited portion of the public who came forward and performed the condition on the faith of the advertisement. Accordingly, the plaintiff recovered the £100.

Using the post

When the buyer and seller transact a sale by post, special rules apply. Generally, when the means of communication is expected to be the post, the acceptance takes place when the letter of acceptance is posted; see *Household Fire & Carriage Insurance Co. v. Grant (1879)*. When the chosen means of communication is instantaneous, such as telephone or fax, the acceptance takes effect when it is actually communicated to the offeror; see *Brinkibon Ltd v. Stahag Stahl (1982)*.

Oral and written contracts

Section 4 provides that the contract of sale "may be made in writing (either with or without seal), or by word of mouth, or it may be implied from the conduct of the parties". Thus the form of the contract is something which is decided by the parties to it, and where the contract is not made in writing, a court may infer the existence of a contract from oral or any documentary evidence tending to show that a contract was made.

The price to be paid

The price to be paid is usually agreed between the parties, but where it is not, *Section 8(2)* provides that "where the price is not determined . . . the buyer must pay a reasonable price". Sometimes, however, the price to be paid for the goods is so fundamental an aspect of the contract that a court will refuse to enforce a contract where none has been agreed. If none has been agreed it may often be the case that the parties have done no more than agree to contract at some later date, and have not concluded an enforceable contract of sale. When deciding upon such issues, the court will look to all the surrounding circumstances to determine the intention of the parties at the time of the agreement in order to determine whether they intended to contract.

Cancelling the contract

As a general rule, once a contract has been concluded it cannot be cancelled. There are certain exceptions under the Consumer Protection (Cancellation of Contracts Conducted Away From Business Premises) Regulations, 1987, SI 1987, No. 2117, whereby customers who contract with unsolicited traders are entitled to a 7-day cooling-off period in which the buyer may cancel the contract. However, the Regulations do not apply where:

(1)   the price is less than £35
(2)   the contract relates to the sale or provision of finance for the sale of land
(3)   the contract relates to building construction or alteration
(4)   the contract relates to the sale of food or drink.

There are also exceptions for certain "distance contracts" where agreements for goods or services are concluded exclusively by "distance communication" – see the Consumer Protection (Distance Selling) Regulations 2000. The cancellation period is usually 7 working days from receipt of the good or conclusion of the contract in the case of services. However, this period may be extended if the supplier does not give the requisite confirmatory information with details about the right to cancel. The cancellation of a contract under the Regulations also has the effect of cancelling any "related credit contract".

Other exceptions apply for certain mail order catalogues where separate rights are set out in the mail order contract. Where the purchase is made by the consumer with the assistance of credit, a separate statutory regime applies in the form of the Consumer Credit Act 1974 and the Consumer Protection Act 1987. This legislation falls outside the scope of this book.

The passing of property

The time at which ownership transfers from the seller to the buyer does not always coincide with the transfer of physical possession from one to another. Often, for example in shipping contracts, property passes before the buyer accepts delivery. It is important to determine when ownership vests in the buyer for a number of reasons:

(1)   The "risk" in the goods, i.e. the risk of them falling in value or perishing passes with ownership.
(2)   The buyer cannot transfer ownership to a third party until such time as he has ownership himself.
(3)   The seller cannot sue the buyer for the price of the goods until ownership has passed.
(4)   If the buyer or seller becomes bankrupt, the rights of the other party will depend on who has ownership.

The rules governing the transfer of ownership are contained in *Sections 16–19*, and their application depends upon whether the goods are specified or unspecified at the time of making the contract. Specified goods are those which are identified and agreed on at the time the contract of sale is made. A branded bottle of cough mixture taken from a display is therefore specific, but 100 grams of aqueous cream taken from a larger quantity is not specific as it cannot be said which 100 grams have been sold.

Section 17 provides that ownership of specific goods passes to the buyer at such time as the parties intended it to be transferred. If no specific provision has been agreed between the parties, then the court will look at all the surrounding circumstances to see what their intention was. If none can be found, the rules in *Sections 16–19* apply.

Section 16 provides that "where there is a contract for the sale of unascertained goods no property is transferred to the buyer unless and until the goods are ascertained". Thus until the goods can be specifically identified as those forming the subject matter of the contract, ownership cannot pass. For example, an English buyer contracts to buy 100 tonnes of senna leaves from the cargo of the ship *Empress* and the ship leaves India with 500 tonnes, 400 of which are first being delivered to Lisbon. If the 100 tonnes is mixed in with the bulk, it does not become ascertained until the 400 tonnes is unloaded. Once the goods are ascertained, ownership passes in accordance with the intention of the parties.

Rules set out in *Section 18* of the Act apply where the intention of the parties cannot be ascertained.

Rule 1. Where there is an unconditional contract for the sale of specific goods, in a deliverable state, the property in the goods passes to the buyer when the contract is made, and it is immaterial whether the time of payment, or the time of delivery, or both be postponed.

Thus, when the goods are specific and ready to be handed over, the buyer becomes the owner the moment the contract is made. However, if the goods are not in a deliverable state and require something to be done to them before delivery, ownership cannot pass until they are in an appropriate condition (see below).

Rule 2. Where there is a contract for the sale of specific goods and the seller is bound to do something to the goods for the purpose of putting them in a deliverable state, the property does not pass until the thing is done, and the buyer has notice that it has been done.

"Notice" means actual knowledge that the goods are in a deliverable state.

Rule 3. Where there is a contract for sale of specific goods in a deliverable state, but the seller is bound to weigh, measure, test or do some other act or thing with reference to the goods for the purpose of ascertaining the price, the property does not pass until the act or thing is done and the buyer has notice that it has been done.

Rule 3 is self-explanatory, but it must be noted that it applies only where the seller is bound to do something to the goods.

Rule 4. When goods are delivered to the buyer on approval or on sale or return or similar terms, the property in the goods passes to the buyer:

(a)   When he signifies his approval or acceptance to the seller or does any other act adopting the transaction.

(b)   If he does not signify his approval or acceptance to the seller but retains the goods without giving notice of rejection, then if a time has been fixed for the return of the goods, on the expiration of that time and, if no time has been fixed, on the expiration of reasonable time.

In ascertaining whether the buyer has signified his approval or acceptance where he has not specifically stated to the seller that he has accepted the goods, he will be taken to have done so if he does something which substantially impedes his ability to return the goods by the end of the period. Pledging the goods to a pawnbroker for a period exceeding the time limit for refusal would satisfy this test. However, if he cannot return the goods because, for example, they have been stolen, this will operate as an excuse and property will not pass.

Rule 5(1). Where there is a contract for the sale of unascertained or future goods by description, and goods of that description and in a deliverable condition are unconditionally appropriated to the contract, either by the seller with the assent of the buyer, or by the buyer with the assent of the seller, the property in the goods then passes to the buyer; and the assent may be express or implied, and may be given before or after the appropriation is made.

Rule 5(2). Where, in pursuance of the contract, the seller delivers the goods to the buyer or to a carrier or other bailee or custodian for the purpose of transmission to the buyer, and does not reserve the right of disposal, he is taken to have unconditionally appropriated the goods to the contract.

Thus, for the operation of Rule 5 it is necessary that the goods complying with the contract be unconditionally appropriated to the contract, i.e. they become specified by one of the parties, and that the other party assents. Returning to the example of the cargo of senna leaves, if the contract was merely for the delivery of 100 tonnes of senna leaves, the goods would not become specified and accepted until the senna leaves were offloaded and accepted by the buyer. When goods have to be dispatched by a carrier, they will normally be unconditionally appropriated when they are handed over to the carrier. However, the same rules apply, and the goods must be specified in order for ownership to pass.

Section 19 provides that, if the seller reserves a right of disposal of the goods until certain conditions are fulfilled, ownership does not pass until those conditions are fulfilled. For example, if a seller dispatches goods to the buyer through a carrier with instructions that the goods cannot be handed over until the buyer has paid, the goods will remain the seller's property until the buyer has paid for them.

The Romalpa clause

In the case of *Aluminium Industrie Vaasen BV* v. *Romalpa Aluminium Ltd (1976)*, the Court of Appeal had to consider the situation where the seller had sold a large quantity of materials to the buyer in the knowledge that the buyer would only be able to pay the seller when the materials had been used to manufacture goods, and the finished product sold. Before full payment was made the buyer became insolvent, some of the materials remained in their raw state, and some had been processed and mixed with other substances. The Court of Appeal upheld the validity of a clause in the contract of sale which reserved the ownership of the materials to the seller until they had been paid for or until they became processed with other materials, and which created a fiduciary duty (binding financial duty) in the buyer to repay the seller out of the proceeds of sale of the manufactured product the price of the raw materials. Thus a seller in such a situation can reserve ownership of the goods until they become transformed or sold onto a third party, and can create a right to be paid out of the proceeds of the buyer's subsequent sale to a third party. Such clauses have become commonly known as Romalpa clauses. They are sometimes found in the standard contracts used by perfume and cosmetic manufacturers.

Transfer of risk

As was stated above, the usual position is that the risk in the goods transfers with ownership unless the parties agree otherwise (*Section 20(1)*). Therefore, if the goods are damaged or stolen, the loss falls on the seller if it occurs before ownership is transferred, otherwise it falls on the buyer.

There are two limitations on this rule. The first is created by *Section 20(2)* which provides that ". . . where the delivery has been delayed through the fault of either the buyer or seller, the goods are at the risk of the party at fault as regards any loss which might not have occurred but for such fault." The second is created by *Section 20(3)* which provides that "nothing in this section shall affect the duties or liabilities of either seller or buyer as a bailee or custodian of the goods of the other party". The effect of this section is that the party in possession of the goods must take reasonable care of them, and if the goods are damaged or lost as a result of his negligence, he will have to bear that loss.

If the buyer has to bear some loss because the risk in the goods has passed to him, he must still carry out all his obligations under the contract. Thus if he withholds some of the purchase price, he is in breach of the contract and can be sued for the remainder by the seller.

Perishing of goods

Section 6 provides that "where there is a contract for the sale of specific goods, and the goods without the knowledge of the seller have perished at the time when the contract is made, the contract is void". There can be no legally constituted contract for goods which have perished before the contract date. "Perish" means more than slight deterioration not sufficient to change the commercial character of the goods. In *Asfar* v. *Blundell (1896)* it was held that dates which had been under water for 2 days and which had been contaminated with sewage had "perished" and were no longer commercially valuable.

Section 7 provides that "where there is an agreement to sell specific goods, and subsequently the goods, without any fault on the part of the seller or the buyer, perish before the risk passes to the buyer, the agreement is avoided". This section applies the common law doctrine of frustration, whereby a contract is declared void if supervening events outside the control of either party render performance of the contract impossible. *Section 7* applies only to specific goods, but the same considerations apply to unspecified goods as applied in the case of goods perishing before the making of the contract. The contract will not be frustrated if the origin of the unspecified goods is not specified.

It follows from this that once the risk in the goods has passed to the buyer, the contract cannot be avoided by *Section 7*, or in the case of unspecified goods at common law by the doctrine of frustration. If the position were to be otherwise, the concept of the passing of risk would be meaningless.

When the contract is either avoided by the operation of *Section 6* or *7* or declared void at common law, the buyer need not pay for the goods and the seller need not deliver them. However, if the parties had provided for the eventuality which occurred, the terms of the contract would take precedence. In the case where the buyer has paid some of the purchase price before the goods perished, if the contract is avoided by operation of *Section 6* or *7*, then the buyer will recover the whole of the sums he has paid over. If the contract is frustrated at common law, i.e. the goods were unspecified, the Law Reform (Frustrated Contracts) Act 1943 empowers the court, before remitting the balance to the buyer, to deduct from the sums already paid to the seller a sum towards expenses incurred by the seller in performing the contract and to deduct any reasonable sum for any benefit the buyer has received under the contract.

Invalid title

The situation often arises where the seller of goods does not have proper title to the goods. This may occur where the goods are not his to sell, or where the contract by which he originally acquired the goods is voidable (discussed below). The general principle is contained in the maxim, *nemo dat quod non habet*, in other words, you cannot give what you do not own. *Section 2(1)* provides that

> . . . where goods are sold by a person who is not their owner, and who does not sell them under the authority or with the consent of the owner, the buyer acquires no better title to the goods than the seller had, unless the owner of the goods is by his conduct precluded from denying the seller's authority to sell.

Generally speaking, a seller cannot transfer to a buyer any better title than that which he already possesses. Where there has been a chain of sales, for example, where B, without authority, sells A's goods to C who in turn sells them to D, C and D have no better title to the goods than B had. In order to retrieve his goods A can take out an action (called an action for conversion) against D for the recovery of the goods. D may then sue C who may in turn sue B for breach of contract, for it will be an implied term of each contract that the seller had full title to the goods.

If, however, A represented by words or conduct that B had authority to sell his goods, then A will be prevented from asserting that the sale was unauthorised. For the representation to have this effect, it must have been made intentionally or negligently, it must have misled the innocent purchaser and the innocent purchaser must have bought the goods. For example, in *Eastern Distributors v. Goldring (1957)*, a customer who wished to raise some money against his van conspired with a motor trader by pretending that he was buying the van from the motor trader. Both of them filled out their portions of the hire purchase forms. The customer subsequently sold the van to a third party and defaulted on the payments to the hire purchase company. The question then arose as to whether the hire purchase company had acquired title from the motor trader or the customer. It was held that as the customer had allowed the motor trader to represent the van as belonging to him, he was prevented from disputing that the title had passed to the hire purchase company.

Where the owner has signed a document purporting to transfer title, the document will usually be taken to have legal effect except in the rare circumstances where the owner can show both that he was radically mistaken about the nature and effect of the document, and where he can show that he was not careless in signing it.

Exceptions to the nemo dat *principle*

Mercantile agents

A mercantile agent is an independent agent to whom someone else entrusts his goods and to whom is usually transferred the authority to sell the goods, consign them or to raise money on the security of the goods. Problems as to title may occur when the owner instructs the mercantile agent that his goods are not to be sold without his express authority. For example, a man may wish to place his sports car in the window of a car showroom to see how many offers may be lodged, and to ascertain the level of offers made. The manager of the showroom may be acting as a mercantile agent on a commission basis, but it may be agreed between the parties that the car is not to be sold without the owner's express permission.

Another exception to the *nemo dat* maxim is created by *Section 2(1)* of the Factors Act 1889, by which a mercantile agent in possession of goods with the authority of the owner, but without the authority to sell, may pass a good title to a purchaser from him if the purchaser buys from him in good faith and without notice that he does not have authority to sell. In this situation the burden is on the purchaser to prove that he was acting bona fide and bought without knowledge of the absence of authority. Thus a purchaser can acquire good title to the sports car if he innocently believes the mercantile agent to be the true owner. The owner must then sue the agent for the market value of the car.

Sale where the owner's title is voidable

An exception to the *nemo dat* rule can occur where the owner's title is voidable. An example of what is meant by voidable title is where B has induced A to enter into a contract of sale by making some misrepresentation, for example that he is a respectable person whose cheque will be honoured, when in fact he is an impostor who has no funds to meet the cheque. Under these circumstances B has falsely induced A to enter into the contract and will acquire only a voidable title. A will retain the right to set the contract aside and claim his goods back. However, if B sells the goods to C before A realises that he has been misled, C will get a perfect title (provided he buys in good faith and without notice of B's dishonesty) by virtue of *Section 23*.

Lawyers distinguish between a voidable contract and one which is void, i.e. not valid from the outset. Where the contract is void, C cannot acquire good title. This will occur when the following two conditions are met:

(1) The identity of the buyer was an essential fact to A when selling to B.
(2) When making the contract, A was intending to deal with someone other than B.

Thus in *Cundy* v. *Lindsay (1878)*, a rogue purchaser ordered goods from the seller, Lindsay, in the name of Blenkarn of 37 Wood Street. The signature was written in such a way that it looked like the name of the reputable firm Blenkirn & Co. Assuming that he was dealing with a reputable firm, Lindsay dispatched the goods to Blenkirn & Co. at 37 Wood Street. Blenkarn received the goods but never paid for them, and sold them to Cundy who knew nothing of the fraud. The House of Lords held that the contract between Lindsay and Blenkarn was void and therefore the goods still belonged to Lindsay.

Seller retaining possession sells to third party

The situation may arise where the seller, A, sells or agrees to sell goods to B and later sells or agrees to sell them to C. The question arises, to whom do the goods belong? Applying *Section 24* of the 1979 Act and *Section 8* of the Factors Act 1889, under certain circumstances C may acquire title to the goods following a previous sale to B. The conditions are as follows:

(1)   A must have been in possession of the goods or documents of title at the time of the sale to C. The point of this condition is that B could have safeguarded his position by taking immediate possession of the goods or documents of title.
(2)   There must be delivery to C of the goods or documents of title.
(3)   C must be acting in good faith and acting without notice of the previous contract with B.

The purpose of these provisions is to safeguard the position of C. B obviously retains the right to sue A for breach of contract when the goods are not delivered.

Buyer in possession without ownership sells to third party

The buyer usually has ownership of goods when he takes possession, but in some circumstances he may have possession without ownership. For example, a buyer may take delivery, but the agreement is that ownership does not pass until payment is made. What is the position of the third-party purchaser who buys before the original buyer has paid the original seller and thereby acquired title? The answer is that by operation of *Section 25* of the 1979 Act and *Section 9* of the Factors Act 1889, the subsequent purchaser will acquire good title where certain conditions are satisfied as follows:

(1)   The person selling must be someone who has bought or agreed to buy the goods. Purchasing an option or purchasing goods on hire purchase is not sufficient for this condition to be met.
(2)   The person selling the goods must have been a buyer in possession, in other words he must have obtained possession of, or documents of title to, the goods with the consent of the seller.
(3)   There must be a delivery or transfer of the goods or documents of title to the innocent sub-purchaser.
(4)   The buyer in possession must have acted in the normal course of business of a mercantile agent. In other words the transaction with the sub-purchaser must be carried out in such a way as it would be carried out by a mercantile agent. This is a little absurd as the buyer in possession may not be a mercantile agent, but the requirement is implicit in the statutory section.
(5)   The sub-purchaser must be acting bona fide and unaware that the original seller has any rights in respect of the goods.

All the above requirements must be fulfilled in order for the sub-purchaser to acquire a good title.

Misrepresentation

A misrepresentation occurs when one party is induced into entering a contract as a result of something which has been represented by the other party which is in fact false. Statements amounting to a misrepresentation may be made orally or in writing; the essential factor is that it operates on the mind of the other party. A distinction must be drawn between mere statement of opinion or trader's "puff" and a genuine misrepresentation. A statement of opinion is something other than a statement of fact. Traders' puffs are, for example, claims that a particular product will "cure smoking", or will "protect against cardiac arrest", or some other serious illness.

The misrepresentation need not have been made fraudulently in order for it to be actionable; it may be made innocently or negligently. Accordingly, this area of the law may be particularly relevant to the community pharmacist who sells a product about which he has no personal knowledge. The misrepresentation must, however, be an influencing factor on the mind of the party induced.

The aggrieved party may succeed in rescinding the contract and/or in obtaining damages. The effect of rescission is to return the parties to the position they were in before the making of the contract. Thus goods and purchase price must be returned. Rescission is not available where to grant it would be unfair to one of the parties. For example:

(1) Where the parties cannot be returned to their pre-contract position, e.g. where the goods have been consumed or used in a manufacturing process.
(2) Where the goods of an innocent third party would be affected, e.g. where the goods have been sold on by the purchaser.
(3) Where an unreasonable length of time has elapsed since the date of the contract.
(4) Where the contract has been affirmed by the aggrieved party, e.g. where the purchaser of an unsound second-hand car restores the vehicle and drives it for 6 months before claiming rescission.

Damages may be available in addition to rescission to compensate any extra loss suffered by the aggrieved party, or they may be awarded as an alternative to rescission. However, damages are not normally allowable where the misrepresentation was wholly innocent, e.g. where the misrepresentation is made upon the basis of information honestly believed to be true and by a person who cannot be expected to have known otherwise. The seller of a nicotine patch who states, in reliance upon the manufacturer's claim, that the patch will cure the purchaser from smoking, would make a wholly innocent representation if in fact the properties of the particular patch have no effect on the purchaser who wishes to stop smoking.

Some contracts seek to exclude liability for misrepresentation by means of exclusion clauses. These are invalid unless they satisfy the requirement of reasonableness in the Unfair Contract Terms Act 1977. The circumstances in which such clauses will be valid will be rare and probably confined to specialized markets where the buyer and seller are both expert in the goods being sold.

Terms of the contract

As a general rule, the parties to a contract will be bound by the terms they agree upon. However, in order for a term to be binding, it must be incorporated into the contract. This is often done by reducing the entire contract to writing, but contracts may be made orally. A written contract may also have terms incorporated into it by oral agreement. The requirement is either that the terms were expressly agreed by the parties, or that the party seeking to rely on the term took all reasonable steps to bring it to the attention of the other party. For example, one of the terms of a theatre-goer's contract with the theatre cloakroom may be that no liability is accepted for loss of or damage to coats. This term may be adequately incorporated by the position of a prominent notice which can be seen by potential customers.

Terms of the contract may be express or implied. Express terms are those specifically set out or agreed by the parties. Implied terms are those implied by operation of law. Terms may be implied by statute (see below), or they may be implied by the court to make sense of a contract, for example, where a contract makes no express stipulation as to the time in which goods must be delivered, a term will be implied whereby they must be delivered within a reasonable time.

Conditions and warranties

Contractual terms are classified as either conditions or warranties. Conditions are terms of the contract which are so fundamental to its performance that breach of the term would go to the root or essence of the contract. Warranties are other terms which, although they must be performed, are not so fundamental that a failure to perform goes to the substance of the contract. For example, if a second-hand car is sold purportedly running in good order, if it is delivered without an engine, the absence of an engine would be fundamental to the contract and would constitute a breach of condition. If, however, it was delivered requiring minor adjustments to the carburettor, this would amount to no more than a breach of warranty. The significance of this difference is that a breach of condition entitles the other party to treat the contract as repudiated, to return the goods and to sue for damages for any further losses incurred, whereas a breach of warranty merely entitles the aggrieved party to sue for compensation in damages, e.g. the cost of employing a mechanic to adjust the carburettor.

Terms implied by statute

In contracts for the sale of goods, *Sections 12–15* of the Sale of Goods Act 1979 imply some important terms into contracts for the benefit of the purchaser. The terms implied are expressly stated to be either conditions or warranties: different remedies apply according to the nature of the term breached.

Section 12(1) implies a condition on the part of the seller that he has a right to sell the goods. *Section 12(2)* implies warranties that

(a)   the goods are free . . . from any charge or encumbrance not disclosed or known to the buyer before the contract is made
(b)   the buyer will enjoy quiet possession of the goods . . . .

We have seen how issues are resolved when a bona fide purchaser buys goods from a seller with a questionable title. If the purchaser acquires ownership through the operation of those rules then there is no dispute with the seller. If, however, the original owner still has ownership, the buyer can sue the seller for breach of condition claiming damages and/or the purchase price.

Where a third party retains any rights over the goods, not amounting to ownership, which have not been disclosed to the buyer, the buyer may sue for damages for breach of warranty. This may occur, for example, where the goods are subject to a repairer's lien, i.e. a party who has carried out repairs to the goods may have acquired ownership of the goods in proportion to the sum outstanding for the cost of repairs carried out by him. In such a case the buyer can sue the seller for the sums still owed to the repairer and any additional sums incurred as a direct result.

Section 13(1) provides that: "Where there is a contract for the sale of goods by description, there is an implied condition that the goods will correspond to the description." This section is designed to cover the situation in which the buyer has not seen the goods for himself but has relied upon a description. Thus, where a car is described as a "Herald, White Convertible 1961" when it emerges after the sale that in fact the vehicle is two cars welded together, one of which is older than 1961, a breach of condition occurs (*Beale* v. *Taylor (1967)*). Most packaged goods sold in pharmacies are sold by descriptions on the label; therefore, if the contents fail to match the label there is a breach of condition.

Section 14 implies two conditions. The first in *Section 14(2)* provides that where the seller sells goods in the course of a business, there is an implied condition that the goods supplied under the contract are of merchantable quality, except that there is no such condition:

(a) as regards defects specifically drawn to the buyer's attention before the contract is made; or
(b) if the buyer examines the goods before the contract is made, as regards defects which the examination ought to reveal.

It is important to note that this section applies only to goods sold in the course of a business. In a private sale, unless such a term is expressly included, there is no such term implying merchantable quality. Further exceptions to the application of the section are included in the section itself, namely that if the buyer examines the goods himself or has the defects drawn to his attention, he cannot then complain that the goods are sub-standard.

"Merchantable quality" is defined in *Section 14(6)* as meaning that the goods must be as fit for the purpose for which goods of that kind are commonly bought as it is reasonable to expect. Thus goods cannot be expected to be in immaculate condition, and the standard to be expected will vary according to the circumstances. For example, a second-hand car sold as "in working mechanical condition" will not be of merchantable quality if the brakes fail immediately after purchase. If, however, the clutch needs replacing 500 miles after the purchase, the car will nonetheless be of merchantable quality as it can only be expected that parts will need to be replaced on second-hand cars.

Section 14(3) provides that

> Where the buyer sells the goods in the course of a business and the buyer . . . makes
> known to the seller . . . any particular purpose for which the goods are being bought,
> there is an implied condition that the goods supplied under the contract are reasonably
> fit for the purpose, whether or not that is a purpose for which such goods are normally
> supplied.

Section 14(3) could be particularly relevant to a pharmacist who counter-prescribes
a product in circumstances where the product is not licensed for the condition in
question.

The section applies to transactions carried out in the course of a business. The
expression "reasonably fit" does not require the goods to be of the highest quality,
merely that they are suitable for the job intended. This can cause difficulties for the
purchaser where, for example, he has bought a washing machine which has cosmetic damage to it but which nonetheless functions perfectly in cleaning clothes.
The retailer may in this situation be able to argue successfully that it is fit for its purpose. If the retailer is successful, the purchaser can then only sue for breach of an
implied warranty that the machine would be in good cosmetic order. (The courts
will only imply a term where it considers that term to have been intended to be
included by the parties, or where the contract would not make sense without the
inclusion of such a term.) It was established in *Slater and Slater* (a firm) v. *Finning Ltd*
(1996) that where a purchaser fails to make known that goods are to be used for
other than their normal purpose, the seller's obligation does not extend to anything
beyond an assurance that the goods are fit for the purpose for which they would
ordinarily be used. There is no breach of the implied condition of fitness where the
failure of the goods to meet the intended purpose arises from an abnormal feature
or idiosyncrasy, not made known to the seller, on the part of the purchaser or the
use to which the goods are to be put.

Section 15 provides that where the contract is a contract for sale by sample, e.g.
where a quantity of senna leaves are bought having examined a sample from the
bulk, there is an implied condition that:

(1)   The bulk will correspond to the sample in quality.
(2)   The buyer will have reasonable opportunity of comparing the bulk with the
      sample.
(3)   The goods will be free from any defect, rendering them unmerchantable, which
      would not be apparent on reasonable examination of the sample.

The bulk must correspond to the sample and, where it does not, the buyer may treat
the contract as repudiated and sue for the price and/or damages.

Implied terms in contracts other than those for sale of goods

The Supply of Goods and Services Act 1982 creates implied terms similar to those
in the Sale of Goods Act 1979, which apply to contracts closely related to the sale
of goods such as barter, contracts for repair and contracts for the provision of
services.

Sections 2–5 of the 1982 Act give to customers in contracts of barter and contracts for repair (e.g. a contract where a roofer repairs a roof and supplies the materials used), rights in relation to title, description, quality and sample which are identical to those conferred by the Sale of Goods Act 1979. These rights relate specifically to the goods/materials supplied under such a contract. *Sections 2–5* of the 1982 Act correspond only to *Sections 12–15* of the Sale of Goods Act 1979, and do not create any further rule concerning, for example, the passing of ownership and risk under a contract of barter.

Sections 6–10 of the 1982 Act imply similar conditions to those in *Sections 12–15* of the Sale of Goods Act 1979 into contracts of hire other than hire purchase agreements. Thus in contracts for the hire of cars or plant, for example, similar terms relating to title, merchantable quality, fitness for purpose and correspondence to sample apply.

Sections 13–15 deal specifically with contracts for the supply of services, and are fairly self-explanatory.

Section 13 implies a term that:

> . . . where the supplier is acting in the course of a business, there is an implied term that the supplier will carry out the service with reasonable care and skill.

Where this term is breached, the customer can sue the supplier for damages, e.g. for the cost of having the defective work made good. A pharmacist would be caught by this section if, for example, he failed to take reasonable care in mixing solutions whilst dispensing a prescription for a patient.

Section 14 provides that where a time for performance of the contract for services is not specified in the contract, there is an implied term that the supplier will carry out the service within a reasonable time.

Section 15 provides that where the price is not specifically stated in the contract for services, there is an implied term that the customer will pay a reasonable price.

Exemption clauses

Clauses which purport to exclude or restrict the liability of one or other of the parties to a contract are termed "exemption clauses". The validity of many such clauses is governed by the Unfair Contract Terms Act 1977, but common law rules also apply.

A clause is of no effect unless it is incorporated as a term of the contract, and incorporation must occur at the time of contracting. If the exemption clause is brought to the attention of the purchaser after the time of contracting, it is of no effect. Thus exemption clauses printed on receipts are usually of no effect.

As with all contractual terms, an exemption clause must be specifically incorporated into the contract to be of effect. Where the contract is written and signed by the buyer, he will be presumed to be bound. Where a clause is contained in an unsigned document, the party seeking to rely upon it must prove that it was brought to the attention of the other party, or that all reasonably necessary steps were taken to draw the other party's attention to it.

Where the exemption clause is displayed on a notice, as in a cloakroom or car park, the clause will only be incorporated if at the time of contracting the customer already knew of the existence of the term, or reasonable steps had been taken to draw it to his attention.

Where there has been a course of dealing between the parties on the same terms, the same terms will be presumed to be incorporated into later contracts, including exemption clauses.

A party other than a party to a contract cannot rely on an exclusion clause in that contract. Thus a manufacturer cannot rely on an exclusion clause incorporated into the contract of sale between a retailer and a consumer.

Exemption clauses are always construed narrowly and against the party seeking to rely upon them. In this respect the law is plainly weighted in favour of the person prejudiced by the operation of the clause.

The Unfair Contract Terms Act 1977 curbs the operation of exemption clauses in many respects.

Section 6 of the Act prevents a seller from avoiding any liability imposed by *Sections 12–15* of the Sale of Goods Act 1979, i.e. the terms as to title, description, merchantable quality, fitness for purpose and sample, where the buyer deals as a consumer. A buyer deals as a consumer where he is not acting in the course of business, but where the seller is, and where the goods are of a type normally supplied for private use. Purchases at auctions or by competitive tenders are excluded.

Where the buyer is not dealing as a consumer, the seller cannot exclude himself from the liability imposed by *Section 12* of the Sale of Goods Act 1979 (implied terms as to title), but he can exclude liabilities imposed by *Sections 12–15* insofar as the exemption clause satisfies the requirement of reasonableness. This is in order that businessmen maintain freedom to contract on whatever terms they choose. Exemption clauses can be unreasonable in certain circumstances, however, especially where the parties are not in equal bargaining positions. Thus in determining the reasonableness or otherwise of such a clause, under Schedule 2 of the Unfair Contract Terms Act 1977, the court can take into account the strength of the bargaining positions of the parties; whether the customer was acting under an inducement to agree to the term; whether the customer knew or ought to have known of the existence of the term; whether, where the term excludes liability for the breach of some condition, it was reasonable at the time of the contract to expect that condition to be complied with; and whether the goods were made specifically to the order or specification of the customer.

Where the clause seeks to exclude liability from terms other than those imposed by the Sale of Goods Act 1979, it will be subject to the requirement of reasonableness, where:

(1) The seller's liability is a business liability.
(2) In buying the goods the buyer deals as a consumer or on the seller's written standard terms of business.

Where neither of the above applies, the exemption clause will be valid. Where either of them do apply, *Section 3* of the Unfair Contract Terms Act 1977 applies, by which the seller cannot:

> . . . when in breach of contract, exclude or restrict any liability in respect of his breach; or . . .

(b) claim to be entitled

(i) to render a contractual performance substantially different from that which was reasonably expected of him; or

(ii) in respect of the whole or any part of his contractual obligation, to render no performance at all,

except in so far as the contract term satisfies the requirement of reasonableness.

The courts have obviously a wide discretion in interpreting the reasonableness of exemption clauses in these circumstances, and each case will have to be considered on its facts bearing in mind the factors listed in Schedule 2 (see above).

Where the contract purports to exclude liability for negligence, *Section 2* of the Unfair Contract Terms Act 1977 provides that liability for death or personal injury caused by negligence cannot be excluded. However, liability for other loss or damage can be excluded, but only insofar as the clause satisfies the requirement of reasonableness.

The Unfair Contract Terms Act 1977 applies to contracts generally, and is not limited in its application to contracts for the sale of goods.

The Unfair Terms in Consumer Contracts Regulations 1999

These Regulations provide that in a contract between a business and a consumer, an "unfair term" will not be binding on the consumer. The Regulations give illustrations of terms which will, prima facie, be regarded as unfair: relevant to clauses fixing damages is "requiring any consumer who fails to fulfil his obligation to pay a disproportionately high sum in compensation (Schedule 2 Paragraph 1(e))". So a consumer will be able to appeal to this standard as well as to the common law on penalties.

Remedies available to the seller and buyer in default

When the buyer is in default, the seller has personal remedies exercisable through the courts and remedies exercisable against the goods.

Personal remedies

The seller has two possible remedies under this head: damages for non-acceptance or an action for the price.

Section 49 of the Sale of Goods Act 1979 allows the seller to sue for the price of the goods where:

(1) The buyer has wrongfully refused or neglected to pay according to the terms of the contract; and

(2) Either the property has passed to the buyer or the price is payable on a certain day irrespective of delivery.

The most important thing to note about the above requirements is that the buyer's refusal to pay must be wrongful. If he has rightfully rejected the goods the seller's action fails. Furthermore, under *Section 28* the buyer is entitled to refuse payment until delivery (unless there has been a contrary agreement). If the specified date for payment has passed, however, the seller may bring an action.

Under *Section 37*, the seller may have a claim where the buyer does not take delivery of the goods within a reasonable time from when he has been informed that the seller is ready and able to deliver, and has been requested to take delivery. If for some reason the seller cannot maintain an action under *Section 49*, he may have a claim for damages under *Section 50* where 'the buyer wrongfully neglects or refuses to accept and pay for the goods'. Usually the damages under this head will be less than the price.

Remedies against the goods

The three possible remedies against the goods are lien, stoppage in transit and resale. These are available to the seller who is owed the whole of the price. The seller's lien is a right to retain possession of the goods when ownership of the goods has passed to the buyer. *Section 41(1)* enables this right to be exercised:

(1)   Where the goods have been sold without any stipulation as to credit.
(2)   Where the goods have been sold on credit, but the term of the credit has expired.
(3)   Where the buyer becomes insolvent.

The seller loses his lien where any of the following occurs:

(1)   The seller is paid by the buyer.
(2)   An innocent third party acquires title under one of the *nemo dat* exceptions (see above).
(3)   The seller delivers the goods to any seller or carrier for the purpose of transmission to the buyer without reserving the right of disposal of the goods. However, even when this occurs, the seller may still exercise his right to stoppage in transit.
(4)   The buyer or his agent lawfully obtains title to the goods.
(5)   The seller waives his lien.

Under *Section 44*, if the buyer has become insolvent and the goods are in transit, the seller can resume possession of the goods and retain them until payment is made. Transit ends when the buyer obtains delivery; the carrier acknowledges that he holds the goods on behalf of the buyer; or when the carrier wrongfully refuses to hand the goods to the buyer. The fact that part of the goods have been delivered does not stop the remainder being stopped in transit.

Under *Section 48*, the seller is allowed to resell the goods where:

(1)   they are of a perishable nature and the buyer does not tender the price within a reasonable time of being told that the unpaid seller intends to resell; or
(2)   the seller expressly reserves the right of resale in case the buyer should default, and the buyer defaults.

When the right of resale is exercised, the contract is rescinded. When it is rescinded, if the title has passed to the buyer, it reverts to the seller. Under *Section 48(2)*, if an unpaid seller resells the goods when he has exercised his seller's lien or stopped the goods in transit, the subsequent buyer acquires a good title to them as against the original buyer. The original buyer then has to bring an action against the seller for non-delivery, provided the seller did not have the right to resell.

Buyer's remedies

Specific performance

Section 52 allows the court to make an order that the goods be delivered to the buyer in the case of a contract to deliver specific or ascertained goods. Such an order can only be made where the specific goods are ascertained and where damages would not be an adequate remedy, e.g. when it is commercially essential that the buyer have the specific goods. When such an order is made, the seller does not have an option to deliver other goods or repay the price.

Rejection of the goods

Where the seller has breached a condition of the contract, as well as a right to damages, the buyer has a right to reject the goods (to treat the seller's breach as a repudiation of the contract). The buyer need not deliver the goods to the seller, but may inform him that he rejects the goods. Any storage expenses reasonably incurred will be recoverable from the seller.

Breach of a warranty will not entitle the buyer to reject the goods, but gives him an action for damages.

Where there has been a breach of condition, the buyer loses his right to reject the goods once he has accepted them. Under *Section 35*, acceptance is constituted when:

(1) The buyer informs the seller that he has accepted the goods.
(2) If after taking delivery, and following a reasonable time in which to examine the goods, the buyer carries out some act inconsistent with the seller being owner of them (e.g. he uses them in a manufacturing process).
(3) The buyer retains the goods for more than a reasonable length of time without telling the seller that he has rejected them.

The buyer may lose his right to reject the goods by waiving the right. This may occur where he knows that the seller is in breach of a condition before the date of delivery, but nevertheless accepts delivery in spite of the breach. If the buyer rejects the goods, he can do so without treating the contract as repudiated, and therefore the seller remains at liberty to re-tender goods in accordance with the contract.

Damages

The buyer can claim damages for non-delivery or for breach of any other condition or warranty. This is in addition to any right to reject the goods and recover the purchase price.

The purchase price can be recovered where there has been a failure on the part of the seller to deliver. Where the buyer has rejected the goods or treated the contract as repudiated, he is entitled to the return of any payment made.

The measure of damages

In general, contract damages compensate any loss naturally arising from the breach, and any loss which, at the time of making the contract, the defendant could have predicted as likely to result from the breach of it. Some specific rules relate to contracts for the sale of goods.

Non-acceptance

Section 50 of the Sale of Goods Act 1979 provides that:

(1) Where the buyer wrongfully neglects or refuses to accept and pay for the goods, the seller may maintain an action against him for damages for non-acceptance.
(2) The measure of damages is the estimated loss directly and naturally resulting, in the ordinary course of events, from the breach of contract.
(3) Where there is an available market for the goods in question, the measure of damages is prima facie to be ascertained by the difference between the contract price and the current market price at the time or times when the goods ought to have been accepted, or at the time of refusal to accept.

The principle behind this section is that if the seller is able to resell the goods he will receive only nominal damages if he could get a good price on resale. This section does not, however, exclude any further loss which was reasonably foreseeable. So, for example, the seller will be able to recover any extra storage expenses he had to incur.

Non-delivery

Section 51 provides that:

(1) Where the seller wrongfully neglects or refuses to deliver the goods to the buyer, the buyer may maintain an action against the seller for damages for non-delivery.
(2) The measure of the damages is the estimated loss directly and naturally resulting, in the ordinary course of events, from the seller's breach of contract.
(3) Where there is an available market for the goods in question the measure of damages is prima facie to be ascertained by the difference between the contract and market price or current price of the goods at the time . . . when they ought to have been delivered . . . or at the time of refusal to deliver.

This is the converse of *Section 50*, and provides that where the buyer may buy the goods elsewhere, his damages are limited to the difference between the contract price and the price elsewhere, plus any other reasonably foreseeable loss.

Anticipatory breach

Where one of the parties to a contract commits an anticipatory breach, e.g., before the date for performance of the contract the seller informs the buyer that he will not deliver, or the buyer informs the seller that he cannot pay, the other party has an option to treat the contract as repudiated immediately and to claim damages, or wait until there has been actual failure to perform and claim damages under the principles in either *Section 50* or *Section 51*. If the former course is adopted, the innocent party is under a duty to minimize his loss by buying alternative goods at the best available price. If the price of the goods is currently rising, the damages will be assessed according to the best price the innocent party could have obtained as soon as reasonably practicable after the acceptance of the repudiation. However, if the innocent party refuses to accept the anticipatory breach as a repudiation, he is not under a duty to minimize his loss, and damages will be assessed according to the normal principles in *Section 50* or *51*.

Late delivery

Late delivery by the seller will normally be a breach of condition. If the buyer rejects the goods for breach of condition, his damages are assessed as in the case of non-delivery. If it is only a breach of warranty or if the buyer accepts the goods, the damages are prima facie assessed according to the difference between the value of the goods on the date they should have been delivered and their value (if lower) when actually delivered.

Breach of warranty

Section 53(2) and *(3)* provides that:

(2) The measure of damages for breach of warranty is the estimated loss directly and naturally resulting, in the ordinary course of events, from the breach of warranty.
(3) In the case of breach of warranty of quality such loss is prima facie the difference between the value of the goods at the time of delivery to the buyer and the value they would have had if they had fulfilled the warranty.

Under this section the buyer has a choice as to claiming his capital loss or his loss of profit. He cannot claim both. In *Cullinane* v. *British Rema (1953)*, the sellers had warranted that a clay pulverising machine would process clay at six tons per hour. In fact it could not do so. The buyer claimed first for capital loss and secondly for loss of profits, being the difference between those profits actually made and those that would have been made had the machine performed as promised. The Court of Appeal held that both claims could not succeed, and disallowed the smaller of the claims. The Appeal Court also stated that loss of profits could have been claimed for the whole of the useful life of the machine. *Subsection 3* provides that only the prima facie amount can be claimed. In addition to the losses discussed above, the buyer may also claim any loss which could reasonably have been predicted by both parties as likely to occur in the event of the breach. The question is, "had the seller been aware of the defect at the time of the contract, what type of damage could the seller at the time of contract have reasonably predicted?"

In *Parsons* v. *Uttley Ingham (1978)*, the sellers sold a hopper to a farmer for the storage of pig nuts. When it was installed, the ventilator was not opened by the installers. As a result, the pig nuts became mouldy and the pigs died as a result of eating them. The sellers were held liable for the loss of the pigs, the Court of Appeal taking the view that the loss of the pigs was a reasonably foreseeable consequence of the failure to ensure that the ventilator was working correctly. Under *Section 55(1)*, the buyer may set off damages due to him for breach of warranty against the price he owes the seller, but retains the right to sue for any excess.

Mitigation of loss

In all cases of breach of contract, whether or not in a contract for the sale of goods, the innocent party is under a duty to take reasonable steps to minimize his loss. Failure to do so will result in the loss which could have been avoided being deducted from the damages. The requirement is one to act reasonably in the particular circumstances. For example, if the seller delivers defective goods but offers to buy them back at a reasonable price, the buyer will normally be under a duty to accept the offer. This does not prejudice his claim for the excess. The seller cannot force the buyer to accept defective goods. If the buyer rejects the goods and the market price is climbing, the buyer will usually be under an obligation to minimize his loss by purchasing alternative goods as soon as reasonably practicable. However, if alternative goods are not available, e.g. the goods were being made especially for the buyer, the buyer cannot reasonably be expected to buy alternative goods which will not suit his purpose.

Penalty clauses

Some contracts contain a clause which stipulates how much is to be paid by the party in breach; e.g. £50 for every day payment fails to be made after the due date. The general rule is that such a clause is binding on the party in breach if it is a genuine attempt by the parties to estimate the actual loss which will be caused to the innocent party during the period of breach. Thus, if the sum claimed is extravagant and unconscionable in comparison with the amount of the actual loss, the clause will be of no effect. However, if the penalty clause is void, the innocent party may nevertheless sue for his loss in the normal way.

Product liability

Fundamental to the English law of contract is the doctrine of privity of contract. This means that no one other than a party to a contract can sue on it. This has particular implications where damage has been caused by a product to a consumer or a third party. If damage is caused to a consumer, he can sue the retailer under one of the implied terms in the Sale of Goods Act 1979. He cannot, however, sue the manufacturer under normal contractual principles as he has no contract with him. In any event, the measure of damages under the contract is limited to putting the parties back into the positions they would have enjoyed had the contract never been made. If the product is, for example, a defective medicine, contractual damages will not cover damages for personal injury and loss of earnings incurred by the consumer. Furthermore, if the person harmed is someone other than the buyer, he has no right to sue on the contract of sale at all. The traditional remedy for such an occurrence was to sue for negligence in the law of tort. Damages in negligence compensate the aggrieved party for all the reasonably foreseeable losses incurred as a result of the negligence. The main problem for the consumer, however, is that he bears the burden of proving that the manufacturer was negligent, a task which is often by no means easy.

Consumer Protection Act 1987

The law in this area was considerably advanced by the Consumer Protection Act 1987, which implemented an EC (now EU) Directive on product liability. Under the Act, any person who is injured by a defective product can sue the manufacturer for compensation whether or not the manufacturer was negligent.

To succeed the consumer must establish four things:

(1)   that the product contained a defect
(2)   that the plaintiff suffered damage
(3)   that the damage was caused by the defect
(4)   that the defendant was producer, own-brander or importer into the EU of the product.

A product is defective if its safety is not such as persons generally are entitled to expect. Safety includes not only safety in the context of death or personal injury, but also the risk of damage to property. In determining the defectiveness of the product, *Section 39(2)* of the Act requires that the nature of the product, any instructions, what use might reasonably be expected for the product and the time when the product was supplied by the producer must all be considered. The term "product" is very wide and covers everything which can be considered a product, including gas and electricity. There are exceptions relating to land, some agricultural produce and game.

Under the 1987 Act damages may be claimed for death, personal injury or damage to property (including land) which is ordinarily intended for private use, occupation or consumption; and intended by the person suffering the loss or damage mainly for his private use, occupation or consumption. Thus damage to business property cannot be claimed under the Act (and must therefore be claimed for in negligence). Furthermore, only claims worth over £275 can be entertained. The final qualification is that under the Act a claim cannot be made for the cost of the defective product itself – this must be made under the contract of sale.

Claims can be brought against the manufacturer or, in the case of products which are abstracted from the earth such as coal, the abstracter. An "own-brander" is someone who holds themselves out as a producer. Pharmacies which carry their own brand name on goods fall into this category. The only importers who are liable are those who import the goods from outside the EU into the EU.

Defences

Section 4 of the Act provides the following defences which, if relied upon, must be proved by the defendant:

(1) The defect is due to compliance with a statutory regulation or EU rule.
(2) The defendant did not supply the product.
(3) The defendant supplied the product otherwise than in the course of business and did not produce it with a view to profit, e.g. the defendant gave to friends a bottle of his home-made wine which had become contaminated.
(4) The defect did not exist in the product at the time of supply.
(5) The defect is in the design of the overall product and the defendant is merely the manufacturer of a component.
(6) The defect was such "that the state of scientific and technical knowledge at the relevant time was not such that a producer of products of the same description as the product in question might be expected to have discovered the defect if it had existed in his products while they were under his control". This "state of the art" defence protects the producer who can show that the defect was not such that it could have been discovered at the time the product was made, abstracted or imported.

Furthermore, it is open to the producer to argue that part of the damage was due to the contributory negligence of the consumer, e.g. when the purchaser of a lawn mower fails to read the safety instructions and suffers an injury which he would not have suffered if he had read the instructions. If this is proved, then the damages will be reduced in proportion to the culpability of the consumer. Under the Act the producer is prohibited from excluding liability imposed by the Act. However, any claim must be made within 3 years of the date of the injury or damage occurring, and in any event within 10 years of the producer supplying the product.

Chapter 30

Employment Law

The contract of employment

A pharmacist needs to be aware of the basic principles of employment law. He may employ members of staff, perhaps a locum pharmacist, dispenser or shop assistant; or alternatively he may himself be an employee of a limited company, sole trader or partnership.

A contract of employment is approached legally in the same way as any other commercial contract. Over the years, however, there have developed particular regulations relating to the formation of such a contract, the conditions of service and termination of the contract. Much of the law in this area is contained in the Employment Rights Act 1996 (ERA), though some common law rules remain. Thus contracts of employment are subject to rigorous controls from the beginning to the end of the employment. The rules are complex, and they need to be examined in considerable detail in order for their application to be fully grasped.

Statutory controls on the contents of the contract

Statute law used to confine itself generally to termination of the contract of employment i.e. unfair dismissal, redundancy and takeovers and to certain specific areas which cover employment as one among several areas of human activity, i.e. discrimination and health and safety.

The position has now changed considerably. In the National Minimum Wage Act 1998 and the Working Time Regulations 1998, we have for the first time a general statutory control of the two most basic elements of the contract of employment: how much employees are paid and how long they can be required to work in return. In addition "family-friendly" measures have been introduced by the Employment Relations Act 1999 and the Employment Act 2002.

Contract of service or contract for services?

There is a fundamental difference between a contract of service (employment) and a contract for services, i.e. between the existence of an employer–employee relationship, and the relationship between a party and a self-employed contractor. This distinction is important as most of the relevant legislation applies only to the employer–employee relationship. The system of taxation is also different. The duties of the employer towards his employee are far more onerous. There are certain terms which are only implied into a contract of employment and which are not implied into a contract for services. Further, in some situations where the employee has committed an unlawful act, his employer will be vicariously liable for his wrongdoing; no such principle applies where the contract is merely one for services.

The distinction is not always an easy one to draw, and in the past the courts have experienced difficulty in devising a satisfactory test to discern the difference. Having tried tests which look to the level of control exercised by the employer, or the extent to which the employee is integrated into the employer's business, a three stage "economic reality" test has been developed.

In *Ready Mix Concrete Ltd v. Minister of Pensions and National Insurance (1968)*, the court held that a contract of employment can only exist where:

(1)   the employee agrees to provide his own work and skill;
(2)   there is some element of control exercisable by the employer; and
(3)   the other terms of the contract are not inconsistent with a contract of employment.

This case involved the question of whether the driver of a lorry who had obtained it on hire-purchase from the plaintiff company was an employee. He was required to paint the lorry in the company livery, but could use substitute drivers if he was unwell or away. The court found that the provision for the use of substitute drivers rendered the driver an independent contractor.

Form of the contract of employment

There is no formal requirement that the entire contract of employment be evidenced in writing: therefore valid contracts can be made orally. However, *Section 1* of the ERA 1996 requires the employer to produce a written statement within 2 months of the commencement of employment containing the following information:

(1)   the names of the parties and the date upon which the period of employment began
(2)   the rate of remuneration and the method for calculating it
(3)   the intervals at which remuneration is to be paid
(4)   the terms relating to hours of work
(5)   the terms concerning entitlement to holiday
(6)   terms relating to provision for inability to work through sickness and details of sick pay arrangements
(7)   the periods of notice required for either party to terminate the contract
(8)   the terms concerning pension arrangements
(9)   the job title/description.

The employee must also be provided with details of:

(1)   any applicable disciplinary rules
(2)   the person to whom he can apply should he be unhappy with the operation of any disciplinary procedure

(3) the person to whom he can apply if he has any grievance with his employment generally

(4) whether a contracting-out certificate (under the provisions of the Social Security Pensions Act 1975) is in force in relation to that employment.

All the above information may be included in one document to which the employer may then draw the employee's attention. The written statement is not itself the contract of employment, but is strong prima facie evidence of the terms agreed upon by the parties. There is nothing to prevent the parties from altering the terms set out in the statement at a later date, in which case the subsequent agreement will take precedence.

Terms of the contract of employment

Apart from the conditions implied by statute, the contract of employment will usually consist of a written or an oral agreement between the parties setting out the basic conditions of employment. Express statements made prior to the contract may also be incorporated, and deviation from such statements will constitute breach of contract unless there has been specific agreement to be contrary. Attempts to vary the terms or conditions of employment after the contract has been made will only be effectual if they are specifically agreed to by the parties.

Collective agreements

Many contracts of employment consist partly or wholly of terms which have been arrived at collectively by means of negotiations with a trade union. Such collective agreements may be incorporated into the contract of employment by express incorporation, or may be implied by statute. For example, under the ERA 1996 there is provision for collective agreements to replace the statutory provisions for the right to claim unfair dismissal or the right to claim statutory redundancy payment. Should the S of S approve the collective agreement, the terms negotiated between the trade union and the employers will replace those created and implied by statute.

Company rules

Where there is a company rule book, those rules may be incorporated into the individual contract of employment subject to the following principles.

(1) If the employee agrees before the making of the contract that the rules are to form part of the contract, then they are expressly incorporated into the contract.

(2) The rules may be incorporated if he is given other notice, i.e. the posting of a large notice, that they are to be included in the contract. However, the matter is usually decided as a matter of custom and practice.

(3) Not all rules automatically become terms of the contract. This may be so where, for example, rules have become out of date. It is a matter of construction of the specific rules as to whether they are terms of the contract or merely guidelines as to how the work should be performed.

The nebulous nature of this area of law is further emphasized by the part which custom plays in determining terms of the contract of employment. In *Marshall* v. *English Electric Co. Ltd (1945)* it was stated as a matter of general principle that "established practice at a particular factory may be incorporated into a workman's contract of service, and whether he knew it or not, it must be presumed that he accepted employment on the same terms as applied to other workers in the same factory". The range of customs is potentially wide and may even relate to such matters as dismissals procedure. Examples of the incorporation of custom can be seen in case law. In *Sagar* v. *Ridehalgh and Son Ltd (1931)*, it was held that the customs of the Lancashire weaving trade were incorporated into the contract of employment of an individual weaver. Therefore customary deductions for faulty workmanship were held to be lawfully deductible. *Davson* v. *France (1959)* shows the operation of the principle in the converse manner. A musician who had received one week's notice to quit was held to have been wrongfully dismissed as the customary period in the trade was 14 days.

Continuity of employment

Once an employee has commenced employment, he acquires various rights if continuity of employment is maintained. For example, although an employee is always entitled to sue for breach of his contract of employment in an action for wrongful dismissal (i.e. dismissal that is in breach of the terms of the contract of employment), the right to complain to an industrial tribunal for unfair dismissal (a much wider concept the conditions for which are contained in the Industrial Tribunals Act 1996 (ITA) and discussed below) is only acquired after 1 year's continuous employment. The length of time an employer has spent with his employer has always been an important factor in determining whether or not he qualifies for unfair dismissal rights. The present position is contained in the Unfair Dismissal and Statements of Reasons for Dismissal (Variation of Qualifying Period) Order 1999, which reduced the qualifying period from 2 years to 1 year.

Part XIV of the ERA 1996 deals with the continuity of employment, and *Section 218(2)* prescribes that:

> If a trade or business, or an undertaking (whether or not established by or under an Act) is transferred from one person to another –
>
> (a) the period of employment of an employee in the trade or business or undertaking at the time of the transfer counts as a period of employment with the transferee, and
> (b) the transfer does not break the continuity of the period of employment.

Special categories of employee

There are several categories of employee to whom special considerations apply.

Company directors

Company directors are usually considered as employees if they have a written service contract with the company, but non-executive directors are usually not. The question as to whether such a person is or is not an employee is always a matter of law to be decided upon the test for the incidents of employment (see above). Where, for example, a non-executive director did not have anything in writing referring to him as an employee, and where he had not been paid remuneration for a period due to the financial condition of the company, the Employment Appeal Tribunal would be unable to find that he was an employee.

Partners

Partners in a firm are not employees. However, those employed by partnerships may be employees.

Civil servants

Civil servants were long thought not to be employees, but the position now seems to be that they enjoy a relationship similar to that created under a contract of employment, subject to the right of the Crown to dismiss its servants at its pleasure. This is not as harsh as it sounds, as many of the legal protections accorded to other employees, including the ERA 1996 provisions for unfair dismissal, apply equally to Crown servants. Police officers and prison officers are exceptions to this, however, and cannot claim unfair dismissal. Similarly, members of the armed forces are specifically excluded from statutory protection.

Minors

Minors (i.e. persons under the age of 18) are bound by the contract of employment subject to the same proviso affecting any other contract, that it must be substantially for their benefit when taken as a whole. This is a matter to be decided by the court, and is a measure designed to stop an unfair advantage being taken of young persons.

Children under the age of 13 cannot be employed. Between the ages of 13 and 16 a minor may work part-time subject to a strict limit on hours. "Young persons" between the ages of 16 and 18 may work subject to various restrictions, e.g. those contained in the Factories Act 1961, which limit the hours of work and the nature of work which may be undertaken.

Temporary staff

Temporary workers, who are drafted into replace regular employees who are absent through illness or maternity leave, are not normally regarded as unfairly dismissed if the regular employee returns to work.

Probationary staff

Probationary employees can be dismissed in accordance with the conditions of their probation, but if the probationary period extends to 1 year of continuous employment, the statutory rights will be acquired and the employer will be subject to the statutory requirement of showing that the dismissal was fair.

Retirement age

Section 109 of the ERA provides that employees who have reached the "normal retirement age" for the position which they hold are unable to claim unfair dismissal and, that in any other case, they are over the age of 65. So many companies may have, for example, 55 as their stated retirement age. A few may even have an age greater than 65, at least for some senior employees. In each case the "normal retirement age" needs to be established. A comparator employee is not required.

These provisions were interpreted by the House of Lords in *Northman* v. *Barnet London Borough (1979)*. It decided that the employee had to be below the normal retirement age (if there was one) or 65 (if there was the normal retirement age) in order to claim. Thus, if the normal retirement age for a particular employee is 70 then unfair dismissal rights will continue until that age. If the normal retirement age is 55, unfair dismissal rights will cease at that point. Prior to this case it had been thought that the maximum age would be 65 in all cases.

It is, however, important to note that 65 is the maximum age for statutory redundancy payments rights. Under *Section 156* of the ERA an employee does not have any right to a redundancy payment if before the relevant date he has attained the normal retiring age (which is the same for men and women) for the organisation in which they work or, in any other case, the age of 65.

Employee's duties under the contract of employment

The duties upon the employee which are commonly implied into the contract of employment by historical operation of the common law are the duties:

● to be ready and willing to work
● to use reasonable care and skill
● to obey lawful orders
● to take care of the employer's property and
● to act in good faith.

The duty to be ready and willing to work needs little explanation. It is the duty of the employee to present himself for work and to abide by the terms of his employment. If the employee fails to attend for work, it constitutes a breach of the contract of employment and the employer may act accordingly. The employer may withhold pay with just cause if the employee is failing in his contractual duties, but withholding pay for no just cause is a breach of contract which gives the employee the option to repudiate the contract and sue for damages.

Reasonable care

The duty to use reasonable care and skill can be described as a twofold duty, i.e. not to be unduly negligent and to be reasonably competent. Where a third party takes an action against an employer for the negligent act of an employee, the employer will be vicariously liable (liable on the employee's behalf), but if the employer can prove that the employee was in breach of the implied term in his contract not to be unduly negligent, the employee may be held liable to the employer for all or a portion of the damages. The duty to be reasonably competent requires that the employee is able and competent at the job. Therefore if someone holds himself out as skilled in a trade in which he has no experience, the employer will be entitled to claim that the employee has breached his duty of competence.

Lawful orders

Disobedience to orders which are in the scope of the contract of employment can amount to a breach of contract and may in certain circumstances justify summary dismissal. However, in order for such action to be justified, the order must have been within the scope of the contract. Although employees are not obliged to obey orders falling outside their contract, they will be obliged to adapt to new machinery and working techniques if the appropriate training is given. Whether the extent of the change is unreasonable is a matter which can only be decided in specific circumstances. An employee may lawfully disobey an order which is prima facie within the scope of his contract if either the execution of the order involves exceptional danger for which there is no extra payment, or the execution of the order constitutes a criminal offence. (Most cases involving dismissal for disobedience to an order come before the industrial tribunal. Under the ERA 1996 the employer must show that the dismissal was reasonable, therefore the nature of the order will be subject to the test of reasonableness – see below.)

Care of the employer's property

The duty to take care of the employer's property is self-explanatory. Where the employee's breach of the implied term to take care of the employer's property results in the employer sustaining loss, the employee is liable to indemnify him.

Act in good faith

The duty to act in good faith towards an employer has several aspects. There is a duty not to make a secret profit which entails an obligation on the employee not to make a personal profit in the course of his employment. If such profits are discovered, the employee will be liable to repay them.

There is a duty to disclose certain information. For example, in an action by the widow of an epileptic building worker, the court found that the employee had breached his duty to inform his employer of his condition. As the employee's death resulted from his suffering a fit at height, the claim for compensation failed.

There is a general duty on the employee not to disclose confidential information gained from his employer. Information is confidential if the owner believes that the release of the information could be injurious to him and if the information is not publicly known. Whether particular information satisfies these requirements will depend on the particular circumstances, including the availability of the information within the profession and generally. Contracts of employment relating to work in areas where confidential information is handled will usually contain a specific term dealing with the duty not to disclose. Problems often arise when employees leave their employment and seek to use information gained whilst employed. The duty not to disclose confidential information does extend to ex-employees, but it is not so wide as to extend to "know-how". In *Faccenda Chicken* v. *Fowler (1986)*, the Court of Appeal stated that the distinction between confidential information and know-how is based on:

(1) The nature of the employment, i.e. whether information known to be secret is dealt with by the employee.
(2) The nature of the information, i.e. whether it is such as to constitute a trade secret.
(3) Whether the employee was informed by the employer that the information was confidential.
(4) Whether the confidential information was easily distinguishable from other information which the employee was free to disclose.

These are common-sense principles which will be applied to each specific situation.

Restraint of trade covenants

Employers are often keen that the employee does not use the expertise gained whilst in employment to aid competing concerns when he leaves his employment. Thus covenants in restraint of trade may be included in the contract of employment, whereby the employee promises:

- Not to establish a competing business within a certain distance from his former employer, or within a specified period of time from terminating his employment; or
- Not to use his expertise to the benefit of a competing concern within a certain period of the termination of his employment.

Such covenants (which are merely terms of the contract which have continuing effect after the termination of the period of employment) are subject to the requirement of reasonableness. If an employer sues a former employee for breach of his covenant, the issue of reasonableness will be decided by reference to the following factors:

(1) *Time* – the covenant will be held invalid if it purports to run for an excessive period of time.
(2) *Area* – the covenant must normally be limited to the area within which the former employee worked. (An action for breach of an express or implied term forbidding the former employee from using confidential information is distinct from an action for breach of restraint of trade covenant. In the former case the duty will attach notwithstanding the whereabouts of the former employee.)
(3) *Nature of the competing business* – the covenant must be limited to similar business in competition with the former employer.
(4) *The public interest in not fettering the activities and marketability of a skilled man* – thus a balance always has to be struck between the gaining of an unfair advantage by an employee, and the public interest in free trade and availability of services.

If an employee is thought by the former employer to be in breach of his covenant, an application may be made to the courts for an injunction restraining the employee from acting in continuing breach of the covenant.

If during the period of employment the employer breaches the contract of employment by unfairly dismissing the employee, the employee may thereafter disregard the effect of the restraint of trade clause.

Employer's duties under the contract of employment

Both common law and statute have created a variety of obligations which must be fulfilled by the employer. The main obligations are as follows:

(1) The duty to pay remuneration.
(2) The duty to pay sick pay.
(3) The duty to treat the employee with trust and confidence.
(4) The duty not to require the employee to work beyond agreed hours or hours prescribed by statute.
(5) The duty to allow time off work for the purpose of carrying out certain public functions.
(6) The duty to indemnify legitimate expenses.
(7) The duty to provide a safe working environment.

Remuneration

This is normally determined by reference to the contract. Failure to pay the agreed rate is a breach of contract which may entitle the employee in certain circumstances to claim constructive dismissal (see below under "unfair dismissal").

Minimum pay

The adult rate of the minimum wage (for workers aged 22 and over) increased from its present hourly rate of £4.85 to £5.05 in October 2005, and to £5.35 in October 2006. The 2006 increase is subject to confirmation by the Commission in February 2006, to check that the economic conditions continue to make it appropriate.

The development rate (for workers aged 18–21 inclusive) increased from the present hourly rate of £4.10 to £4.25 in October 2005 and £4.45 in October 2006. The National Minimum Wage Act 1998 provides for a statutory minimum wage of £4.85 an hour before deductions for most workers. Those aged between 18 and 21 are only entitled to £4.10 an hour.

Although there are some exceptions (such as apprentices and 16- and 17-year-olds) the Act's application to "workers" goes beyond the unfair dismissal legislation in applying to home workers and agency temps. In the context of community pharmacy, this means that the legislation will apply to collection and delivery drivers who may not be employed by a pharmacy under a formal contract of employment.

Workers paid less than the minimum wage will be able to complain of an unauthorised deduction in the industrial tribunal or bring a civil action for breach of contract. Workers are entitled to access to records and the right not to be victimised for asserting their rights under this legislation in good faith. The Act also provides for enforcement by government agency and for criminal penalties. The detailed provisions are complex and may be found in the National Minimum Wage Regulations 1999. They address situations where workers are paid by reference to output rather than time, are on standby, etc.

Sick pay

The contract of employment will normally specify the terms relating to the payment of sick pay. If it does not do so, terms may be implied. There is no general presumption that sick pay is to be paid, but the court or industrial tribunal will attempt to construe the intentions of the parties at the time of contracting. However, under the Social Security and Housing Benefits Act 1982, as amended by Schedule 2 Paragraph 13 of the ERA 1996, all employers are obliged to pay their employees up to 8 weeks sick pay in any one tax year. To qualify for statutory sick pay the employee must be

(1) At least 16 years of age and gainfully employed.
(2) He must have been incapable of work for a period of at least 4 days.
(3) The claim must be made for a period when the employee would have been working but for the incapacity.

The current rates of Statutory Sick Pay (SSP) are

   The weekly rate of SSP for the 2005/06 tax year is £68.20 but it is computed at a daily rate. The daily rate may vary for different employees. It is calculated by dividing the weekly rate by the number of qualifying days in a week. For example an employee with a 5-day working week would normally have a daily rate of £13.23 (£13.64 2005/06). Only QDs qualify for SSP and the first 3 days (WDs) do not qualify. The maximum entitlement is 28 weeks in each period of sickness or linked PIW.
   Should the employer fail to pay statutory sick pay, a complaint may be made to the employer. Should the employer fail to give adequate reasons for failing to pay, the matter may be referred to an insurance officer, whose decision can be in turn appealed to the DSS.

Trust and confidence

This duty has grown up as a result of case law involving constructive dismissal, i.e. a claim by the employee that the behaviour of the employer was such that it left no reasonable alternative but to leave the employment. In *Courtalds Northern Textiles Ltd v. Andrew (1978)*, the Employment Appeal Tribunal held that in a contract of employment there was an implied term that an employer "would not without reasonable cause, conduct (himself) in a manner calculated to be likely to destroy or seriously damage the relationship of trust and confidence between the parties". Breach of such a term is likely only to be argued in a dismissal claim; in other words, when the relationship between the employer and the employee has broken down.

Hours of duty

The hours to be worked will be included in the contract of employment. However, there are statutory maxima which apply to limit the total hours allowable.

Minimum hours

The Working Time Regulations 1998 provide for:

(a) a minimum daily rest period of 11 consecutive hours
(b) an additional minimum weekly rest period of 24 hours
(c) a rest break in any working day over 6 hours
(d) maximum average working week of 48 hours (over a 4-month reference period)
(e) minimum 4 weeks' annual paid holiday
(f) night workers' normal working hours should not exceed 8 in 24.

The average weekly working time is normally calculated over 17 weeks. This can be longer in certain situations (26 weeks) and it can be extended by agreement (up to 52 weeks). Workers can agree to work longer than the 48-hour limit. An agreement must be made in writing and signed by the worker. This is generally referred to as an opt-out. It can be for a specified period or a indefinite period. Workers can cancel the opt-out agreement whenever they want, although they must give their employer at least 7 days' notice, or longer (up to 3 months) if this has been agreed.

The Working Time Regulations 1998 provide for enforcement by the Health and Safety Executive and local authorities. However, in *Barber* v. *RJB Mining (UK) Ltd (1999)* the High Court held that employees may also seek a declaration and injunction restraining their employer from requiring them to work an average of 48 hours per week.

Time off for public functions

These include being a magistrate; a member of a local authority; a member of a statutory tribunal; a member of an HA; a member of the governing body of a local authority maintained establishment; or being a member of a water authority. Time off must also be allowed for jury service. Under *Section 55* of the ERA 1996 a pregnant employee must also be allowed a reasonable amount of time off for the purposes of receiving ante-natal care.

Incurred expenses

There is a duty on employers to indemnify employees for expenses incurred in executing their duties.

Safe working environment

Control of Substances Hazardous to Health Regulations 1988

The Control of Substances Hazardous to Health (COSHH) Regulations 1988 came into force on 1 October 1989. They affect the use of hazardous substances in a work situation, by laying down measures which an employer must take to control hazardous substances and to protect people who are exposed to such substances. Regulation 6 requires that an employer may not carry on any work that is liable to

expose any person to any substance hazardous to health, unless a suitable and sufficient assessment of the risks has been made.

Hazardous substances

A substance hazardous to health is defined as "any natural or artificial substance: solid,
liquid, gas, vapour or hazardous micro-organism, and certain dust levels".
   Substances hazardous to health can include:

(1)   Any substance classed under the Chemicals (Hazard Information and
      Packaging) Regulations 1994, SI 1994 No. 3247 as "toxic, very toxic, harmful,
      corrosive, irritant, carcinogenic, mutagenic, toxic for reproduction, sensitizing".
(2)   Any micro-organism.
(3)   Any dust.
(4)   Any substance which has a prescribed maximum exposure limit, e.g. formalde-
      hyde.
(5)   Any other substance which can adversely affect the health.

In other words, any substance used or present at work.
   Helpfully, the COSHH Regulations state that a substance is not hazardous when it
is at a level that nearly all the population can be exposed to it, repeatedly, without ill
effect.

Exclusions

Certain situations are specifically excluded from COSHH:

(1)   Those covered by the Control of Lead at Work Regulations 1980.
(2)   Those covered by the Control of Asbestos at Work Regulations 1987.
(3)   When the hazard is radioactivity.
(4)   When the hazard is the explosive or flammable properties of the substance.
(5)   Underground mines.
(6)   Medicines administered to patients.

Employer's duties

The employer must first of all decide whether or not any substance is potentially
hazardous. This must be done by a competent person. The employer must then:

(1)   Assess the risk to health from the use of the substance in the workplace.
(2)   Decide what precautions are needed.
(3)   Introduce appropriate measures to control the risk.
(4)   Inform and train employees about the risks and about the precautions to be
      taken.
(5)   Ensure the measures are actually taken.
(6)   In some cases, monitor any exposure of workers to hazardous substances.

Detailed guidance on such assessment is given in the Management of Health and Safety at Work Regulations 1992, SI 1992 No. 2051 which require all employers to assess the risk to employees while at work, and are made under the Health and Safety at Work, etc. Act 1974.

Records

All records should be available for inspection by the Health and Safety Executive.

The Manual Handling Operations Regulations 1992

These require the employer to take steps to avoid hazardous manual handling operations; to assess the safety of any operations which are necessary; to reduce the risk of injury from those operations so far as is reasonably practicable. Employees are required to follow specified systems of work.

The Electricity at Work Regulations 1989

These require employers to take all reasonably practicable steps to avoid danger from electrical installations. The Regulations do not specifically require annual tests of equipment, although this is one way of minimizing risk.

The Health and Safety (Display Screen Equipment) Regulations 1992

These implement a European Directive 90/270/EEC on health and safety. They require an employer to assess the risks in the use of computers, and to minimize those risks. This is to be done by ensuring that equipment, including desks, hardware and software is suitable and appropriate. Eyesight tests are to be provided for employees on request.

The Safety Representative and Safety Committee Regulations 1977

An employer must consult with all staff, either directly or where appropriate through a recognised trade union, on health and safety matters. This includes telling staff about new measures, and taking account of their views. A "competent person" must be appointed to liaise with staff.

Wages issues

Deductions

The Wages Act of 1986 regulated the payment of wages, and created a system based upon the contract of employment. The Act abolished the old requirement that wages be paid in cash, thus permitting cashless payment. Now subsumed by Part II of the ERA 1996, deductions from wages can only be made in order to comply with a statutory provision (e.g. tax or national insurance), or by prior agreement.

Itemized pay statement

An employee has a right to an itemized pay statement giving particulars of the amount of gross pay and deductions made.

Lay-off periods

During periods when an employee is laid off because there is no work, Part III of the ERA 1996 provides for a system of guaranteed payments during the period of the lay-off. In order to be eligible for such a payment the employee must have been continuously employed for at least 1 month when the lay-off occurs; he must have been laid off for the whole of his normal working hours on a day he is normally required to work; he must not have refused a reasonable offer of alternative employment; he must comply with any requirements imposed by the employer with a view to ensuring that his services are available; he must not have been laid off as a result of industrial action; and he must have been available for employment on the day.

If the above conditions are fulfilled, then the employee is entitled to be paid for the number of hours per day for which he was laid off, or £18.40 per day, whichever is the lesser sum. Failure to pay the guaranteed payment may be made the subject of a complaint to the industrial tribunal.

If an employee is suspended from work as a result of the operation of certain statutory provisions (listed in *Section 64(3)* of the ERA 1996), for example, if his workshop is temporarily closed as a result of a notice served under the Health and Safety at Work Act 1974, he is entitled to remuneration. To qualify, the employee must have been continuously employed by the employer for 1 month, he must not be incapable of work through sickness; he must not have unreasonably refused suitable alternative work; and he must not have refused to comply with reasonable requirements imposed by the employer with a view to ensuring that his services are available. The maximum period for such pay is 26 weeks.

Maternity issues

Maternity pay

In order to qualify for maternity pay an employee:

- must have been employed by the same employer without a break for at least 26 weeks into the 15th week before the week the baby is due.
- must have ceased to work for the employer wholly or partly because of pregnancy or confinement (it is no longer necessary that she ceases work "wholly or partly because of pregnancy or confinement." (EA 2002, *Section 20*)

Her normal weekly earnings for the period of 8 weeks ending with the work immediately preceding the 14th week before the expected week of confinement must be not less than the lower limit for the payment of National Insurance contributions (currently £79) (SSCBA 1992, *Section 164(1)* and *(2)*).

Statutory maternity pay is payable for a 26-week period. For the first 6 weeks it is at the rate of 90% of normal weekly earnings. For the remaining 20 weeks it is either

90% of normal weekly earnings or a prescribed rate reviewed annually (currently £106.00 per week) whichever of these is the lowest.

A complaint about non-payment may be made to the industrial tribunal. (An employer who has paid maternity leave in accordance with these provisions is entitled to recover the full amount from the Maternity Pay Fund which is maintained by class 1 social security contributions.)

Return to work

The employee has the right to return to work after the birth if at least 21 days prior to her absence (or as soon as reasonably practicable thereafter), she informs the employer in writing of her expected absence; of her intention to return to work; and of the expected week of confinement. Not later than 49 days after the start of the week of confinement, the employer may write to the employee asking for written confirmation of the intention to return to work. Confirmation must be made within 14 days of the request.

The right to return to work may be exercised before the expiration of 29 weeks from the actual week of confinement, and includes the right to return to the same job on terms no less favourable than those previously enjoyed. If the employer can prove that by the time the employee intended lawfully to return there was no suitable position, she will be entitled to a redundancy payment. There will be no such entitlement if she refuses a suitable vacancy.

Unlawful dismissal

If, in breach of her right to return, the employee is not allowed to return to work, or if she has been made redundant and not been offered a suitable available alternative position, the employee may claim to have been unlawfully dismissed, subject to the employer's defence that he acted reasonably because of something which happened in the employee's absence.

Postponed return

The employer has the right to postpone the return of the employee for up to 4 weeks. The employee may postpone her return if either she is ill (in which case the postponement can be for up to 4 weeks), or if there is an interruption in work (such as a strike), which renders it unreasonable to expect the employee to return to work on that day.

Maternity leave

Until the amendments under ERA 1999, the rules on maternity leave had become very complicated. We now find in Schedule 4 of ERA 1999 a complete replacement of Part VIII of ERA 1996, and in particular new *Sections 71–75* setting out the structure of maternity leave. In addition one needs to take account of the Maternity and Parental Leave Regulations 1999 (MPL Regulations 1999) as amended in 2002 which enlarge on the statutory framework.

Irrespective of any entitlement to maternity pay, *Section 71* of ERA 1996 as amended establishes a general right to 26 weeks' maternity leave for all employees, regardless of length of service, hours of work or size of firm, during which an employee is entitled to the benefit of all her normal contractual rights, except for remuneration, which is specifically excluded. This right to maternity leave was introduced in 1993, implementing the requirements of a European Directive on the introduction of measures to encourage improvements in the safety and health at work of pregnant workers and workers who have recently given birth or are breast-feeding.

Under ERA 1996, *Section 73*, employees whose service with the employer is 26 weeks or more at the 14th week before expected week of childbirth are entitled to additional maternity leave. This is the right to return up to 26 weeks after the birth. The employee is required to give no notice of her intention to return if she returns at the end of the 26-week period but must give 28 days' notice of an intention to return early (Regulation 11). A statement of her intention to return at all can be required by the employer in a prescribed written form, in which event the woman must reply in writing (MPL Regulation 12).

An employee with a separate contractual right to maternity leave is entitled to exercise a "composite" right by taking advantage of whichever right is, in any particular respect, the more favourable. However, the rights and duties of the parties during additional leave are much reduced. There is no right to remuneration or to fringe benefits. Under MPL Regulations 1999, Regulation 17(1), the only terms of the contract that apply for the benefit of the employee are the right to notice, the right to redundancy pay, access to disciplinary or grievance procedures and the employer's implied obligation of good faith and by any acceptance of gifts and her participation in any business.

Under MPL Regulations, Regulation 18, the employee is entitled to return after additional maternity leave to do the same job or if it is not reasonably practicable for the employer to permit her to do that, to a job which is both suitable for her and appropriate for her to do in the circumstances and her terms and conditions of employment are to be the same as would have applied to her if she had not been absent. Her seniority on the day she returns is to be the same as it was when she started the additional leave. Thus the period of additional leave, unlike ordinary leave, does not count towards continuity of service in relation to any contractual right, e.g. service-related holidays. It counts under ERA 1996, *Section 212* towards continuity for statutory purposes.

Insolvent employer

If an employer becomes insolvent, Part XII of the ERA 1996 provides that the employee becomes a preferential creditor in respect of up to 4 months' wages, or such limit as may be set by the S of S. Other payments such as guarantee payments and payments for time off during ante-natal care are also classed as preferential debts. The employee may claim from the S of S certain sums due from his employer, comprising arrears of up to 8 weeks' wages, 6 weeks' holiday pay and wages during the statutory minimum period of notice. The employee also has the right to ask the S of S to pay pensions contributions which have not been paid due to the employer's insolvency. If the employee does not receive the sums to which he believes he is entitled from the S of S, he has the right to make a complaint to an industrial tribunal.

Equal pay and discrimination

Equal pay

Article 141 of the Treaty of Rome, the Treaty which was signed by the UK on joining the then EEC, provides that:

> Each member state shall . . . maintain the application of the principle that men and women should receive equal pay for equal work.
>
> For the purpose of this Article, "pay" means the ordinary basic or minimum wage or salary and any other consideration, whether in cash or in kind, which the worker receives, directly or indirectly, in respect of his employment from his employer.

The spirit of Article 141 is now embodied in the Equal Pay Act 1970 (as amended by the Equal Pay (Amendment) Regulations 1983, SI 1983 No. 1794).

The Act is broadly designed to ensure that men and women employed in similar work receive equal remuneration.

By *section 1(1)* of the Act an "equality clause" is implied into a woman's contract of employment if one has not already been included. A woman thus has the right to equal pay with men in three situations:

(1) Where the woman is carrying out "like work" with a man in the same employment (*Section 1(2)(a)*).
(2) Where her work is "rated as equivalent" to that done by a man following a job evaluation study (*Section 1(2)(b)*).
(3) Where her work is of "equal value" in terms of the demands made upon her, to that of a man in the same employment.

Each of these situations must be examined in turn.

Like work

Where a woman claims to be entitled to equal pay on the grounds that her work is "like work" with a man in the same employment, she must show that the work done by them both is of a broadly similar nature, and that any differences are not of practical importance in relation to terms and conditions of employment. The nature and extent of any differences will have to be closely examined in each individual case. However, the Act is so worded as to prevent irrelevant or insignificant differences in jobs from precluding equal pay. For example, in *Coombs Holdings* v. *Shields (1978)* a female teller in a betting shop claimed equal pay with a male employee doing the same job. On behalf of the employer it was urged that the male employee deserved greater remuneration because he was expected to deal with any trouble that arose. The tribunal found that the difference did not justify a finding that they were not doing like work.

Rated as equivalent

A claim for equal pay based on a finding that the work carried out by the woman is rated as equivalent to that carried out by a male employee invariably follows a job evaluation study. An employer is not obliged to authorize or commission such a study, but once he does he will be bound by the findings.

Section 1(5) of the Act provides that:

> A woman is to be regarded as employed on work rated as equivalent with that of any men if, but only if, her job and their job have been given an equal value, in terms of the demands made on the worker . . . or would have been given an equal value but for the evaluation being made on a system setting different values for men and women on the same demand under any heading.

Equal value

By an amendment made in 1983, *Section 1(2)(c)* of the 1970 Act states that an equality clause is to be implied into a contract of employment:

> Where a woman is employed on work which . . . is, in terms of the demand made on her (for instance under such headings as effort, skill and decision), of equal value to that of a man in the same employment.

This clause is operative only where the provisions relating to like work and work rated as equivalent have no application, for example, where a cook in a shipyard canteen claims to be entitled to equal pay with male shipyard workers (*Hayward* v. *Cammell Laird Shipbuilders Ltd (1984)*). In order to adjudicate on this matter the industrial tribunal must first be satisfied that there are reasonable grounds for determining that the work is of equal value. If there are not, the claim will automatically be dismissed. Secondly, the tribunal must require a panel of experts (to be appointed by the Advisory, Conciliation and Arbitration Service (ACAS)) to compile a report on whether the work is of equal value. The tribunal will then consider the findings in the report in deciding whether the work is of equal value.

The general approach is for the work of the complainant to be compared with that of the "comparator" male, with whom the complainant alleges she is entitled to equal pay. Percentage points are awarded, taking the output of the comparator as 100%. For example, in *Wells* v. *F. Smales and Son (Fish Merchants) Ltd (1985)*, there were 14 female applicants. The ACAS assessor said that nine of them scored higher than the comparator, but five scored lower (between 79 and 95% of the comparator's score). The tribunal found that they all scored so closely that they should all be entitled to equal pay.

The House of Lords in *British Coal Corporation* v. *Smith (1996)* ruled that common terms and conditions meant terms and conditions which were substantially comparable on a broad basis. It is sufficient for the applicant to show that her comparators at another establishment and at her establishment were or would be employed on broadly similar terms.

Employer's defences

Section 1(3) of the 1970 Act provides a defence to an employer against a claim for equal pay where he can prove that the variation in pay is genuinely due to a material factor which is not the difference of sex. That factor must be a material difference between the woman's case and the man's, except where work is alleged to be of equal value, in which case the difference may be such a material difference. In other words, where there is a claim based on an allegation of equal value the employer may be able to base his defence arguments on economics. For example, where there are existing females doing a skilled job and, in order to attract other skilled workers into the job, the employer offers more money to new employees who happen to be male, the employer may successfully defend the disparity in wages on the grounds of economic necessity. In the case of *Bilka-Kaufhaus GmbH* v. *Weber von Hartz (1986)*, the European Court of Justice held that the disparity in pay must be objectively justified, and must be reasonably necessary in order to cope with a particular set of circumstances (like those previously described). Therefore matters of mere convenience are prevented from justifying a departure from equal terms in a woman's contract. An employee wishing to make a complaint must do so by making an application to the industrial tribunal. If the tribunal finds in the employee's favour, it may make a declaration to the effect that equal pay must be paid, and up to 2 years of back pay may be awarded.

Sex discrimination

The Sex Discrimination Act 1975 outlaws discrimination on the grounds of sex and/or the fact that a person is married. There are certain exceptions to the prohibition on discrimination contained in the Act as follows:

(1)   "Special treatment" of women on the grounds of pregnancy and childbirth (*Section 2*).
(2)   Discrimination in favour of members of a sex of which in the previous year there were few or no members in the particular job (*Section 48*).
(3)   Discrimination in selection, promoting or training where being a man or a woman is a "genuine occupational qualification".
(4)   Discrimination in certain specified professions such as the police and prison service (*Sections 17–20*).
(5)   Discrimination in respect of provisions relating to death or retirement.

In relation to (5) above there is still a certain amount of uncertainty. Until recently the position was that if there was a fixed retirement age for men with a particular employer, a woman could not be compelled to retire at a lower age. An exemption from SDA 1975 in respect of those employing five or less employees was repealed in 1986 and the Act now applies to all employers regardless of number of employees.
   The Act covers the following areas of employment:

(1)   The selection, interviewing and offering of a job (*Section 6(1)(a)*).
(2)   The terms upon which employment is offered (as opposed to the terms of employment once it has commenced) (*Section 6(1)(a)*).

(3) Access to promotion, training, transfer or any other benefit, facility or service (*Section 6(2)(a)*).
(4) Dismissal or the subjecting of any person to any detriment (*Section 6(2)(b)*).

Under *Section 38(1)* it is unlawful to publish any advertisement which might reasonably be taken as displaying an intention to commit an act which is contrary to the Act. Job descriptions which specify the sex of candidates are therefore unlawful.

The categories of discrimination

There are two categories of discrimination in the Act.

Direct discrimination
Less favourable treatment on the grounds of sex or being married. For this to be shown, a direct comparison between the treatment of men and women in the same employment must be possible.

Indirect discrimination
A person discriminates against a woman if:

he applies to her a requirement which he applies or would apply to a man but

(i) which is such that the proportion of women who can comply with it is considerably smaller than the proportion of men who can comply with it, and
(ii) which he cannot show to be justifiable irrespective of the sex of the person to whom it is applied, and
(iii) which is to her detriment because she cannot comply with it.

An example of indirect discrimination would be where candidates are required to be at least 65 kg in weight where that requirement cannot be shown to be justifiable in order to fulfil (ii) above. For example, in *Price* v. *Civil Service Commission (1978)* a condition that all job applicants be under 28 years of age was held to be discriminatory as many women have time off to have children in their late twenties.

Direct discrimination is unlawful *per se*, but indirect discrimination is not unlawful if it can be shown to be justifiable. "Justifiable" was defined in *Panesar* v. *Nestle Co. Ltd (1980)* as "reasonable commercial necessity" and not "absolutely necessary".

In *Ojutiku* v. *Manpower Services Commission (1982)* Lord Keith said: "I decline to put any gloss on the word 'justifiable' ... except that I would say that it clearly applies a lower standard than the word 'necessary'. There should be sound and tolerable reasons." Thus commercial considerations will often be capable of defeating a claim based on an allegation of indirect discrimination.

Financial compensation

When the sex and race discrimination legislation was enacted, Parliament provided that financial compensation may not be awarded in cases of indirect discrimination unless it is established that the discrimination was intentional. The law has been developed further in respect of sex discrimination by virtue of the Sex Discrimination and Equal Pay (Miscellaneous Amendments) Regulations 1996. These Regulations provide that industrial tribunals in indirect sex discrimination cases may now award compensation regardless of whether or not the indirect sex discrimination is intentional or not. The Regulations respond to recent criticism that the law was out of line with the requirements of the EC Equal Treatment Directive 76/207. As a consequence the provisions of the Sex Discrimination Act 1975 which preclude the award of damages in cases of unintentional indirect sex discrimination must now be read as amended by the Regulations.

Discrimination on the grounds of race

The Race Relations Act 1976 renders unlawful discrimination on grounds of "colour, race, nationality or ethnic or national origin". As with the Sex Discrimination Act 1975 there are defences available to an employer, for example, where it can be proved that being a member of a certain racial group is a "genuine occupational qualification". Thus it would not be unlawful for the owner of an Indian restaurant to discriminate against applicants for the job of a waiter where the aim of the restaurant is to create a particular ambience (see *Section 5(2)* of the 1976 Act).

A person who wishes to make a complaint may complain to the industrial tribunal. If the tribunal finds in the applicant's favour, it may make a declaration of rights of the respective parties, and may order compensation. The employer may also be ordered to take certain steps to reduce the effect of the discrimination on the complainant.

The Commission for Racial Equality

The Commission for Racial Equality has extensive investigatory powers, and may conduct formal investigations of employers. Where appropriate the Commission may issue a non-discrimination notice against the employer it has investigated, requiring him to take steps to remedy the situation. Where the notice is not acted upon, the Commission may seek a High Court injunction to enforce compliance. The Commission may issue codes of practice for employers to encourage compliance with the terms of the Act. It also encourages employers to adopt an equal opportunities policy. The position is slightly different under various Acts with respect to Northern Ireland, where in some types of employment employers are obliged to discriminate positively in favour of persons belonging to certain religious groups.

Disability discrimination

The Disability Discrimination Act 1995 introduced new rights for disabled people where discrimination occurs during the course of employment. All employers (as of 1 October 2004, there is no exemption for small employers from the provisions of DDA 1005 (Amendment Regulations), Regulation 6) are placed under a statutory duty to accommodate the needs of a disabled person at work, by considering what adjustments are needed for a particular individual. The duty applies to the situation where a person becomes disabled during the course of his employment, as well as to the situation where an employer interviews a disabled person at the recruitment stage.

A disabled person is one who has "a physical or mental impairment which has substantial and long-term adverse affects on his or her ability to carry out day-to-day activities". An "impairment" will be regarded as affecting normal daily activities if it affects mobility, dexterity, coordination, continence, ability to carry, speech, hearing, eyesight, memory, ability to concentrate, and perception of the risk of personal danger. This will include depression since it is a recognised clinical illness causing impairment.

Self-induced illnesses are specifically excluded from the Act. These include abuse of an addictive substance (alcohol, drugs, nicotine) and complications resulting from deliberate disfigurement (tattoos, body piercing).

In addition to accommodating the needs of a disabled person, the Act provides that reasons for dismissing an employee must not be discriminatory on the grounds of disability. However, this does not mean that employment can never be terminated on grounds of ill-health. If, for example, an employee developed multiple sclerosis or Parkinson's disease, it would be acceptable for an employer to terminate the employment, but only where the illness made it impossible for an employee to perform the main functions of his job and it was not reasonable and practical for an employer to make an adjustment.

In this context the kind of adjustments that an employer should consider include adjustments to premises, re-allocating some of the disabled employee's duties to another employee, altering the employee's working hours, assigning the employee to a different place of work or a different activity at work, allowing the employee reasonable time away from work for rehabilitation and treatment, acquiring or modifying equipment, and where necessary providing supervision. As of 1 October 2004, a failure to make reasonable adjustments cannot be justified.

Exceptions

Whilst there are certain exceptions under RRA 1976 and SDA 1975 where the nature of the job required a particular kind of person there are no equivalent exceptions under DDA 1995. The only exception remaining after 1 October 2004 is the armed forces.

Disability-related discrimination

Under the present legislation, an employer engages in disability-related discrimination if, for a reason which relates to the disabled person's disability, he treats that person less favourably than he treats a person not having that particular disability whose relevant circumstances, including his abilities, are the same as, or not materially different from, those of the disabled person.

A reason relating to disability may include, the disabled person's poor time-keeping due to lack of mobility. In *Clark* v. *Novacold Ltd (1999)*, the Court of Appeal confirmed that for a disabled person to establish that there has been less favourable treatment for a reason relating to disability there is no need to identify an able-bodied comparator (or a person with a different disability) who has or would have been treated differently. All that a disabled person has to show is that, for a reason related to his disability, he was treated less favourably than another to whom that reason, i.e. the reason for the treatment, does not apply.

Defence of justification

As of 1 October 2004, the defence of justification is only available in cases of disability-related discrimination. Direct discrimination, on the other hand, on the grounds of a person's disability where the relevant circumstances are the same or not materially different can never be justified.

In order to establish the defence of justification, the employer must show that the reason for the treatment in question of the disabled person is both material in the circumstances and substantial (DDA 1995, *Section 3A(3)*).

The case of *Matty* v. *Tesco Stores*, IDS Brief 609, is an example of a case where a defence of justification has been accepted: A failure to employ a diabetic as a fitter at a distribution centre was justified as the risk of injury to a diabetic employee in the low-temperature environment could not be reduced by supplying or modifying equipment.

Discrimination against part-time workers

A part-time worker may complain to an industrial tribunal where an employer discriminates against him because he is part-time. Regulation 5 of the Part-time Workers (Prevention of Less Favourable Treatment) Regulations 2000 gives a part-time worker a right not to be treated less favourably than the employer treats a comparable full-time worker as regards the terms of his contract, or by being subjected to any other detriment by any act or deliberate failure to act. The starting point for assessing whether a part-time worker is being treated less favourably is to determine who the correct comparable full-time worker should be. The regulations state that a full-time worker is comparable to a part-time worker if, at the time when the treatment alleged to be less favourable to the part-time worker takes place, both workers have been employed by the same employer doing the same work with similar levels of qualification, skills and experience.

The definition of a worker for the purposes of the regulations is sufficiently wide to include a self-employed worker who does not genuinely run his own business. Moreover, there is no prescribed maximum number of hours to be worked by a part-time worker before he can be said to become a full-time worker for the purposes of the regulations. A worker is full-time if he is paid wholly or in part by reference to the time he works, and, having regard to custom and practice of the employer in relation to workers employed by him under the same type of contract, is identified as a full-time worker. There is no minimum number of hours to be worked before a worker qualifies as a part-time worker. Examples of where an employer in a pharmacy might treat a part-time worker less favourably are:

- where a part-time worker's workload is re-organised and he is given more or less work on a pro rata basis
- where a part-time worker is not considered as a candidate for promotion because he is part-time
- where a part-time worker's pay is less pro rata
- where a part-time worker is not afforded equivalent contractual sick pay and maternity pay
- where a part-time worker does not have equal access to an occupational pension scheme, or other benefits such as health insurance, staff discounts, etc
- where a part-time worker is not given equal access to training

- where a part-time worker is selected for redundancy because he is part-time
- where a part-time worker is not afforded his statutory entitlement to annual leave and parental leave.

Bringing the employment to an end

Dismissal

The position at common law is that an employer could lawfully dismiss an employee by giving notice in accordance with the period prescribed by the contract of employment. To a certain extent this still remains the case but, as will be seen below, in a few circumstances an employee will be entitled to compensation for loss of his job even though notice was given.

The requisite period of notice required to effect a dismissal may be expressly stated in the contract of employment, or may be implied into the contract by custom in the trade or profession. Where no such period can be implied, a court may arrive at a reasonable period which will be determined by taking all the surrounding circumstances into account, including the age of the employee and the length of service. As a fall-back, *Section 86* of the ERA 1996 provides a minimum period of notice of one week for an employee who has been continuously employed for between 1 month and 2 years, and for an employee who has been employed for over 2 years, the period is 1 week for every full year of employment. However, after an individual has been employed for 13 years the minimum notice of entitlement is 12 weeks. The statutory minimum period of notice therefore has a ceiling of 12 weeks.

Of note, the term "not less than [x weeks]" is used under *Section 86*. This leaves the courts and tribunals open to awarding "reasonable notice" instead of the minimum period. However, the courts will only turn to reasonable notice where either the contract has been unclear or the facts have been extreme.

Waiving rights to notice

The parties are also free to agree to give shorter notice than would normally be required or even to waive notice. Provided such variations are genuine there will be no breach of contract and no damages to pay: *Baldwin* v. *British Coal Corporation (1995)*.

Summary dismissal

Where an employer dismisses an employee without notice, it is termed "summary dismissal". If there is no justification for the dismissal it is wrongful, and an action for damages may be brought in the county court for breach of the contract of employment. Alternatively, the dismissal may be sufficiently unjustified to merit a complaint of unfair dismissal to an industrial tribunal (although both actions cannot be taken in respect of the same incident).

As a general rule, summary dismissal is only justifiable where the conduct of the employee is such that it prevents "further satisfactory continuance of the relationship". For example, in the case of *Sinclair* v. *Neighbour (1967)*, the manager of a betting shop borrowed some money from the till, without attempting to hide the fact and with every intention of paying it back. His summary dismissal was nevertheless justified as he was also fully aware that the practice was forbidden.

Employers sometimes attempt to set out a right to dismiss without notice on the occurrence of certain events, other than gross misconduct. This is questionable practice in itself; but, certainly, the wording of such clauses will be construed *contra proferentem*: *T & K Improvements Ltd* v. *Skilton (2002)*, where a clause allowing dismissal "with immediate effect" on failing to reach sales targets was held not to permit dismissal without notice.

Resignation

If the employee wishes to leave his employment, he must also comply with the notice procedures. An employee may resign at any time by giving proper notice under the contract. The minimum (*Section 86*) period is one week; and this does not alter with length of service. The contract may set any notice requirement.

In a situation where an employee feels forced to leave immediately through the behaviour of his employer, he may make a claim for "constructive dismissal" (see below). The employment may be terminated by agreement, in which case the termination will not qualify as a dismissal for the purposes of an unfair dismissal or redundancy claim, although to achieve this result the employment must not be terminated as a result of pressure being applied to the employee to encourage him to leave. Further, the employment may come to an end where it is "frustrated", i.e. where sickness or imprisonment prevent the employee from returning to work. However, the negative effect of finding a contract of employment frustrated through sickness is that frustration brings a contract to an end: therefore, the employee will not be entitled to statutory sick pay from his employer, and will have to rely on state benefits.

Action for wrongful dismissal

Where an employee alleges that he has been wrongfully dismissed, i.e. where he has been unjustifiably dismissed without, or without the requisite period of, notice by his employer, he may bring an action in the civil courts for wages lost through insufficient notice being given. For this purpose the wages are calculated in accordance with the amount the employee could reasonably be expected to have earned in the notice period (including income such as commission which does not come directly from the employer). Deductions will be made for:

(1) Other sums earned in alternative employment during the dismissal period.
(2) Any state benefits received during the same period.
(3) Sums representing the tax and national insurance contributions that would have been paid out of the wages in the notice period.

Unfair dismissal

The most common form of action taken against an employer is an action for unfair dismissal in the industrial tribunal. Section 94 of the ERA 1996 gives every employee the right not to be unfairly dismissed. This applies whether the dismissal was in accordance with the contract of employment or not. (This procedure is open to all employees except for a few categories, the most important of which are persons over retiring age, policemen, employees on certain "fixed term" contracts, share fishermen and employees who mainly work outside the UK.).

Proving unfair dismissal

In order to prove unfair dismissal, the employee must first show that there was a dismissal. In most cases this will be obvious. In some cases, however, the employee will have to allege "constructive dismissal", i.e. the behaviour of the employer was such that the employee could not reasonably be expected to have continued in the employment.

For some time an industrial tribunal would only find constructive dismissal where the employer could be shown to have breached the terms of the contract of employment. However, this was not adequate to cover situations where employers "squeezed out" employees without committing any specific breach. The modern approach is therefore to imply a term that the employer will not breach the "relationship of trust and confidence" between himself and the employee and to find constructive dismissal where that term is breached. In the case of *Woods* v. *W.M. Car Service (1981)* it was said that

> ... an employer who persistently attempts to vary an employee's conditions of services with a view to getting rid of the employee or varying the employee's conditions of service, does an act in a manner calculated to destroy the relationship of confidence and trust between [them].

Such an employer has therefore breached an implied term.

Unfairness

Having established dismissal, the tribunal must then decide the issue of unfairness. In order to determine the unfairness or otherwise of the dismissal, the reasonableness of the employer's actions are examined. It is for the employer to establish the reasons for the dismissal. *Section 98(4)* of the ERA 1996 provides that the tribunal must then decide whether:

> in the circumstances (including the size and administrative resources of the employer's undertaking) the employer acted reasonably or unreasonably in treating it as a sufficient reason for dismissing the employee; and that question shall be determined in accordance with the equity and substantial merits of the case.

Thus the employer is under a duty to act reasonably both substantively and procedurally. In determining the reasonableness of the dismissal, the tribunal must consider the surrounding circumstances and the provisions of the ACAS code of conduct Disciplinary Practice and Procedures in Employment. The Code generally recommends the use of informal action to resolve matters followed by formal action and provides for various steps to be taken before dismissal such as warnings for offences which are not of the utmost gravity, and a fair hearing before dismissal.

Reasonableness of the dismissal

The employer may rely on one of five categories of reasons to justify the dismissal as reasonable.

Capability or qualifications

The employer may show that the employee was incompetent or not suitably quali-fied for the employment, but even where this is proved, the employer remains under a duty to comply with the procedural requirements for dismissal in order to render the dismissal reasonable.

Conduct

Where there has been misconduct on the part of the employee, the employer may act reasonably in dismissing him. The ACAS code of practice deals with the procedures which should be adopted by employers, and provides, for example, that only "serious misconduct" justifies dismissal for a first breach of discipline. The categories of misconduct are wide, but would include, for exam-ple, drunkenness, dishonesty, sexual harassment and criminal convictions out-side the employment.

Redundancy

This is discussed in further detail below, but where an employer can show that the reason for the dismissal was that the employee had genuinely been rendered redun-dant, the dismissal will not be unfair. Dismissal for redundancy may be rendered unfair in certain situations where the procedure for choosing specific employees for redundancy in similar occupations may have been carried out unfairly. Thus employers are obliged to operate redundancy criteria, and to apply the criteria fairly. Such criteria are often decided in conjunction with trade unions, and where this is the case they may be considered by the tribunal.

Illegality of continued employment

Where it would be illegal for an employee to carry on his employment, e.g. where a solicitor has lost his practising certificate and so can no longer act for clients, dismissal may be justified on the ground of reasonableness. The ERA 1996, *Section 98(2)(d)*, states that such occurrences provide a fair reason for dismissal where the employee "could not continue to work in the position which he held without contravention (either on his part or on that of his employer) of a duty or restriction imposed by or under an enactment" (thus statutory instruments are included in the definition). It is also now a criminal offence under *Section 8* of the Asylum and Immigration Act 1996 to employ a person who does not have permission to work in the United Kingdom.

Other substantial reasons

This is an open category to accommodate particular circumstances. Thus dismissal has been held as justified in cases where employees have unreasonably refused to agree to alterations in working arrangements and hours; where there has been an insurmountable conflict of personalities between employer and employee; and where the work was only of a temporary nature and came to an end.

Pregnancy

A dismissal on the grounds of pregnancy alone will be unfair. The employer can only justify a dismissal in such circumstances where he can show that the employee is, or will have become incapable of doing the work required, or that the employee will not be able to do the work without contravening a legal requirement.

Trade union membership

Except in certain limited circumstances, it is unfair to dismiss an employee for belonging to a trade union. However, membership of trade unions in specific employment is illegal, e.g. the security services.

Procedure

An employee who wishes to allege that a dismissal has been carried out unfairly must make a complaint to the industrial tribunal on form IT1 within 3 months of the termination of employment (although this period is extendible at the discretion of the tribunal). A copy of the complaint is then sent to the employer who may contest the allegation by replying within 14 days. ACAS is also informed of the complaint, and an attempt to organize a reconciliation between the parties without the need for a formal hearing is made. The procedure governing applications to the industrial tribunal is set out in the Industrial Tribunals Act 1996.

Powers of the tribunal

When a finding of unfair dismissal has been made, the tribunal has a number of remedies available. When the finding has been made, the employee has the option (where practical) to be reinstated (in the same job), or re-engaged (in similar employment). Where it is practicable to make such an order for re-instatement or re-engagement, and the employer only partially complies or fails to comply with the order, the tribunal may make an award of compensation of between 13 and 26 weeks' pay (or 52 weeks' pay in the case of sexual or racial discrimination). The existence of such compensatory awards is designed to encourage the employer to comply with the terms of the order.

Where re-instatement or re-engagement are not appropriate, an award of compensation will be made. The compensation will consist of a basic award and a compensatory award.

Basic award

The amount of the basic award will, in most cases, be the same as that of a statutory redundancy payment; the principle difference is that in the case of redundancy payment employment prior to the 18th birthday is not counted. It depends upon basic weekly pay, length of service and age.

The maximum amount of a week's pay for the purpose of the calculation is £270 (for dismissals taking place after 1 February 2004) and the maximum number of years to be taken into account is 20. A week's pay is calculated in accordance with ERA 1996, *Sections 221–229* and is based on gross pay. The Employment Relations Act 1999 provides that the maximum amount of the basic award is calculated by reference to the period, ending with the effective date of termination, during which the employee was continuously employed, by starting at the end of that period and reckoning backwards the number of complete years of employment falling within that period and allowing for the following: Age of Employee Amount of Award (calculated in weeks' pay for each year of continuous employment).

18–21 0.5
22–40 1
41–65 1.5

Compensatory award

The compensatory award will invariably be larger, and is subject to a current maximum of £55,000. However, there is no maximum in health and safety cases (ERA 1996, *Section 100*), protected disclosure cases (ERA 1996, *Section 103A*), selection for redundancy on protected disclosure grounds (ERA 1996, *Section 105(6A)*). In the case of a refusal to reinstate or reengage, the tribunal may exceed the normal maximum to the extent necessary fully to reflect the sums which would have been payable under its original order (ERA 1996, *Section 124(4)*).

The heads of loss compensated are as follows:

(1) Expenses directly incurred as a result of the dismissal including loss of perks and fringe benefits.
(2) Lost earnings up to the hearing date.
(3) Estimated future loss of earnings.
(4) The manner of the dismissal, i.e. if the manner of the dismissal will have made the employee less attractive to subsequent employers, compensation may be awarded.
(5) Loss of the protection afforded against unfair dismissal by two years of continuous employment, i.e. the risk of being unfairly dismissed during the first two years of subsequent employment without the protection of the ERA 1996 may be compensated for in small amount.
(6) Loss of pension rights.

There is no upper limit for the compensatory award in unfair dismissal proceedings where the dismissal is attributable to discrimination under the EEC Directive for equal pay and equal treatment for men and women, as regards access to employment, vocational training and working conditions; see *Marshall* v. *Southampton and SW Hampshire AHA (1993)*.

The employee is under a duty to minimize his loss by taking all reasonable steps to find and accept offers of reasonable alternative employment. Further, if the tribunal finds that the employee contributed to the loss of his employment, it may make a deduction from the overall sum of the compensatory award.

Maximum awards

The maximum basic award is $20 \times 1\frac{1}{2} \times £270 = £8100$.

The maximum compensatory award is £55,000.

For dismissals prior to 25 October 1999, the maximum additional award which may be made in respect of non-compliance with an order is £5750, or £11,440 in cases of race or sex discrimination.

An employee may also receive an award in respect of unfair dismissal which is increased by £540 to £1080 under EA 2002, *Section 38*.

The maximum amount of a "week's pay", which determines the maximum amount of a basic award, is revised annually and linked to the RPI.

Redundancy

Under the ERA 1996, all persons who work under a contract of employment are entitled to an award on being made redundant with exceptions as follows:

(1) Employees of less than 2 years' standing.
(2) Persons over retirement age.
(3) Persons under 18 years.
(4) Share fishermen.
(5) Persons on "fixed term" contracts of longer than 2 years who have agreed in writing to forgo their right to a redundancy payment.
(6) Persons normally working outside the UK.
(7) Those covered by an approved redundancy agreement.

An employee can only claim to have been made redundant where he can be shown to have been dismissed. Once dismissal has been proved, there is a presumption by virtue of *Section 163(2)* of the ERA 1996 that the reason for the dismissal was redundancy. It is then for the employer to show that the dismissal was for some reason other than redundancy (e.g. misconduct). By *Section 139(1)* of the ERA 1996, there is a redundancy where the dismissal is attributable to:

(a) the fact that the employer has ceased, or intends to cease, to carry on the business for the purposes of which the employee was employed by him; . . .

(or)

(b) the fact that the requirements of that business for employees to carry out work of a particular kind . . . have ceased or diminished or are expected to cease or diminish.

Where the employer has asked for volunteers for redundancy, and the employee accepts a redundancy package voluntarily, the right to claim a redundancy payment under the ERA 1996 is lost.

Where an employee is laid off or put on short time, and there is no provision for such an eventuality in the contract of employment, the employee is entitled to claim to have been made redundant. If the contract of employment does make provision for such eventualities, but the employee is laid off or on short time for

4 consecutive weeks or for 6 of the preceding 13 weeks, the employee may claim redundancy.

This is done by sending written notice of intention to claim redundancy to the employer. The employer then issues a counter notice within 7 days stating that there is a reasonable chance within the following 4 weeks that the employee will commence a period of 13 weeks' consecutive employment. If the promise is not fulfilled, the employee is entitled to a redundancy payment. If an employee is offered suitable alternative employment by his employer, he will lose his right to a redundancy payment if he unreasonably refuses it.

Redundancy awards

An employee who considers that he has been made redundant must make a written claim for a payment to his employer. If the employer refuses to make the payment, the employee can refer the matter to the industrial tribunal within 6 months of the termination of the employment. The amount of the award is calculated in accordance with the table set out above which is also used for calculating the basic award in unfair dismissal proceedings. However, for each month a claimant is over the age of 64, the overall amount is reduced by one-twelfth for each complete month worked and the maximum weekly figure for earnings used in calculating the payment is £270, and the maximum number of years for which payment can be claimed is 20.

Some large employers agree their own schemes for redundancy with employees and trade unions. With the consent of the S of S, they can thereby contract out of the legislation.

Where the employee is a member of an independent trade union, the employer is usually under a duty to discuss proposed redundancy with a union representative. Particular rules requiring consultation apply when the number of employees facing redundancy is greater than 20. It is a statutory duty for an employer to consult employee representatives collectively under TURLCA 1992, *Section 188*, and any failure to do so may make individuals' dismissals unfair.

If the employer fails to carry out the necessary consultation process, the trade union may make a complaint to the industrial tribunal and seek a declaration of the parties' respective rights. The tribunal may also make a "protective award" whereby the employees concerned must be paid during a specific period not exceeding 90 days. This is designed to protect the employees' interests during the consultation period. If the employer fails to comply with an order for a protective award, the employee may make a complaint to the tribunal as an individual.

There is therefore fairly comprehensive provision for compensatory payments to employees who are made redundant, but unless the employee has been working for many years, the size of the statutory award is likely to be relatively small. An employee who has been notified of forthcoming redundancy is entitled to reasonable time off work in order to look for alternative employment, but only if he has been in continuous employment for 2 years.

Human rights at work

One of the areas forecast to be most affected by the Human Rights Act 1998 is employment law. Although the Act does not create direct obligations by an employer to an employee, industrial tribunals will be required to interpret existing UK employment law in line with the principles of the European Convention on Human Rights and its associated case law.

Employee privacy is a key area, since Article 8 of the Convention provides for the right to respect for private and family life, home and correspondence. Interference with this right is only permitted if it is "in accordance with the law" and "necessary in a democratic society" and is effected for a legitimate purpose, such as the prevention of crime or the protection of health.

The case law under the Convention makes it clear that employees cannot complain if they are made aware that their employer reserves the right to conduct monitoring of telephone, e-mail and other communication facilities. Since working in a pharmacy exposes a dishonest employee to a vista of temptations (viz. unlawful sales of medicines, fraudulent prescription claims, etc.) pharmacists would be well advised to insert a clause to this effect in an employee's contract of employment.

The use of CCTV and other monitoring equipment may be permitted; however, a crucial point is that measures conflicting with the right to privacy can only be taken where "proportionate", in the sense that the interference must be reasonable and justifiable in the circumstances. Indiscriminate monitoring may not be permitted.

Dress codes are frequently discussed in the light of Article 10 of the Convention, which guarantees freedom of expression. One of the leading cases on this point concerned an employee who was dismissed for insisting upon wearing a number of badges to work proclaiming that she was a lesbian. Her unfair dismissal claim failed on the basis that the employer could decide, after sensible consideration, what was likely to offend fellow customers and employees. The result of this case is unlikely to be different now that the Human Rights Act 1998 is in force. Community pharmacists have reasonable grounds to impose a sensible dress code to operate their pharmacy, provided that the code is reasonable and justifiable, or proportionate, in all the circumstances.

Forced/compulsory labour under Article 4 of the European Convention of Human Rights

No forced labour claim has succeeded to date, and speculations that working conditions, long hours and compulsory overtime amount to such a breach are not convincing. The employment relationship is a contractual one which both parties can terminate and, even within the relationship, existing legislation on working time, harassment, etc. cover these areas adequately.

Only time will tell how much the principles of the Act will affect the approach of industrial tribunals to their application of UK employment law. Although many of the issues covered by the Act are already addressed by domestic law, inevitably there will be some cases where the Human Rights Act 1998 will give rise to some expanded arguments on the part of an aggrieved employee.

Chapter 31

Human Rights

The Human Rights Act 1998 creates a statutory general requirement that all legislation be read and given effect in a way that is compatible with the ECHR. In all cases in which Convention rights are in question, the Act gives "further effect" to the Convention, whether the litigants are private persons or public authorities. There is no doubt that community pharmacists, alongside everybody else in the United Kingdom, will be affected by the Human Rights Act 1998, and accordingly it is most important that pharmacists know all about it. The Act takes effect in three ways:

(1) By obliging courts to decide all cases before them (whether brought under statute or the common law) compatibly with Convention rights unless prevented from doing so either by primary legislation, or by provisions made under primary legislation which cannot be read compatibly with the Convention (*Section 6(1)–(3)*);

(2) By introducing an obligation for courts to interpret existing and future legislation in conformity with the Convention wherever possible (*Section 3*);

(3) By requiring the courts to take Strasbourg case law into account in all cases, in so far as they consider it relevant to proceedings before them (*Section 2(1)*).

Human rights and privacy

The incorporation of Article 8 of the European Convention on Human Rights (the Convention) into UK law by the Human Rights Act 1998 (HRA) creates a general right to respect for privacy where none previously existed. Article 8 offers general protection for a person's private and family life, home and correspondence from arbitrary interference by the State in the following terms:

> Everyone has the right to respect for his private and family life, his home and his correspondence.

> There shall be no interference by a public authority with the exercise of this right except such as is in accordance with the law and is necessary in a democratic society in the interests of national security, public safety or the economic well-being of the country, for the prevention of disorder or crime, for the protection of health or morals, or for the protection of the rights and freedoms of others.

The duty of public authorities

The requirement on public authorities, such as the NHS, to act compatibly with Article 8 of the Convention is contained in *Section 6 of the HRA. Section 6* provides that central government, local government and other public bodies such as the police and the courts must all act compatibly with human rights.

Horizontal effect of the HRA 1998

Not only will the HRA 1998 affect public companies *per se*, but it will also affect the relationship between private companies (which are not public bodies) and individuals, because many of the protected rights have horizontal effect. For example, by reason of the horizontal effect, Article 8 will protect confidentiality of messages between Internet users (e-mail, etc.).

Interferences with rights to privacy

This right affects a large number of areas of life. However, the right to respect for these aspects of privacy under Article 8 is qualified. This means that interferences by the State can be permissible, but such interferences must be justified and satisfy certain conditions.

Article 8(2) provides that there can be no interference by a public authority with the rights protected by Article 8(1), except such as in accordance with the law and is necessary in a democratic society. An applicant, alleging a violation of Article 8, needs to show, first, that there has been an interference and, secondly, that the interference was by a public authority. An interference can be due to either an act of a public authority or its failure to act but establishing an interference will depend on the facts of each individual case.

The nature and extent of each interference must be judged against the end it is meant to achieve. Thus, any interference with rights under Article 8 that goes further than is necessary may well be unlawful. The more severe the infringement of privacy, the more important the legitimate objective in each case will need to be. In most cases, the interference will be judged against whether it meets a pressing social need, and the extent to which an alternative, less intrusive interference would achieve the same result.

In addition any interference must be in the interests of the legitimate objectives identified in Article 8(2). These objectives are widely drawn and it will often be possible for an interference to be categorised as being in pursuit of one of these legitimate objectives.

More difficult questions arise where there are competing interests at issue, such as balancing privacy rights. In some cases it will be important to distinguish between a lawful interference in someone's private life in the public interest, as opposed to an unlawful one which has occurred merely because it is something in which the public might be interested.

Human rights and patient confidentiality

Patient confidentiality is a key example. The Access to Health Records Act 1990 was passed as a result of the case of *Gaskin* v. *United Kingdom (1990)*, where the European

Court of Human Rights held that the UK's refusal to grant a right of access by a patient to his health records was in breach of Article 8 of the European Convention. This has now been replaced by the Data Protection Act 1998.

The Data Protection Act 1998 has been designed to protect the right of individuals to privacy with respect to the processing of personal data. Under the Data Protection Act 1998, individuals are entitled to access their patient medication records or other personal information about them and can contact their pharmacist in order to do this. However, any right of access to medical records is subject to certain exclusions.

The public expects pharmacists and their staff to respect and protect privacy. This duty extends to any information relating to an individual, which pharmacists or their staff acquire in the course of their professional activities. Confidential information includes personal details and medication, both prescribed and non-prescribed.

Pharmacists must ensure that the confidentiality of information acquired about an individual in the course of their professional activities is respected and protected, and is disclosed only with the consent of the individual other than in the circumstances defined below in (2). It may be appropriate to disclose information without the patient's consent in the following circumstances:

- Where the patient's parent, guardian or carer has consented to the disclosure and the patient's apparent age or health makes them incapable of giving consent to disclose;
- Pharmacists should not normally disclose information about services provided to adolescent patients to their parents.
- Where disclosure of the information is to a person or body empowered by statute to require such disclosure (e.g. the RPSGB inspector or a Controlled Drugs Inspector).
- Where disclosure is directed by a coroner, judge or other presiding officer of a court, Crown Prosecution Office in England and Wales.
- To a police officer or NHS Fraud Investigation Officer who provides in writing confirmation that disclosure is necessary to assist in the prevention, detection or prosecution of serious crime;
- Where necessary to prevent serious injury or damage to the health of the patient, a third party or to public health.

Pharmacists should not disclose information relating to the prescribing practices of identifiable prescribers or their practices, for example to sales representatives, other than for the necessary purposes of the NHS or other health care provider, unless the prescriber has given his written informed consent to the disclosure. This does not interfere with a pharmacist's right to disclose information to an appropriate body where he has reasonable concerns for the well-being of a patient or the public.

Access to confidential information within the pharmacy must be restricted to those who require access to that information and who are themselves subject to an obligation of confidentiality.

The requirements of data protection legislation for data collection and use must be complied with. Confidential information must be protected effectively against improper disclosure when it is stored, transmitted, received or disposed of.

Pharmacy computer and manual systems which include patient-specific information must incorporate access control systems to minimise the risk of unauthorised or unnecessary access to the data. Pharmacy computer systems, which include patient-specific information and which are linked to the Internet or other networks must incorporate measures such as encryption to eliminate the risk of unauthorised access to confidential data.

Human rights and employment issues

The important articles of the HRA 1998 which are most likely to have an impact in the employment field include Article 4 (right not to be held in slavery and to be protected against forced or compulsory labour), Article 5 (right to liberty and security of the person), Article 6 (right to a fair and public hearing within a reasonable period of time), Article 8 (right to respect for private and family life), Article 9 (freedom of religion), Article 10 (right to freedom of expression), Article 11 (right to peaceful assembly and the freedom of association with others) and Article 14 (prohibition of discrimination).

Many of the rights and fundamental freedoms under the Convention have exceptions, (e.g. Articles 8–11) and as such many cases have failed because of the exceptions – e.g. for public safety or for the protection of health.

Under the Convention employment cases have not been particularly successful. Future developments will depend on a number of factors including more flexible courts. Article 6 (right to a fair and public hearing within a reasonable period of time) may be the most useful in challenging the conduct of court and tribunal processes. This is because "public authorities" are defined to include courts and tribunals.

However, Article 6 does not usually apply to internal disciplinary hearings though it may apply to those held by professional bodies which can affect a worker's right to practice unless there is a subsequent right of appeal to a court (see *Tehrani* v. *UK Central Council for Nursing, Midwifery and Health Visiting (2001)* and *Preiss* v. *General Dental Council (2001)*).

Human rights and property interests

Under the Convention, the human right relating to property is not a right to have or acquire property but a right to the protection of a person's existing property. By protecting property rights as a human right, the Convention, and the HRA 1998, empower an individual to utilise the judicial arm to seek to prevent interferences with property which may be aimed at advancing the public interest.

Protocol 1, Article 1, ECHR protects peaceful enjoyment of possessions:

> Every natural or legal person is entitled to the peaceful enjoyment of his possessions. No one shall be deprived of his possession except in the public interest and subject to the conditions provided for by law and by the general principles of international law.

> The preceding provisions shall not, however, in any way impair the right of a State to enforce such laws as it deems necessary to control the use of property in accordance with the general interest or to secure the payment of taxes or other contributions or penalties.

The term 'possessions' in Protocol 1, Article 1 has a very wide meaning, including all property and chattels and also acquired rights with economic interest such as:

- Leases
- Planning consents
- The vested interests of a doctor in private practice
- Goodwill (e.g. the ability to retain clientele or the goodwill of customers).

In order to show that Protocol 1, Article, has been violated, it must be shown that:

- The peaceful enjoyment of the applicant's possessions has been interfered with (Rule 1); or
- The Applicant has been deprived of possessions by the state (Rule 2); or
- The Applicant's possessions have been subject to control by the state (Rule 3).

The essence of Article 1, Protocol 1 is that it provides a guarantee for the right of property. It provides both a positive guarantee to the peaceful enjoyment of possessions, which embraces the right to own, possess, use, lend or dispose of the property, but also a negative guarantee that no one shall be deprived of their possessions by the state except in certain circumstances. This is clearly a valuable protection that all community pharmacists who have a freehold or leasehold ownership of a property should be aware of.

Freedom of information

The Freedom of Information Act (FOIA) was passed on 30 November 2000. It is challenged with the task of reversing the working premise that everything is secret, unless otherwise stated, to a position where everything is public unless it falls into specified excepted cases.

From 1 January 2005 the Freedom of Information Act 2000 has obliged pharmacies to respond to requests about information that it holds about NHS Pharmaceutical Services, and creates a right of access to that information, subject to some exemptions, which have to be taken into consideration before deciding what information it can release.

The FOIA 2000 recognises that members of the public have the right to know how public services are organised and run, how much they cost and how the decisions are made. In addition to accessing the information identified in the Publication Scheme, members of the public are entitled to request information about an individual pharmacy under the NHS Openness Code 1995.

The Freedom of Information Act does not, however, change the right of patients to the protection of their patient confidentiality in accordance with HRA 1998 Schedule 1 Article 8, the Data Protection Act 1998 and at common law.

Types of information that can be requested under the FOIA 2000

The type of information that can be requested must be the type that authorities believe will not cause significant harm. For example, *Section 38* of the Act provides a qualified exemption from the duty to provide information if its disclosure under the

Act would, or would be likely to endanger the physical or mental health of any individual, or endanger the safety of any individual.

Insofar as the information under request involves living individuals it will be covered by *Section 49* relating to personal information. The focus of *Section 38* will be on other information whose disclosure might pose a risk and this may include:

- Information about sites of controversial scientific research which may be targets for sabotage. There may be well-founded fears that if the location of such sites were disclosed to individuals or groups opposed to the research there would be risks to the physical safety of staff;
- Information relating to the dead (not therefore covered by the personal information exemption) whose disclosure might endanger the mental health of surviving relatives;
- Information whose disclosure might have an adverse effect on public health.

In such cases, the information will be withheld under the appropriate exemption of the code of practice. It also places a number of obligations on public authorities about the way in which they provide information. Subject to the exemptions, anyone making a request must be informed whether the public authority holds the information and, if so, be supplied with it – generally within 20 working days. There is also a duty to provide advice or assistance to anyone seeking information (e.g. in order to explain what is readily available or to clarify what is wanted).

Complaints procedure

The best policy is to be as open as possible and supply the information that has been requested. If the release of that information is considered to cause significant harm then the information may be withheld. The Information Commissioner might later force the disclosure of the information.

In the case where information is requested and there are sections of the information that are exempt then the document should be clearly marked to show where exempt information is withheld. If all information is withheld, then the public body will have to give full reasons as to why the information has been withheld. If the person requesting access is not satisfied with the reasons, they have the right to appeal. They may also appeal if they think that the charges for information are unfair. The Freedom of Information Act will be enforced by the Information Commissioner, formerly, the Data Protection Registrar.

FOI is openness with teeth. The maximum sentence punishable under the FOI Act is 2 years imprisonment for the accountable officer of the public body. A practice recommendation can be issued that outlines the steps to help the authority with compliance. These must be given in writing and refer to the relevant section of the Codes of Practice with which the authority does not comply.

If a member of the public feels that they have not had their request for information dealt with in accordance with the Act, they may apply to the Commissioner for a decision. If the complainant has exhausted all internal procedures, the Commissioner either informs the complainant that no decision will be made and the reason for that, or serve a decision notice on the complainant and the public authority.

When the Commissioner has received an application for a decision notice or requires more information to consider whether compliance has been achieved with the Codes of Practice and the Act, he can serve an information notice. This is time limited and again must be in writing and must say why the notice has been issued.

If the authority fails to comply with any of its duties under the Act, he may serve an enforcement notice. Failure to comply with a notice may result in the Commissioner certifying this to the Court who may ultimately deem non-compliance as Contempt of Court.

Index

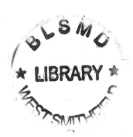